1998
YEAR BOOK OF
PSYCHIATRY AND
APPLIED MENTAL HEALTH®

Statement of Purpose

The YEAR BOOK Service

The YEAR BOOK series was devised in 1901 by practicing health professionals who observed that the literature of medicine and related disciplines had become so voluminous that no one individual could read and place in perspective every potential advance in a major specialty. In the final decade of the 20th century, this recognition is more acutely true than it was in 1901.

More than merely a series of books, YEAR BOOK volumes are the tangible results of a unique service designed to accomplish the following:

- to *survey* a wide range of journals of proven value
- to *select* from those journals papers representing significant advances and statements of important clinical principles
- to provide *abstracts* of those articles that are readable, convenient summaries of their key points
- to provide *commentary* about those articles to place them in perspective

These publications grow out of a unique process that calls on the talents of outstanding authorities in clinical and fundamental disciplines, trained literature specialists, and professional writers, all supported by the resources of Mosby, the world's preeminent publisher for the health professions.

The Literature Base

Mosby and its Editors survey more than 1,000 journals published worldwide, covering the full range of the health professions. On an annual basis, the publisher examines usage patterns and polls its expert authorities to add new journals to the literature base and to delete journals that are no longer useful as potential YEAR BOOK sources.

The Literature Survey

The publisher's team of literature specialists, all of whom are trained and experienced health professionals, examines every original, peer-reviewed article in each journal issue. More than 250,000 articles per year are scanned systematically, including title, text, illustrations, tables, and references. Each scan is compared, article by article, to the search strategies that the publisher has developed in consultation with the 270 outside experts who form the pool of YEAR BOOK editors. A given article may be reviewed by any number of editors, from one to a dozen or more, regardless of the discipline for which the paper was originally published. In turn, each editor who receives the article reviews it to determine whether the article should be included in the YEAR BOOK. This decision is based on the article's inherent quality, its probable usefulness to readers of that YEAR BOOK, and the editor's goal to represent a balanced picture of a given field in each volume of the YEAR BOOK. In addition, the editor indicates when to include figures and tables from the article to help the YEAR BOOK reader better understand the information.

Of the quarter million articles scanned each year, only 5% are selected for detailed analysis within the YEAR BOOK series, thereby assuring readers of the high value of every selection.

The Abstract

The publisher's abstracting staff is headed by a seasoned medical professional and includes individuals with training in the life sciences, medicine, and other areas, plus extensive experience in writing for the health professions and related industries. Each selected article is assigned to a specific writer on this abstracting staff. The abstracter, guided in many cases by notations supplied by the expert editor, writes a structured, condensed summary designed so that the reader can rapidly acquire the essential information contained in the article.

The Commentary

The YEAR BOOK editorial boards, sometimes assisted by guest commentators, write comments that place each article in perspective for the reader. This provides the reader with the equivalent of a personal consultation with a leading international authority—an opportunity to better understand the value of the article and to benefit from the authority's thought processes in assessing the article.

Additional Editorial Features

The editorial boards of each YEAR BOOK organize the abstracts and comments to provide a logical and satisfying sequence of information. To enhance the organization, editors also provide introductions to sections or individual chapters, comments linking a number of abstracts, citations to additional literature, and other features.

The published YEAR BOOK contains enhanced bibliographic citations for each selected article, including extended listings of multiple authors and identification of author affiliations. Each YEAR BOOK contains a Table of Contents specific to that year's volume. From year to year, the Table of Contents for a given YEAR BOOK will vary depending on developments within the field.

Every YEAR BOOK contains a list of the journals from which papers have been selected. This list represents a subset of the more than 1,000 journals surveyed by the publisher and occasionally reflects a particularly pertinent article from a journal that is not surveyed on a routine basis.

Finally, each volume contains a comprehensive subject index and an index to authors of each selected paper.

The 1998 Year Book Series

Year Book of Allergy, Asthma, and Clinical Immunology: Drs. Rosenwasser, Borish, Gelfand, Leung, Nelson, and Szefler

Year Book of Anesthesiology and Pain Management®: Drs. Tinker, Abram, Chestnut, Roizen, Rothenberg, and Wood

Year Book of Cardiology®: Drs. Schlant, Collins, Gersh, Graham, Kaplan, and Waldo

Year Book of Chiropractic®: Dr. Lawrence

Year Book of Critical Care Medicine®: Drs. Parrillo, Balk, Calvin, Franklin, and Shapiro

Year Book of Dentistry®: Drs. Meskin, Berry, Jeffcoat, Leinfelder, Roser, Summitt, and Zakariasen

Year Book of Dermatologic Surgery®: Drs. Greenway, Papadopoulos, Whitaker, and Barrett

Year Book of Dermatology®: Dr. Thiers

Year Book of Diagnostic Radiology®: Drs. Osborn, Groskin, Dalinka, Maynard, Pentecost, Rebner, Ros, Smirniotopoulos, and Young

Year Book of Drug Therapy®: Drs. Lasagna and Weintraub

Year Book of Emergency Medicine®: Drs. Wagner, Dronen, Davidson, King, Niemann, and Roberts

Year Book of Endocrinology®: Drs. Bagdade, Braverman, Horton, Kannan, Landsberg, Molitch, Morley, Nathan, Odell, Poehlman, Rogol, and Ryan

Year Book of Family Practice®: Drs. Berg, Bowman, Davidson, Dexter, and Scherger

Year Book of Gastroenterology®: Drs. Aliperti and Fleshman

Year Book of Geriatrics and Gerontology®: Drs. Beck, Burton, Ostwald, Rabins, Reuben, Roth, Shapiro, and Whitehouse

Year Book of Hand Surgery®: Drs. Amadio and Hentz

Year Book of Hematology®: Drs. Spivak, Bell, Ness, Quesenberry, Wiernik, and Horowitz

Year Book of Infectious Diseases: Drs. Keusch, Barza, Bennish, Poutsiaka, Skolnik, and Snydman

Year Book of Medicine®: Drs. Klahr, Cline, McCallum, Frishman, Utiger, Malawista, Mandell, and Jett

Year Book of Neonatal and Perinatal Medicine®: Drs. Fanaroff, Maisels, and Stevenson

Year Book of Nephrology, Hypertension, and Mineral Metabolism: Drs. Schwab, Bennett, Emmett, Hostetter, Kumar, and Toto

Year Book of Neurology and Neurosurgery®: Drs. Bradley and Gibbs

Year Book of Nuclear Medicine®: Drs. Gottschalk, Blaufox, Neumann, Strauss, and Zubal

Year Book of Obstetrics, Gynecology, and Women's Health: Drs. Mishell, Herbst, and Kirschbaum

Year Book of Occupational and Environmental Medicine®: Drs. Emmett, Frank, Gochfeld, and Hessl

Year Book of Oncology®: Drs. Ozols, Eisenberg, Glatstein, Loehrer, Tallman, and Wiersma

Year Book of Ophthalmology®: Drs. Wilson, Augsburger, Cohen, Eagle, Grossman, Laibson, Maguire, Nelson, Penne, Rapuano, Sergott, Spaeth, Tipperman, Ms. Gosfield, and Ms. Salmon

Year Book of Orthopedics®: Drs. Morrey, Beauchamp, Currier, Tolo, Trigg, and Swiontkowski

Year Book of Otolaryngology–Head and Neck Surgery®: Drs. Paparella and Holt

Year Book of Pathology and Laboratory Medicine®: Drs. Raab, Cohen, Olson, Sirgi, and Stanley

Year Book of Pediatrics®: Dr. Stockman

Year Book of Plastic, Reconstructive, and Aesthetic Surgery®: Drs. Miller, Bartlett, Garner, McKinney, Ruberg, Salisbury, and Smith

Year Book of Psychiatry and Applied Mental Health®: Drs. Talbott, Ballenger, Frances, Lydiard, Meltzer, Schowalter, and Tasman

Year Book of Pulmonary Disease®: Drs. Jett, Maurer, Ryu, Strollo, and Wenzel

Year Book of Rheumatology®: Drs. Panush, Hadler, LeRoy, Liang, Reichlin, Simon, and Weinblatt

Year Book of Sports Medicine®: Drs. Shephard, Drinkwater, Eichner, Torg, Alexander, and Mr. George

Year Book of Surgery®: Drs. Copeland, Bland, Deitch, Eberlein, Howard, Luce, Seeger, Souba, and Sugarbaker

Year Book of Thoracic and Cardiovascular Surgery®: Drs. Ginsberg, Wechsler, and Williams

Year Book of Urology®: Drs. Andriole and Coplen

Year Book of Vascular Surgery®: Dr. Porter

1998

The Year Book of PSYCHIATRY AND APPLIED MENTAL HEALTH®

Editor in Chief

John A. Talbott, M.D.

Professor and Chair, Department of Psychiatry, University of Maryland School of Medicine; Director, Institute of Psychiatry, University of Maryland Medical System, Baltimore, Maryland

Mosby

St. Louis Baltimore Boston Carlsbad Naples New York Philadelphia Portland London Madrid Mexico City Singapore Sydney Tokyo Toronto Wiesbaden

Mosby
Dedicated to Publishing Excellence

A Times Mirror
Company

Publisher: Theresa Van Schaik
Developmental Editor: Jaime Chatman
Manuscript Editor: Amanda Maguire
Project Supervisor, Production: Joy Moore
Production Assistant: Laura Bayless
Manager, Literature Services: Idelle L. Winer
Illustrations and Permissions Coordinator: Steve Ramay

1998 EDITION

Printed in the United States of America
Composition by Reed Technology and Information Services, Inc.
Printing/binding by Maple-Vail

Editorial Office:
Mosby, Inc.
11830 Westline Industrial Drive
St. Louis, MO 63146
Customer Service: customer.support@mosby.com
www.mosby.com/Mosby/CustomerSupport/index.html

International Standard Serial Number: 0084–3970
International Standard Book Number: 0–8151–9733-0

Editors

James C. Ballenger, M.D.
Professor and Chair, Department of Psychiatry and Behavioral Sciences; Director, Institute of Psychiatry; Executive Director, Center for Drug and Alcohol Programs, Medical University of South Carolina, Charleston, South Carolina

Richard J. Frances, M.D., F.A.C.P., F.A.P.A.
Clinical Professor, New York University; Adjunct Professor, University of Medicine and Dentistry of New Jersey; President and Medical Director, Silver Hill Hospital, New Canaan, Connecticut

R. Bruce Lydiard, Ph.D., M.D.
Professor of Psychiatry and Behavioral Sciences, Medical University of South Carolina; Director, Clinical Psychopharmacology Research Division, Institute of Psychiatry, Medical University of South Carolina, Charleston, South Carolina.

Herbert Y. Meltzer, M.D.
Professor of Psychiatry and Pharmacology; Director, Division of Psychopharmacology, Vanderbilt University Medical Center, Nashville, Tennessee

John E. Schowalter, M.D.
Albert J. Solnit Professor of Child Psychiatry and Pediatrics, Yale Child Study Center, New Haven, Connecticut

Allan Tasman, M.D.
Professor and Chair, Department of Psychiatry and Behavioral Sciences, University of Louisville School of Medicine, Louisville, Kentucky

Table of Contents

Journals Represented

Mosby and its Editors survey more than 1,000 journals for its abstract and commentary publications. From these journals, the Editors select the articles to be abstracted. Journals represented in this YEAR BOOK are listed below.

Acta Neurologica Scandinavica
Acta Psychiatrica Scandinavica
American Journal of Drug and Alcohol Abuse
American Journal of Health Promotion
American Journal of Human Genetics
American Journal of Hypertension
American Journal of Industrial Medicine
American Journal of Medicine
American Journal of Orthopsychiatry
American Journal of Psychiatry
American Journal of Psychotherapy
American Journal of Public Health
Annals of Emergency Medicine
Archives of Family Medicine
Archives of General Psychiatry
Archives of Pediatrics and Adolescent Medicine
Australian and New Zealand Journal of Psychiatry
Behaviour Research and Therapy
Biological Psychiatry
Brain
British Journal of General Practice
British Journal of Psychiatry
British Journal of Urology
British Medical Journal
Bulletin of the American Academy of Psychiatry and the Law
Canadian Family Physician
Canadian Journal of Psychiatry
Circulation
Clinical Orthopaedics and Related Research
Community Mental Health Journal
Comprehensive Psychiatry
Developmental Medicine and Child Neurology
Digestive Diseases and Sciences
Drug and Alcohol Dependence
European Journal of Obstetrics, Gynecology and Reproductive Biology
Family Planning Perspectives
General Hospital Psychiatry
Harvard Review Psychiatry
International Journal of Group Psychotherapy
Journal of Adolescent Health
Journal of Affective Disorders
Journal of Behavior Therapy and Experimental Psychiatry
Journal of Child Psychology and Psychiatry and Allied Disciplines
Journal of Clinical Endocrinology and Metabolism
Journal of Clincal Pharmacology
Journal of Clinical Psychiatry
Journal of Clinical Psychopharmacology

Journal of Consulting and Clinical Psychology
Journal of Developmental and Behavioral Pediatrics
Journal of General Internal Medicine
Journal of Nervous and Mental Disease
Journal of Pediatrics
Journal of Pharmacology and Experimental Therapeutics
Journal of Psychiatric Research
Journal of Psychotherapy Practice and Research
Journal of the American Academy of Child and Adolescent Psychiatry
Journal of the American Geriatrics Society
Journal of the American Medical Association
Lancet
Medical Care
Nature
Neurosurgery
New Directions for Mental Health Services
New England Journal of Medicine
Pediatrics
Pharmacotherapy
Proceedings of the National Academy of Sciences
Psychiatric Services
Psychiatry
Psychiatry Research
Psychological Medicine
Psychosomatic Medicine
Psychotherapy and Psychosomatics
Schizophrenia Bulletin
Science
Southern Medical Journal

Standard Abbreviations

The following terms are abbreviated in this edition: acquired immunodeficiency syndrome (AIDS), cardiopulmonary resuscitation (CPR), central nervous system (CNS), cerebrospinal fluid (CSF), computed tomography (CT), deoxyribonucleic acid (DNA), electrocardiography (ECG), health maintenance organization (HMO), human immunodeficiency virus (HIV), intensive care unit (ICU), intramuscular (IM), intravenous (IV), magnetic resonance (MR) imaging (MRI), and ribonucleic acid (RNA).

Note

The Year Book of Psychiatry and Applied Mental Health® is a literature survey service providing abstracts of articles published in the professional literature. Every effort is made to assure the accuracy of the information presented in these pages. Neither the editors nor the publisher of the Year Book of Psychiatry and Applied Mental Health® can be responsible for errors in the original materials. The editors' comments are their own opinions. Mention of specific products within this publication does not constitute endorsement.

To facilitate the use of the Year Book of Psychiatry and Applied Mental Health® as a reference tool, all illustrations and tables included in this publication are now identified as they appear in the original article. This change is meant to help the reader recognize that any illustration or table appearing in the Year Book

OF PSYCHIATRY AND APPLIED MENTAL HEALTH® may be only one of many in the original article. For this reason, figure and table numbers will often appear to be out of sequence within the YEAR BOOK OF PSYCHIATRY AND APPLIED MENTAL HEALTH®.

Publisher's Preface

With this edition of the YEAR BOOK, we say good-bye to two distinguished colleagues, Alan F. Breier, M.D., and John E. Schowalter, M.D. Dr. Breier decided to step down from the editorial board after the publication of the 1997 YEAR BOOK. The 1998 YEAR BOOK will be Dr. Schowalter's last volume. We extend our deepest appreciation to Drs. Breier and Schowalter for their years of service, as well as their unending support and enthusiasm for this publication. Although we will miss them, we wish them the very best in all future endeavors.

We are pleased to welcome R. Bruce Lydiard, Ph.D., M.D., to the board. We know you will find Dr. Lydiard's commentary to be insightful and thought-provoking.

Peter S. Jensen, M.D., will join the editorial board commencing with the 1999 edition of the YEAR BOOK. Please join us in welcoming Dr. Jensen to his new role.

Mosby, Inc.

1 Genetics and Mental Health

Introduction

Genetics is perhaps the most rapidly moving field in medicine. Genetic findings bear down like an avalanche on researcher, clinician, and lay person alike. The trick, of course, is how to be able to separate quality from quantity. It is almost customary for findings to be announced with fanfare as a breakthrough, only to be later modified or disproven.

One such modification was the finding that the so-called Alzheimer's gene, apoE-4, is not responsible as was supposed for 50% of cases of Alzheimer's disease, but only for about 10% of early-onset sufferers.[1] Interestingly, within two months, authors of another study claimed the discovery of defects in two mitochondrial genes that encode cytochromec oxidase, an enzyme crucial to the metabolism of oxygen, which they predict are linked to 60% to 70% of Alzheimer's disease cases.[2] This group also hopes that their findings can lead to a simple diagnostic test for Alzheimer's disease. There is some question, however, whether the authors' findings are a cause or a consequence of Alzheimer's disease.

How to use genetic screening well is becoming an increasingly difficult question, and psychiatry is one of the most sensitive areas for this dilemma. We know we should not order a test if we do not know how to use the results. Just because we can do something does not mean we should do it, but the temptations rise as the possibilities rise. One study showed that one third of the physicians who referred patients for genetic testing then misinterpreted the results.[3] Until recently, genetic testing was only associated with research studies, but with stepped-up availability and advertising, testing is tantalizingly more available to everyone. Patients are more wary about genetic screening than are physicians. One study of families having members with genetic disorders and associated with the Human Genome Education Model Project showed that 47% of those who were asked about genetic diseases or disabilities on a health insurance application were subsequently turned down.[4] Eighty-three percent of the respondents were, if tested positive, unwilling to share the results with their insurers, and 87% of this group did not want their employers to know the results.

A Swedish adoption study casts doubt on the theory that there are two types of alcoholism, one that is not primarily hereditary (type 1) and one that is (type 2).[5] This study showed that both types of alcoholism can occur in the same family. Type 1 individuals are thought to be of both genders, while type 2 individuals are mainly men who have an earlier age of onset and more social and legal problems. In this study, type 1 alcoholism was slightly more common in families with a type 2 genetic background than with a type 1 background.

There have been a number of studies that have ruled out a genetic link. One shows that eight of the known 13 subunits of Gamma-Aminobuytric Acid type A are not associated with panic disorder.[6] The December 1996 issue of the *American Journal of Psychiatry* presents a group of articles on the genetics of schizophrenia, and James Kennedy provides a helpful editorial comment which begins, "The voyage toward genetic answers for schizophrenia has been fraught with false starts and murky passages."[7] However, he points out that current researchers are much more careful about their methods and their claims.

Some informative positive genetic findings have also recently come to light. One points to an association between a polymorphic gene involved in serotonin transport and with personality traits.[8] Although interesting, this is hardly "the anxiety gene," since the polymorphism accounts for less than 10% of the genetic contribution to the anxiety-related traits. Two studies show loci on chromosomes 12 and 13, which are associated with primary nocturnal enuresis.[9, 10]

A very fascinating study was carried out with Turner Syndrome patients (persons with a single X chromosome). The patients were divided into those whose X chromosome came from their mothers and those whose X chromosome came from their fathers.[11] Those subjects who were sex–chromosome-linked to their fathers showed much better social skills, verbal skills, and higher-order executive function skills. Although seemingly counterintuitive, all boys receive their X chromosome from their mothers, so although many people, particularly women, complain about the propensity of males to be boors, it may be that their mother's gene makes them do it. Females, on the other hand, obtain one X chromosome from each parent. It may be that females are typically more socially adroit than males because ot their fathers' chromosomes, not that the Xs did the fathers much good. Needless to say, the above extrapolation of findings from patients with Turner disorder to the general population is speculative to say the least.

It is impossible to close without mentioning the first cloning of an adult mammal.[12] The researchers are from the Roslin Institute in Scotland. They extracted the nucleus of a cell from an adult female white-faced sheep and transferred it into an egg taken from a black-faced sheep. That egg was then reimplanted into the uterus of the black-faced sheep. In the fullness of time, presto, out came a white-faced lamb. Hello Dolly, and who needs males! Ethicists and media pundits now have the opportunity for a most interesting debate about the pros and cons of cloning humans. Federal, but not private, funding for human embryo research is banned in the United States.

John E. Schowalter, M.D.

References

1. Blacker D, Haines JL, Rodes L: ApoE-4 and age of onset of Alzheimer's disease: The NIMH genetics initiative. *Neurology* 48: 139–147, 1997.
2. Davis RE, Miller S, Herrnstadt C, et al: Mutations in mitochrondial cytochrome C oxidase genes segregate with late-onset Alzheimer disease. *Proc Natl Acad Sci USA* 94:4526–4531, 1997.
3. Giardiello FM, Brensinger JD, Peterson GM, et al: The use and interpretation of commercial APC gene testing for familial adenomatous polyposis. *N Engl J Med* 336:823–827, 1997.
4. Lapham V, Kozma C, Weiss J: Genetic discrimination: perspectives of consumers. *Science* 272:621–624, 1996.
5. Sigvardsson S, Bohman M, Cloninger RC: Replication of the Stockholm adoption study of alcoholism: Confirmatory cross-fostering analysis. *Arch Gen Psychiatry* 53:681–687, 1996.
6. Crowe RR, Wang Z, Noyes R Jr, et al: Candidate gene study of eight $GABA_A$ receptor subunits in panic disorder. *Am J Psychiatry* 154:1096–1100, 1997.
7. Kennedy JL: Schizophrenia genetics: The quest for an anchor. *Am J Psychiatry* 153:1513–1514, 1996.
8. Lesch KP, Bengel D, Heils A, et al: Association of anxiety related traits with a polymorphism in the serotonin transporter gene regulatory region. *Science* 274:1527–1531, 1996.
9. Eiberg H, Berendt, I, Mohr J: Assignment of dominant inherited nocturnal enuresis (ENUR1) to chromosome 13q. *Nat Genet* 10:354–356, 1995.
10. Arnell H, Hjalmas K, Jagervall M, et al: The genetics of primary nocturnal enuresis: Inheritance and suggestion of a second major gene on chromosome 12q. *J Med Genet* 34:360–365, 1997.
11. Skuse DH, James RS, Bishop DVM, et al: Evidence from Turner's syndrome of an imprinted X-linked locus affecting cognitive function. *Nature* 387:705–708, 1997.
12. Wilmut I, Schnieke AE, McWhir J, et al: Viable offspring derived from fetal and adult mammalian cells. *Nature* 385:810–813, 1997.

► The papers that follow reflect the importance of knowledge of both the specifics of gene action and the broader implications of gene/environment interaction.

John E. Schowalter, M.D.

Genetic Influences on Life Events in Childhood

Thapar A, McGuffin P (Univ of Wales, Cardiff)

Psychol Med 26:813–820, 1996 1–1

Objective.—Life events are not random as previously believed. They appear to have a strong genetic influence. Life events affecting twins aged 8–17 years, and the relationship of those events to genetic factors and to parent ratings of events were investigated.

Methods.—A questionnaire was sent to the mothers and to 376 twin pairs born between 1976 and 1984 and registered in the Cardiff Twin Register. Zygosity, life event scores, and total phenotypic variance were recorded. Traits were analyzed statistically for fit with genetic or environmental factors. The models used were the ACE model, additive genetic effects, shared environmental, and nonshared environmental effects; the CE model, shared environment; AE model, additive genes only; or E model, no familial transmission.

Results.—The questionnaire was returned by 287 parents and 126 twin pairs. There were 113 monozygotic pairs, 85 same-sex dizygotic pairs, and 81 opposite-sex dizygotic pairs. Positive impact scores were significantly related to age and were higher among males than among females. Negative impact scores were significantly higher among females than among males, and higher among dizygotic twins than monozygotic twins. Parent-rated negative impact scores were significantly lower than female twin-rated scores. For total life score, the CE model fit 83% of males and 76% of females. For independent life events, the ACE model fit best for both sexes. Transmission of negative impact scores is best explained by the ACE model for both sexes. The best-fitting model for positive impact scores is ACE for males and CE for females. The AE model provides the best fit for self-rated total life event scores for both sexes.

Conclusion.—Self-reported and parent-reported life events in childhood and adolescence are influenced by genetic factors. The extent of the influence varied by sex and by whether the children or the parent reported the life event. External as well as internal characteristics affect an individual's perception, and therefore reporting, of life events.

▶ This is indeed a far-out twist on increasingly acknowledged gene-environment interactions. Just when clinicians have come to understand that our genes can lead us into environments that reinforce the original genetic propensity, we now learn that how those environmental experiences are remembered may be genetically influenced. This twist requires more substantiation before it becomes less far out, but it is fascinating.

J.E. Schowalter, M.D.

Using MZ Differences in the Search for Nonshared Environmental Effects

Pike A, Reiss D, Hetherington EM, et al (Inst of Psychiatry, London; George Washington Univ, Washington, DC; Univ of Virginia, Charlottesville)

J Child Psychol Psychiatry 37:695–704, 1996 1–2

Background.—In the field of behavioral genetics, the term "nonshared environment" refers to the environmental factors that work to make siblings in the same family grow up different from each other, rather than similar. One research goal in this field is to identify specific environmental influences that give rise to these differences.

Objective.—A study investigated which nonshared environmental influences may underlie associations between parental treatment of adolescents and the adolescents' adjustment. Identical (monozygotic) twins were selected as participants so that nonshared environment could be investigated independent of genetic influences.

Methods.—The data reported here were collected as part of a larger study on nonshared environment and adolescent adjustment. The selected data concerned 93 pairs of identical (monozygotic) twins (mean age, 13.71 years; age range, 10 to 18 years; approximately equal numbers of girls and boys; 94% white; all middle class). The twins and their parents had been interviewed twice, approximately 2 weeks apart. All had completed questionnaires about negative parenting (e.g., conflict, anger/hostility, yielding to coercion), depressive symptoms of the adolescents, and antisocial behavior of the adolescents. In addition, in dyads (4 parent-child dyads and 1 sibling dyad) they had been videotaped having 10-minute conversations. The videotapes had been rated for negative parenting, depressive symptoms of the adolescents, and antisocial behavior of the adolescents.

Results.—Within twin pairs, differences in antisocial behavior correlated significantly with differences in the twins' reports of their parents' negativity.

Conclusions.—A large portion of these identical twins do not experience similar environments. Of course, differences in parental treatment are not necessarily the *cause* of differences in the twins' behavior. Differences in behavior may lead to differences in parental treatment, or a third variable may underlie the associations.

► The MZ (monozygotic)-difference model for studying the influence of nonshared environments is of interest because it allows for a relatively easy within-family approach that also maintains genetic control. As a psychoanalyst, I would be fascinated to know the purported reasons why parents react more negatively toward 1 twin. It might be because of negative expectations (the twin was named after a disliked family member), or perhaps the 1 twin's behavior is truly more unlikable, or something in between. Cause and effect are almost always debatable.

J.E. Schowalter, M.D.

Genetic and Environmental Influences on the Covariation Between Hyperactivity and Conduct Disturbance in Juvenile Twins

Silberg J, Rutter M, Meyer J, et al (Virginia Commonwealth Univ, Richmond; Inst of Psychiatry, London; Inst for Behavioral Genetics Boulder, Colo; et al)

J Child Psychol Psychiatry 37:803–816, 1996 1–3

Background.—Numerous studies have reported a high rate of co-occurrence of hyperactivity/attention deficit disorders and oppositional/conduct disorders. This rate of co-occurrence is so high that some authors have questioned the distinction between these disorders. According to other authors, there are meaningful differences between hyperactivity and conduct disturbances. The distinctiveness of separate diagnostic conditions needs to be determined by the extent to which they differ in their patterns of association with correlates external to the symptoms that comprise them, such as psychosocial factors, responsiveness to treatment, and long-term outcome. The association between hyperactivity and antisocial behavior was studied in juvenile twins.

Methods.—Structural equation models were applied to data from 265 monozygotic and 163 dizygotic male-male twin pairs, to 347 monozygotic and 160 dizygotic female-female twin pairs, and to 262 male-female twin pairs. The subjects were between 8 and 16 years of age and were participants of the Virginia Twin Study of Adolescent Behavioral Development.

Results.—Significant additive genetic influences and contrast effects were observed for hyperactivity. Significant additive genetic and shared environmental effects or positive comparison effects were observed for oppositional/conduct disorders, especially in the girls. The covariation between hyperactivity and oppositional/conduct disturbances in both younger and older boys and girls is almost completely attributable to genetic factors, as shown by bivariate model fitting. In younger boys and girls, the same set of genes explains all the variation in hyperactivity and conduct disturbance. In older subjects, at least some of the genetic effects are behavior-specific and gender-specific.

Discussion.—These findings indicate that the role of genetic factors in the expression of hyperactivity and conduct disturbances in these subjects is significant. These results are consistent with those of other studies that support a strong genetic component to these behavioral problems. The other significant finding in this study was the influence of genetic factors on co-morbidity.

▶ It is extremely difficult to distinguish sibling interaction from rater bias in twin studies. This all-star–authored article is important, in part because it highlights rather than hides the many potential etiologic influences for conduct disorder and for hyperactivity. Genetic influences seem more straightforward for younger children. With advancing age, nonshared environments, and, perhaps "switched on" genes, make influences more murky.

J.E. Schowalter, M.D.

B Lymphocyte Antigen D8/17: A Peripheral Marker for Childhood-onset Obsessive-Compulsive Disorder and Tourette's Syndrome?

Murphy TK, Goodman WK, Fudge MW, et al (Univ of Florida, Gainesville; Rockefeller Univ, New York)

Am J Psychiatry 154:402–407, 1997 1–4

Purpose.—Tourette's syndrome has been linked to some forms of obsessive-compulsive disorder. Sydenham's chorea, a major manifestation of rheumatic fever, is a movement disorder that may serve as a useful medical model for certain types of obsessive-compulsive disorder. Almost all patients with rheumatic fever have expanded expression of a B-lymphocyte antigen identified by the monoclonal antibody D8/17. This antigen may mark a trait toward susceptibility to Sydenham's chorea. D8/17 expression was investigated in patients with obsessive-compulsive disorder and Tourette's syndrome.

Methods.—The study included 31 patients with childhood-onset obsessive-compulsive disorder and/or Tourette's syndrome or chronic tic disorder. Twenty-one healthy subjects were studied as controls. All subjects in both groups were free of rheumatic fever or Sydenham's chorea. The percentage of B cells positive for D8/17 was evaluated in each patient, as were levels of antineuronal antibodies and streptococcal antibodies.

Results.—In the patient group, an average 22% of B cells expressed D8/17, compared with 9% in the control group. When 1 standard deviation or greater above normal was used as the cutoff point, 100% of patients vs. 5% of controls tested positive for D8/17. The presence of antineuronal antibodies and the levels of streptococcal titers were similar in the 2 groups. There were no differences in D8/17 values within the various patient subgroups.

Conclusion.—B-cell D8/17 expression is above normal in patients with childhood-onset obsessive-compulsive disorder or Tourette's syndrome. As it is for rheumatic fever or Sydenham's chorea, D8/17 may be a useful marker for some forms of childhood-onset obsessive-compulsive disorder and Tourette's syndrome. Further studies of D8/17 are needed.

► Back to "real" medicine. When I was training in pediatrics and in child psychiatry and Sydenham's chorea was more prevalent, it was these patients' aggressivity that was often a challenging management problem. It will be fascinating to follow the various post–streptococcal infection research projects now in progress.

J.E. Schowalter, M.D.

Autism or Atypical Autism in Maternally but Not Paternally Derived Proximal 15q Duplication

Cook EH Jr, Lindgren V, Leventhal BL, et al (Univ of Chicago; Univ of California at San Diego, La Jolla)

Am J Hum Genet 60:928–934, 1997 1–5

Background.—Although genetic factors are involved in autism, the genetic basis and mode of transmission are unknown. Patients with autistic disorder and mental retardation have duplications of proximal 15q, often in the form of a supernumerary inverted duplicated—or isodicentric—chromosome 15. Other patients have intrachromosomal duplications. A family with autism associated with maternal, but not paternal, proximal 15q duplication was reported.

Methods and Results.—The findings were based on genotyping studies of patients with autistic disorder and their parents. Microsatellite analysis detected intrachromosomal duplication of proximal 15 q in the mother at the positional candidate locus D15S122. Of this mother's 3 children, 2 had autism or atypical autism. Further analysis of this pedigree showed that the 2 affected children inherited a 15q11–q13 duplication from their mother. This duplication was not present in the third child, who did not have autism. The mother's 15q11–q13 duplication arose de novo in her father.

Discussion.—In this family, a paternally inherited 15q11–q13 duplication leads to a normal phenotype, whereas a maternally inherited duplication leads to autism. The findings demonstrate the significance of parental origins for 15q chromosome duplications.

► Although a study of 3 patients makes one hunger for more patients and more families, the finding of maternal inheritance of the duplication does fit well with previous investigations. It now seems worthwhile to examine proximal 15q in cytogenetic studies of patients with autism or atypical autism.

J.E. Schowalter, M.D.

X Chromosome and Infantile Autism

Petit E, Hérault J, Raynaud M, et al (CHU Bretonneau, Tours, France)
Biol Psychiatry 40:457–464, 1996 1–6

Objective.—Genetic factors appear to be involved in the etiology of autism, the developmental disorder which affects more boys than girls. Chromosomal analyses were conducted in families with autistic children to determine if the syndrome is an X-linked dominant disorder.

Methods.—Extensive developmental, psychiatric, psychological, and neurologic examinations were carried out on 90 autistic children and young adults (27 female), aged 2–20 years, and a control group. Genetic factors, including family history and somatic signs were evaluated, and genomic DNA extracted from ethylenediamineletraacetic acid anticoagulated blood was analyzed for fragile X syndrome. Allele frequency was calculated and proportions were compared statistically.

Results.—Clinical results showed 30 children with isolated peculiarity, dysmorphology, and/or malformations; 5 children with probable genetic disease, and 6 children with proven genetic disease. Control and autistic groups had different allelic distributions for the marker DXS287. These differences were most marked for children with significant autistic behavior but with the least cognitive impairment.

Conclusion.—These preliminary results indicate the involvement of the X chromosome in the etiology of autism. Additional research must be done to confirm this locus and to elicit other causative factors in autism.

► These are very preliminary data, but, as the authors note, the X chromosome makes sense as a possible etiologic risk factor in some children with autism. Because a high-resolution map for the X chromosome has now been completed, it has become increasingly clear just how influential this giant grandmother of DNA—some 160 million chemical units in length—is for so many of the basic building blocks of what makes us who we are.[1]

J.E. Schowalter, M.D.

Reference

1. Nagaraja R, MacMillan S, Keer J, et al: X chromosome map at 75-kb STS resolution, revealing extremes of recombination and GC content. *Genome Res* 7:210–222, 1997.

2 Disorders of Intelligence and Learning

Introduction

As noted in the selections below, the past year has had a rich yield of interesting papers.

Three articles that pertain to decreased IQ also caught my interest. One is an excellent overview paper that highlights the spectrum of autism, including mental retardation which is found in approximately 75% of individuals.[1] Another is a longitudinal study which continues to show a dose-related relationship between dentine lead levels measured at ages 6 to 8 years and poorer educational performance at age 18.[2] The third study describes nonspecific mental retardation over three generations in a family with X-chromosome markers which overlap with 5 loci found by previous researchers in Xq28.[3]

Also interesting have been studies which focus on intelligence development or improvement. A study of twins over the age of 80 suggests that genetic influence continues to contribute about 50% of variance for intelligence even at this advanced age.[4] Another group of investigators turned its nature-nurture attention on the mother's womb environment as a more-important-than-thought variable for IQ.[5] They postulate that similar uterine experiences are more responsible and genetic similarity is less responsible than usually supposed for twins' similarity in IQ.

In conclusion, an Israeli study of preadolescents' breakfast patterns and their cognition suggests that students who had their testing within two hours of consuming sugared cornflakes and milk scored better against personal baselines than those who had breakfast earlier at home or no breakfast at all.[6] A short-term increase in blood glucose is the believed mechanism. Maybe candidates should take a candy bar to their board examinations.

John E. Schowalter, M.D.

References

1. Rapin I: Autism. *N Engl J Med* 337:97–104, 1997.
2. Fergussion DM, Horwood LJ, Lynskey MT: *J Child Psychol Psychiat* 38:471–478, 1997.
3. DesPortes V, Billuart P, Carriè A, et al: A gene dominant nonspecific X-linked mental retardation is located in Xq28. *Am J Hum Genet* 60:903–909, 1997.
4. McClean GE, Johansson B, Berg S et al: Substantial genetic influence on cognitive abilities in twins 80 or more years old. *Science* 276:1560–1563, 1997.
5. Devlin B, Daniels M, Roeder K: The heritability of IQ. *Nature* 388:468–471, 1997.
6. Vaisman N, Voet H, Akivis A, et al: Effect of breakfast timing on the cognitive functions of elementary school students. *Arch Pediatr Adolesc Med* 150:1089–1092, 1996.

In Utero Problems and Beyond

► These infants were born with actual or potential disabilities and are followed up to show their various outcomes.

John E. Schowalter, M.D.

Neuromotor Development of Cocaine-exposed and Control Infants From Birth Through 15 Months: Poor and Poorer Performance

Fetters L, Tronick EZ (Boston Univ; Children's Hosp, Boston)

Pediatrics 98:938–943, 1996 2–1

Objective.—The motor development of infants exposed to cocaine in utero was compared with that of unexposed infants.

Methods.—Mothers and infants were recruited at an urban university hospital between July 1991 and April 1993. The final sample comprised 28 cocaine-exposed infants and a control group of 22 unexposed infants matched for race, family income, and mother's educational level. Among other criteria, infants were required to be free of known major risk factors for developmental impairment, such as fetal alcohol syndrome. On 4 occasions, infants were evaluated with standard clinical instruments by examiners who were masked to group status. The Alberta Infant Motor Scale (AIMS) was used at 1 month of age, the AIMS and the Movement Assessment of Infants inventory were used at 4 months, the AIMS and the Movement Assessment of Infants were used at 7 months, and the Peabody Developmental Motor Scales were used at 15 months.

Results.—Cocaine-exposed infants showed impaired motor development, compared with the control group, at 4 and 7 months but not at 1 or 15 months. A more striking finding was that nearly every infant, regardless of exposure status, had poor motor development at every age, compared with standardized norms. Many needed referrals for intervention.

Conclusions.—A large number of seemingly normal inner-city infants may be at risk for motor problems. This is of grave concern because motor skills are fundamental to infant exploratory behavior. Public health programs should not be targeted only toward high-risk populations.

► This study raises as many questions as it answers. These questions cry out for further follow-ups of the status of these groups at later ages. No one can say that maternal cocaine use is not a risk factor for the fetus, but the infants of other mothers with similar socioeconomic and behavioral factors who did use cocaine show remarkably similar developmental problems during the first 15 months.

J.E. Schowalter, M.D.

Iron-deficiency Anemia and Infant Development: Effects of Extended Oral Iron Therapy

Lozoff B, Wolf AW, Jimenez E (Univ of Michigan, Ann Arbor; Case Western Reserve Univ, Cleveland, Ohio; Hosp Nacional de Niños, San Jose, Costa Rica)

J Pediatr 129:382–389, 1996 2–2

Objective.—Iron-deficiency anemia affects infants' motor and mental development. One study showed improved test scores after iron therapy. Results in anemic and nonanemic infants before and after 3 and 6 months of iron therapy were evaluated.

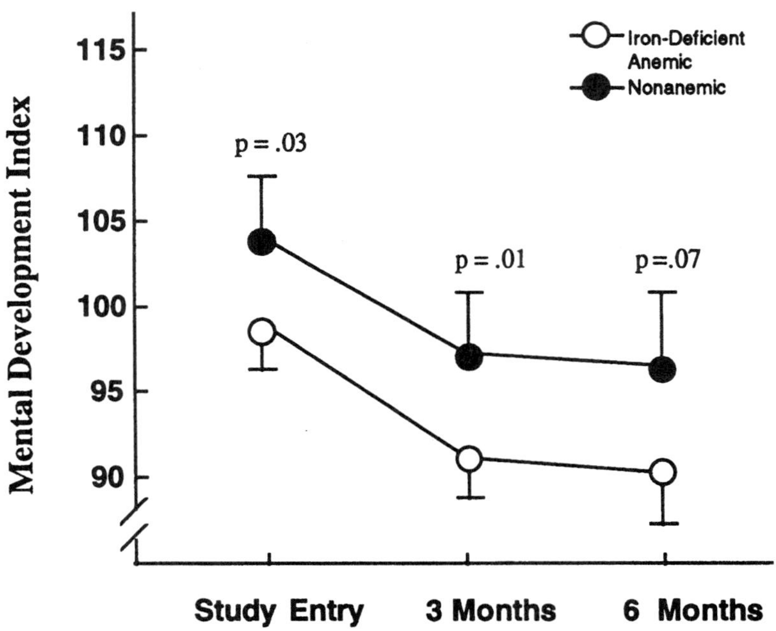

FIGURE 1.—Mental development test scores. The Mental Development Index (adjusted mean ± SEM with age as covariate) of the Bayley Scales of Infant Development are shown for the iron-deficient anemic and nonanemic groups before treatment, after 3 months, and after 6 months. The anemic group's scores were lower than those of the nonanemic group at all 3 time points; statistically significant before treatment and at 3 months, and showing a suggestive trend at 6 months. (Courtesy of Lozoff B, Wolf AW, Jimenez E: Iron-deficiency anemia and infant development: Effects of extended oral iron therapy. *J Pediatr* 129:382–389, 1996.)

Methods.—In Costa Rica between 1986 and 1990, iron status was determined in 54 nonanemic infants receiving either placebo or 3 mg of an oral iron preparation per kilogram twice daily for 6 months and 39 anemic infants receiving the oral iron preparation. Differences in variables between anemic and nonanemic groups were analyzed statistically.

Results.—Baseline hemoglobin levels were 94 g/L for anemic and 132 g/L for nonanemic children. In the nonanemic group, 70% had 1 or more measures of iron deficiency. The average increase in hemoglobin levels for the nonanemic group was 34 mg/L at 3 months and 35 mg/L at 6. The average increase in hemoglobin levels for the anemic group was 7 g/L at 3 months and 10 g/L at 6. Among nonanemic infants with 1 or more measures of iron deficiency, 62% continued to have an iron deficiency at 3 months and 60% at 6 months. Iron-deficient anemic infants had lower mental test scores than nonanemic patients at all 3 time points. (Fig 1). There were no differences in motor scores at any time point (Fig 2). Anemic infants tended to have less well educated mothers, less support at home, and were less likely to be breast fed or were weaned earlier. However, only age was significantly related to anemia in the multiple regression model. Anemic infants were significantly unusually fearful and unhappy and tended to be excessively wary or hesitant.

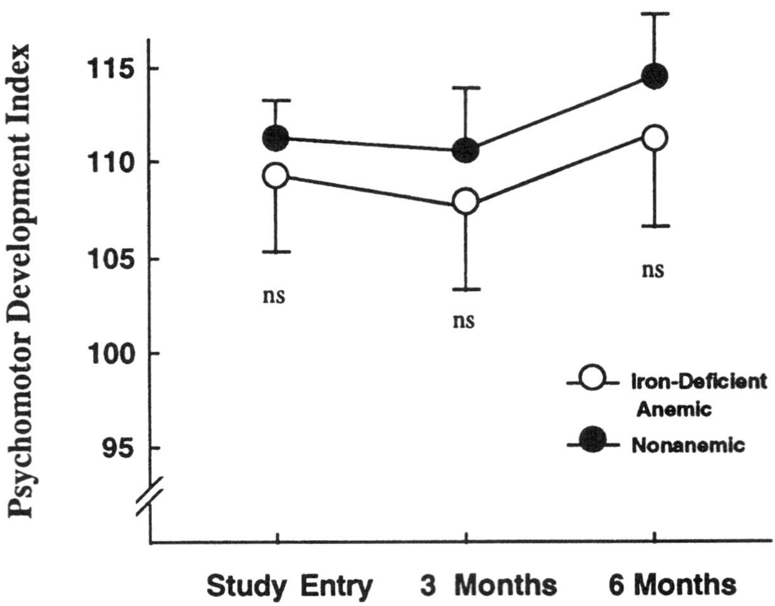

FIGURE 2.—Motor development test scores. The Psychomotor Development Index (adjusted mean ± SEM with age as covariate) of the Bayley Scales of Infant Development are shown for the iron-deficient anemic and nonanemic groups before treatment, after 3 months, and after 6 months. There were no statistically significant differences at any time point. (Courtesy of Lozoff B, Wolf AW, Jimenez E: Iron-deficiency anemia and infant development: Effects of extended oral iron therapy. *J Pediatr* 129:382–389, 1996.)

Conclusion.—Anemic infants continued to have significantly lower mental scores despite iron therapy. Other factors in the home or diet may adversely affect development of these infants.

► I found these findings somewhat surprising. Granted that iron deficiency is usually linked with other environmental deficits, common sense suggests that correcting even one major deficit should allow at least some measurable improvement.

J.E. Schowalter, M.D.

Cognitive and Neurologic Development of the Premature, Small for Gestational Age Infant Through Age 6: Comparison by Birth Weight and Gestational Age

McCarton CM, Wallace IF, Divon M, et al (Albert Einstein College of Medicine, Bronx, NY; Research Triangle Inst, Research Triangle Park, NC; Univ of North Carolina at Chapel Hill)

Pediatrics 98:1167–1178, 1996 2–3

Objective.—The specific developmental effects in premature and small-for-gestational-age (SGA) infants or in premature and appropriate for gestational age (AGA) infants are equivocal. The neurologic and cognitive outcomes of premature SGA infants were compared with those of premature AGA infants from birth to age 6.

Methods.—Developmental evaluations were performed on 130 premature AGA children (43% males) and 129 premature SGA children (44% males) at 1, 2, 3, 5, and 6 years. Results for the 2 groups were compared statistically. Results for children with questionable neurologic status were categorized as suspicious.

Results.—Cognitive scores were significantly related to immaturity at all time points, and were significantly lower at all time points for SGA children. Cognitive scores were significantly related to birth weight at 1, 2, 5, and 6 years for all children. The percentage of AGA children classified as neurologically normal was significantly higher than the percentage of SGA children at all time points. Appropriate for gestational age children had a 2.3–3.3 greater chance of being classified as neurologically normal than SGA children at all time points. The SGA children were 2 times as likely to be classified as abnormal as AGA children at years 1 and 3. When birth weight was taken into account, there was no difference between groups with respect to abnormal neurologic classification. Children with the highest cognitive scores were classified as normal at all time points except 3 years. Neurologic status was significantly related to cognitive status at all time points. The AGA children had higher cognitive scores in all neurologic categories at all time points (Fig 4).

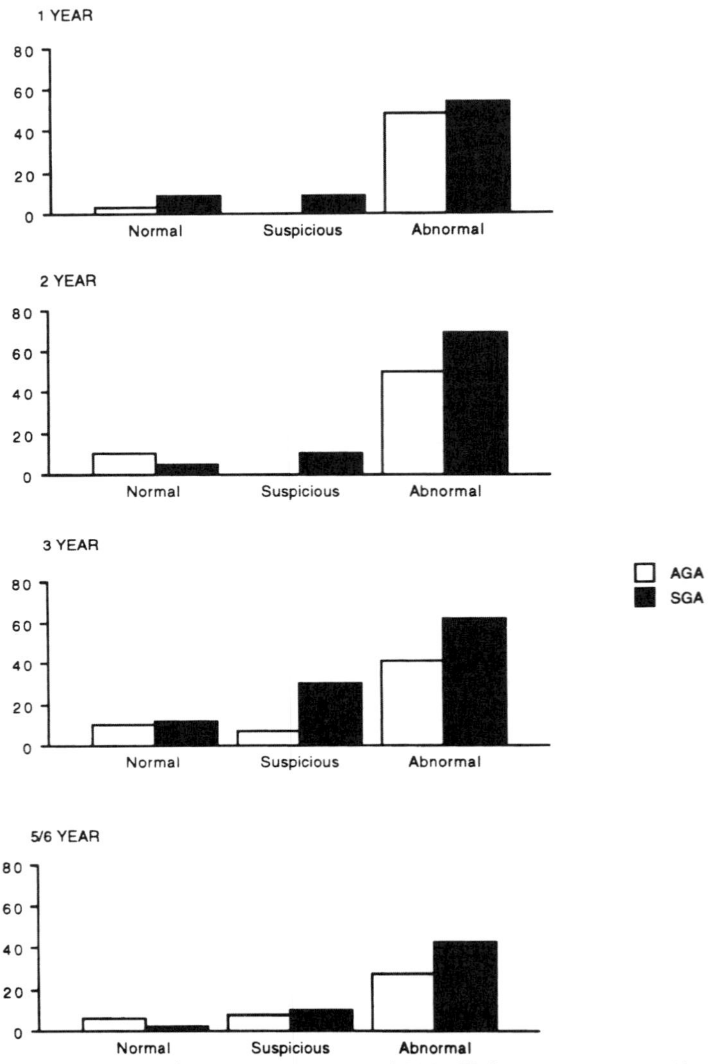

FIGURE 4.—Percentage of AGA (*open squares*) and SGA (*filled squares*) preterms with cognitive retardation as a function of neurologic status. *Abbreviations: AGA*, appropriate for gestational age; *SGA*, small for gestational age. (Reproduced by permission from McCarton CM, Wallace IF, Divon M, et al: Cognitive and neurologic development of the premature, small for gestational age infant through age 6: Comparison by birth weight and gestational age. *Pediatrics* 98:1167–1178, 1996. Copyright 1996.)

Conclusion.—Premature SGA infants are at higher risk than AGA infants of development neurologic and cognitive impairments at every age tested.

► Although difficulties are always present in defining SGA because of possible errors in estimating age and in setting a cutoff criterion, the authors have been open and clear in describing their methodology. The womb is a wonderful environment, and even for embryos of low weight, it seems the longer, the better.

J.E. Schowalter, M.D.

Results at Age 8 Years of Early Intervention for Low-Birth-Weight Premature Infants: The Infant Health and Development Program

McCarton CM, for the Infant Health and Development Program Research Group (Albert Einstein Collge of Medicine, Bronx, NY; Columbia Univ, New York; Research Triangle Inst, Research Triangle Park, NC; et al)

JAMA 277:126–132, 1997 2–4

Objective.—Low–birth-weight (LBW) premature children score lower on global measures of intelligence and other neurodevelopmental assessments than normal birth weight children. The results of a re-evaluation at age 8 years of the intervention in the first 3 years of life of LBW infants by The Infant Health and Development Program multisite randomized clinical trial were discussed.

Methods.—There were 985 children from 8 sites randomly allocated to receive intervention (377 children) or no intervention (608 children) and further stratified into those with birth weights of 2,000 g or less or 2,001–2,500 g. Intervention consisted of home visits through age 3 years, attendance at a special center from ages 1 to 3 years, and parent group meeting every other month during years 2 and 3. All children had periodic developmental and social assessments. Cognitive, academic achievement, and behavioral re-assessments were made in both groups at age 8 years.

Results.—Cognitive outcomes in the heavier LBW intervention group were significantly higher than in the heavier follow-up–only group (4.4 IQ points higher, 4.2 verbal IQ points higher, 3.9 performance IQ points higher). There were no IQ differences among any groups when stratified by maternal education. Results for the lighter LBW intervention group and the follow-up groups were similar. School performance outcomes in mathematics and receptive vocabulary were significantly higher for the heavier LBW intervention group than for the heavier follow-up–only group (4.8 and 6.7 points higher, respectively). There were no differences between the lighter LBW groups. Behavior outcomes were similar among all groups, as were percentages of children with serious behavioral problems. Health outcomes were similar among all groups.

Conclusions.—Heavier LBW premature children at 8 years had retained modest benefits from intervention, whereas lighter LBW premature children seemed to have little to no benefit. Additional intervention strategies to aid these children in a lasting way need to be developed.

► As more and more LBW infants survive, it becomes increasingly important to learn what their long-term developmental outcomes are likely to be. Of particular interest from this follow-up study at age 8 years is the question of whether the progress found at age 3 years was not sustained because different types of interventions must be provided beyond the toddler years. The question of cost-benefit ratio seems repugnant, but if pediatric dollars reach a zero-sum balance, decisions about spending priorities will have to be made, like it or not. From this study, it does seem that money spent on the relatively heavier children has a greater chance to bring sustained change.

J.E. Schowalter, M.D.

Development of a Regional Cohort of Very-Low-Birthweight Children at Six Years: Cognitive Abilities Are Associated With Neurological Disability and Social Background

Dammann O, Walther H, Allers B, et al (Univ Hosp Eppendorf, Hamburg, Germany; Gen Hosp Heidberg, Hamburg, Germany)

Dev Med Child Neurol 38:97–108, 1996 2–5

Objective.—Long-term follow-up data were gathered on the cognitive development of very-low-birth-weight (VLBW) children.

Methods.—The base population in this study was 591 VLBW children who were born during a 3-year period near Hamburg, Germany. Of these, 330 children were traceable at age 6 years, and 317 parents consented to neurologic and psychological testing. Children were not excluded for neurologic disabilities such as cerebral palsy or attention-deficit hyperactivity disorder. However, 19 children were too mentally disabled for psychological testing, so the results reported here are for 298 children.

Results.—On memory and visuomotor skills tests, the mean scores for the whole group were below standardized norms. On language and intelligence tests, the scores for the whole group were not abnormal, but there was a trend toward lower scores for children with cerebral palsy or attention-deficit hyperactivity disorder. Also, on language tests, children from the lower socioeconomic third of the sample scored significantly below the norms, whereas children from the middle and upper socioeconomic thirds scored at or above the norms.

Conclusions.—In this sample of VLBW children, intelligence and language skills were affected more by socioeconomic status than by neurologic deficit. As expected, memory and visuomotor development were subnormal.

▶ The longer we can have for the follow-up of the status of VLBW infants, the more accurate we can be in differentiating the causes for various neurodevelopmental deficits. The importance of this study lies in its large cohort size, its methodological vigor, and its 6-year follow-up.

J.E. Schowalter, M.D.

Mental Retardation

Mental Retardation: Genetic Findings, Clinical Implications and Research Agenda

Simonoff E, Bolton P, Rutter M (Inst of Psychiatry, London; Univ of Cambridge, England)

J Child Psychol Psychiatry 37:259–280, 1996 2–6

Background.—The genetic influences on mental retardation are not as simple and deterministic as once thought. Progress in molecular genetics research has led to a better understanding of the genetic mechanisms involved in mental retardation and the complex links between the abnormal gene, the gene product, and the phenotypic manifestations. It is important to understand how genetic and environmental factors interrelate to produce mental retardation. The role of genetics in mental retardation was reviewed, including some ways in which genes interact with environmental influences in mild mental retardation.

Genetics and Mental Retardation.—The past decade has seen key advances in our understanding of the genetic factors involved in certain types of severe retardation. These include the genetic mechanisms responsible for the fragile X syndrome and the imprinting involved in the Prader-Willi and Angelman syndromes. At the same time, new insights have been gained into the pathogenesis of Down syndrome and phenylketonuria. Nevertheless, the biology of intellectual impairment is poorly understood in almost every case. The identification of abnormal or high-risk genes is highly useful for genetic screening and counseling purposes. However, it has little impact in terms of therapy.

Many cases of mild and severe mental retardation involve genetic defects, including single-gene mendelian disorders and cytogenetic abnormalities. Thus, it is inaccurate to suggest, as was previously done, that severe mental retardation represents a pathologic condition, whereas mild mental retardation is a normal variation. For many patients, no pathologic cause of mental retardation can be identified. Genetic influences seem to play an important role in this group, although the specific genes involved are unknown. The genetic factors interact with environmental factors, and this interaction is not well understood.

Discussion.—A great deal of progress has been made in our understanding of the genetic influences on mental retardation. However, there is a need for more information on how genetic and environmental influences interact to produce intellectual impairment, in particular mild mental retardation. Behavioral genetic studies using direct measures of relevant environmental factors may not only provide insight into the causes of mental retardation but also point the way to targeted interventions.

▶ This is one of those marvelous summary articles published periodically in the *Journal of Child Psychology and Psychiatry*. While concluding that the biological mechanisms that lead to mental retardation are "poorly understood in virtually all cases" and that our genetic clues, to date, have not often led to new treatment approaches, the authors provide a wonderfully written and thorough account of the current understanding of genetic influences in mental retardation. I have always believed that being born smart is dumb luck. An indication of the thoroughness of this article is the bibliography, which contains more than 250 references.

J.E. Schowalter, M.D.

Dopamine Transporters Are Markedly Reduced in Lesch-Nyhan Disease In Vivo

Wong DF, Harris JC, Naidu S, et al (Johns Hopkins Univ, Baltimore, Md; Kennedy-Krieger Inst, Baltimore, Md; Montreal Neurological Inst; et al)

Proc Natl Acad Sci U S A 93:5539–5543, 1996 2–7

Introduction.—Lesch-Nyhan disease (LND) is an X chromosome–linked disease with infantile onset. It is characterized by hyperuricemia, choreoathetosis, dystonia, and compulsive self-injury. The underlying defect is deficiency of an enzyme that is usually present in the brain in greater amounts than in other organs, hypoxanthine-guanine phosphoribosyl transferase (HPRT). Earlier findings suggest that HPRT deficiency is linked to abnormal dopamine (DA) function in patients with LND. The ligand WIN-35,428, which binds to DA transporters, was used to estimate the density of DA-containing neurons in the caudate and putamen of patients with classic LND to determine whether DA deficiency is present in patients with LND.

Methods.—Six patients with classic LND, 3 patients with Rett syndrome, and 10 normal controls underwent 3 methods of positron emission tomographic analysis to estimate DA transporter binding: evaluation of either the caudate- or putamen-to-cerebellum ratio measured in the last 3 frames of PET imaging, kinetic analysis of the binding potential, and graphic analysis of the binding potential.

Results.—When compared with controls, a 50% to 63% (depending on the methods used) reduction in binding to DA transporters in the caudate and a 64% to 75% reduction in the putamen of patients with LND were observed (Fig 2). When patients with LND were compared with patients with Rett syndrome, the reductions in the caudate were 53% to 61%, and reductions in the putamen were 67% to 72%. Patients with Rett syndrome and normal controls differed little in transport binding. A 30% reduction in caudate volume was noted in patients with LND in the volumetric MRI studies. A rigorous partial-volume correction of the caudate time-activity curve was performed to make sure that a reduction in caudate volume would not distort the results. The correction subsequently resulted in a greater decrease in the caudate-cerebellar ratio in patients with LND than in controls.

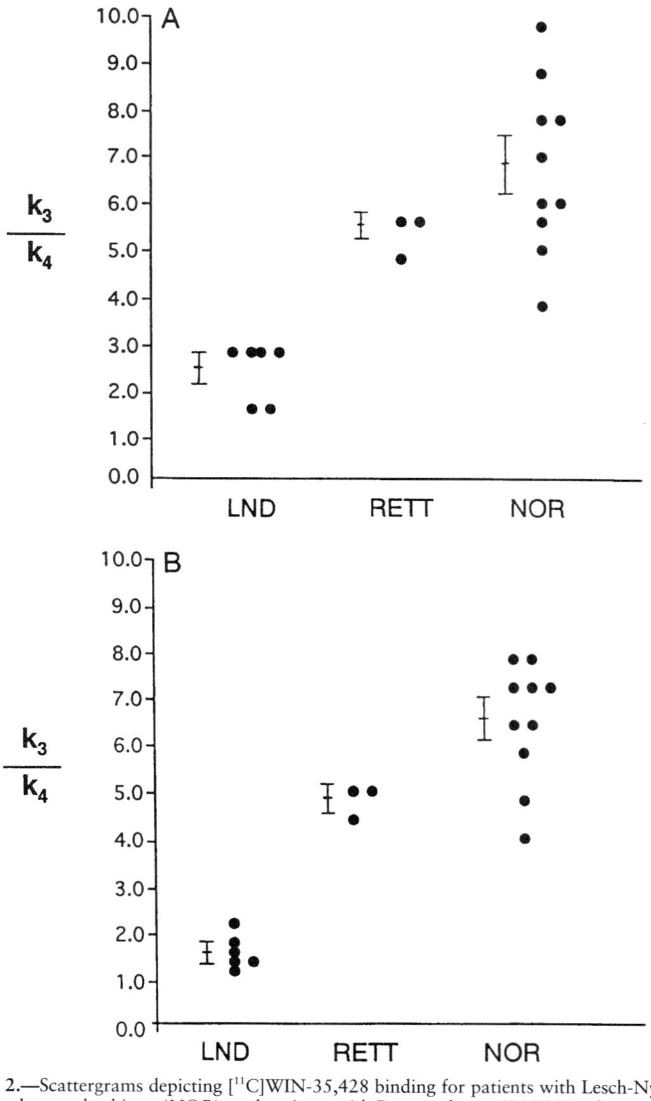

FIGURE 2.—Scattergrams depicting [^{11}C]WIN-35,428 binding for patients with Lesch-Nyhan disease (*LND*), normal control subjects (*NOR*), and patients with Rett syndrome (*RETT*) in the caudate (**A**) and putamen (**B**) by using the k_3/k_4 constrained method. These scattergrams clearly show the absence of overlap of the LND cases with Rett syndrome or normal control subjects. Bars show mean ± SEM. (Courtesy of Wong DF, Harris JC, Naidu S: Dopamine transporters are markedly reduced in Lesch-Nyhan disease in vivo. *Proc Natl Acad Sci U S A* 93:5539–5543, 1996. Copyright 1996 National Academy of Sciences, U.S.A.)

Conclusion.—These findings, reported for the first time, document an in vivo DA reduction in patients with LND. Positron emission tomography can be considered useful in investigating neurodevelopmental disorders.

► In this elegant study, patients with LND were shown in vivo to have substantially decreased dopamine transporter binding function in comparison to normal controls and Rett syndrome controls. Dopamine reduction in patients with LND has earlier been shown in postmortum findings and in spinal fluid analyses. This approach required the as yet complicated interdigitation of findings of positron emission tomography, measurement of ligands that bind to presynaptic or postsynaptic dopamine sites, the help of x-ray CT for positioning, and the use of volumetric MRI of the putamen and candidate. In the future, what was accomplished here will become routine; at present, *elegant* is the word foremost in my mind.

J.E. Schowalter, M.D.

Predictors of Mortality in Children With Severe Mental Retardation: The Effect of Placement

Strauss D, Eyman RK, Grossman HJ (Univ of California, Riverside; Univ of Michigan, Ann Arbor)

Am J Public Health 86:1422–1429, 1996 2–8

Objective.—Whereas immobility, feeding and toileting problems, or severe cerebral palsy are known to be related to mortality in severely retarded children, no studies have examined the relationship of mortality to placement. Predictors of mortality in severely retarded children were studied and risk-adjusted mortality rates for those living in institutions vs. living in the community were compared..

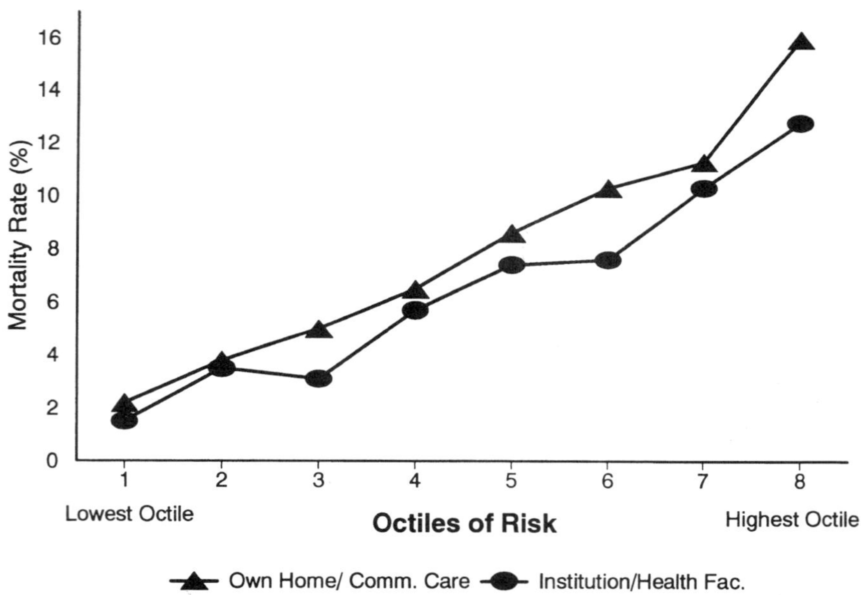

FIGURE 2.—Annual mortality rates, by placement, derived from 7,241 severely retarded California children. (Courtesy of Strauss D, Eyman RK, Grossman HJ: Predictors of mortality in children with severe mental retardation: The effect of placement. *Am J Public Health* 86:1422–1429, Copyright 1996, American Public Health Association.)

Methods.—Information on mobility, feeding, interaction, age, placement, perception, language, and level of retardation was collected for 7,241 children with severe developmental disabilities and in fragile medical condition served by the California Department of Developmental Services between January 1, 1980, and December 31, 1992.

Results.—Those who were tube fed and had the lowest level of mobility had the highest mortality rate. Children in their own home or in community care had a 25% higher risk of death than those cared for in institutions or health facilities (Fig 2).

Conclusion.—Children with severe developmental disabilities who are deinstitutionalized have an increased mortality rate.

▶ This study raises more questions than it answers, but they are valid questions. What seems to me most important is to have all these data available to parents when discussing placement issues. For those parents who still want to have the home experience for themselves and their child, God bless.

J.E. Schowalter, M.D.

Screening, Risk, and Outcome

Utility of the Pediatric Symptom Checklist as a Psychosocial Screen to Meet the Federal Early and Periodic Screening, Diagnosis, and Treatment (EPSDT) Standards: A Pilot Study

Murphy JM, Ichinose C, Hicks RC, et al (Massachusetts Gen Hosp, Boston; Ventura County Depts of Mental Health and Public Health Ventura, Calif; San Mateo County Dept of Mental Health, San Mateo, Calif)

J Pediatr 129:864–869, 1996 2–9

Background.—Since 1989, states in the United States have been under a federal mandate to screen children for psychological and developmental problems during all visits covered under the Medicaid Early and Periodic Screening Diagnosis and Treatment (EPSDT) program. However, few providers actually satisfy this requirement. Recent structural changes in the Medicaid program have made quality indicators critical parameters of capitation and managed care programs. The rate of childhood psychiatric disorders in the United States is reported to be as high as 17% to 22% and may be even higher among poor children. The guidelines for well-child health care under the Medicaid EPSDT program affect about 20% of all children in the United States. The EPSDT program requires that all children receive periodic screenings for various conditions. The Pediatric Symptom Checklist is a useful screening tool and has been validated for a variety of settings.

Methods.—The Pediatric Symptom Checklist was used to screen 379 children between ages 6 and 16 years in 3 health clinics located in a low-income Hispanic community. The checklist was administered in written and oral form and was available in Spanish and English.

Results.—For the entire study population, the Cronbach alpha was high and did not differ for written, oral, Spanish, or English formats. All items on the Pediatric Symptom Checklist were associated with the total score. This checklist identified 10.6% of the study population as being at risk for psychosocial problems; 9.5% of the children were referred for psychological follow up. There was a significant increase of 0.5% to 2.9% in referrals for psychological disorders during the study period in the areas using the Pediatric Symptom Checklist.

Discussion.—The Pediatric Symptom Checklist is valuable for screening children for psychosocial problems during routine health examinations under the Medicaid EPSDT program. Capitation Medicaid programs for poor children should include psychosocial screening, tracking of outcomes, and assessment of cost benefits. Underrecognition of psychosocial problems is a significant danger of managed care programs.

▶ Although the Pediatric Symptom Checklist is, to my mind, the most useful and versatile psychosocial screening instrument available, it is still not known or used sufficiently. Medicaid has highlighted EPSDT standards as a key criterion for assessing managed care organizations' level of functioning. Perhaps the usefulness of the Pediatric Symptom Checklist in this required endeavor will help the checklist to become more widely used.

J.E. Schowalter, M.D.

Mainstreaming Experience in the United States: Is It the Appropriate Educational Placement for Every Disabled Child?

Butler C (Seattle)

Dev Med Child Neurol 38:861–866, 1996 2–10

Objective.—The philosophy of "full inclusion" in special education was discussed.

Definition.—Proponents of "full inclusion" want all students with disabilities, regardless of the severity of type of their disability, to be educated full-time in regular classrooms instead of being removed to special education classrooms for part or all of the day. Some proponents of "full inclusion" want to do away with special education teachers altogether; others want to integrate special education services into the regular classroom.

Origins.—Special education has come under fire for a range of reasons: its concentration on remedial skills instead of helping children keep up with regular class work; the fragmentation of learning that occurs when children are removed to another classroom; and the emotional impact on children who are "labeled" and excluded, at least part of the time, from interacting with their classmates. Many advocates of full inclusion are part of a broader educational restructuring movement in the United States that calls for more aid to all low-achieving schoolchildren (e.g., those who are disadvantaged by poverty or are not fluent in English).

Criticisms.—Critics of full inclusion charge that regular classrooms will actually restrict the opportunities of children who have trouble learning basic skills or controlling their behavior. They want parents and teachers to be able to choose which services are right for a child. There is also concern that "full inclusion" is a euphemism for "dumping" children into regular classrooms to save money.

The Literature.—No study has shown that full inclusion has clear merits over special education. The scant evidence simply suggests that students do no worse in integrated classrooms. Experimental programs have been successful where there has been parent involvement, teacher training, effective collaboration between regular teachers and special education teachers, and student support such as curriculum adaptations and peer tutoring.

▶ I believe that every movement has the capacity to move too far. An interesting situation in my homestate of Connecticut is that an initially family-inspired movement to empty mentally disabled individuals from the state institution has lately run into family opposition. Deinstitutionalization certainly appeals to state officials' budgets, particularly when the institution is almost empty, but the last residents are severely disabled, most with accompanying severe neurologic conditions. These residents' families do not believe that these individuals can be as well cared for outside of the institution.

J.E. Schowalter, M.D.

Self-Sufficiency at Ages 27 to 33 Years: Factors Present Between Birth and 18 Years That Predict Educational Attainment Among Children Born to Inner-City Families

Hardy JB, Shapiro S, Mellits ED, et al (Johns Hopkins Univ, Baltimore, Md)
Pediatrics 99:80–87, 1997 2–11

Background.—An intergenerational, multidisciplinary study was conducted of children born in the 1960s to mothers living in the inner city. This study, the Pathways to Adulthood, identified factors that enable children to overcome the disadvantages of their childhood and become self-sufficient, successful adults. This study identifies key characteristics and events that affect 4 outcome domains of daily living, were identified.

Methods.—There were 2,694 children born between 1960 and 1965 to mothers who lived in the inner city and who were enrolled in the Johns Hopkins Collaborative Perinatal Study. Neurologic and cognitive development, health, behavior, and family and neighborhood socioeconomic characteristics from birth to age 8 years were observed prospectively. Interviews were conducted with 1,758 of these children at ages 27–33 years and with 1,552 of the mothers. Significant factors affecting outcome in the areas of education, physical and mental health, a lifestyle free of self-destructive and unlawful behavior, and independence of public financial assistance were identified.

Results.—Of these study children born between 1960 and 1965, 79% had a successful outcome in education (high school diploma or equivalent), 60% had a successful health outcome, 70% had a successful lifestyle outcome, and 76% had a successful outcome in the area of financial independence. A more favorable outcome was seen in black subjects for education and lifestyle and in white subjects for financial independence. Health outcome was similar for both races. Independent variables predictive of attainment of adult education were the mother's education level when the child was born, the child's attainment of honor roll, average or better reading skills at age 8, nonuse of tobacco, no pregnancy before age 18, and not repeating a grade in school.

Discussion.—Although the educational attainment of the children in this study was higher than that of their mothers, the children still had reading and language skills well below average at ages 7 and 8 years. Language and reading are strongly associated with educational outcome and success in adulthood. Young children should be given more attention in these areas.

► I found this to be a fascinating study. It would be an ideal multicity study. The idea of "family values" was and still is kidded about because some high-profile politicians wrapped themselves in the concept, while not particularly practicing the values personally. Research makes it clear, however, that loving and stable caretakers, education, and the avoidance of dangerous behaviors are wonderful protective factors for all children, regardless of race or social status.

J.E. Schowalter, M.D.

Risk and Protective Factors Affecting the Adjustment of Siblings of Children With Chronic Disabilities

Fisman S, Wolf L, Ellison D, et al (Univ of Western Ontario, London, Ont, Canada; McMaster Univ, Hamilton, Ont, Canada)

J Am Acad Child Adolesc Psychiatry 35:1532–1541, 1996 2–12

Background.—Although many studies have described the effects of chronic disability on affected children and their mothers, few have reported the effects on siblings. Such children may be at a greater risk for emotional and behavioral disorders than the general population. The adjustment of the nondisabled siblings of disabled children was investigated.

Methods.—The 3-year longitudinal study included 46 siblings of children with pervasive developmental disorder (PDD), 45 siblings of children with Down syndrome, and 46 siblings of developmentally normal children. Preliminary information collected from primary caregivers, teachers, and the siblings was analyzed.

Findings.—The siblings of children with PDD had significantly more problems than did the other 2 groups. Different correlates of adjustment

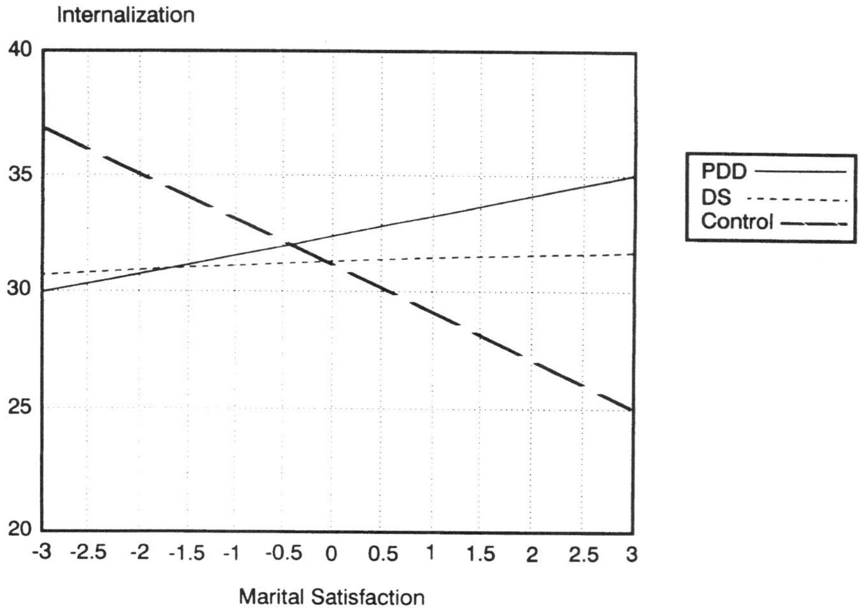

FIGURE 1.—Parent internalizing problems as a function of marital satisfaction and group. (Courtesy of Fisman S, Wolf L, Ellison D, et al: Risk and protective factors affecting the adjustment of siblings of children with chronic disabilities. *J Am Acad Child Adolesc Psychiatry* 35:1532–1541, 1996.)

were noted in the siblings of disabled children, compared with nondisabled children. Mediating factors differed in parent and teacher reports of internalizing problems in the siblings of children with PDD. Protective factors for the siblings of normal children and those with Down syndrome were parental marital satisfaction, lack of parental depression, a cohesive family, and a warm and nonconflictual relationship between siblings. These factors were not protective for the siblings of children with PDD (Figs 1 and 2).

Conclusions.—The siblings of children with PDD are at risk. A transactional mechanism, rather than the identification of single risk or protective factors, is important in predicting sibling adjustment. Subsequent analysis of the data collected in this longitudinal study will better define these mechanisms and enable improved intervention strategies.

► I am sure it is impossible for those who have never parented a child with PDD to fully comprehend the pain of not being acknowledged, whether entirely or only partially, by a son or daughter.

J.E. Schowalter, M.D.

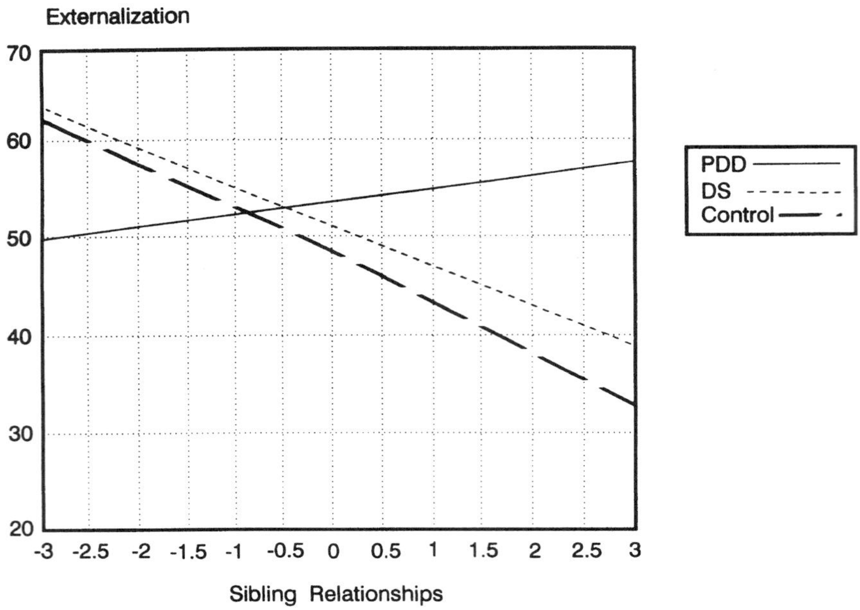

FIGURE 2.—Teacher externalizing problems as a function of sibling relationships and group. (Courtesy of Fisman S, Wolf L, Ellison D, et al: Risk and protective factors affecting the adjustment of siblings of children with chronic disabilities. *J Am Acad Child Adolesc Psychiatry* 35(11):1532–1541, 1996.)

Speech and Language Outcomes

Long-term Consistency in Speech/Language Profiles: I. Developmental and Academic Outcomes
Beitchman JH, Wilson B, Brownlie EB, et al (Clarke Inst of Psychiatry, Toronto)
J Am Acad Child Adolesc Psychiatry 35:804–814, 1996 2–13

Introduction.—Few attempts have been made to evaluate the relationship between demographic, cognitive, behavioral, academic, and psychiatric status and specific speech/language competencies. Psychiatric measures and speech/language competencies were identified in a cohort of 169 5-year-old children. These measures were re-evaluated when the children were 12.5 years old. The association between speech/language clusters and linguistic, cognitive, and academic measures was compared at ages 5 and 12.5.

Methods.—Of the 169 children evaluated at 5 years of age, 124 children were re-evaluated at 12.5 years of age. At both times, the children underwent a series of tests of speech/language and cognitive, developmental, and demographic measures. Academic measures were evaluated at age 12.5. Outcomes of both times were compared to determine whether children's scores remained stable over time.

Results.—Four linguistic groups were identified: high overall, poor comprehension, poor articulation, and low overall. Children with language problems at age 5 had difficulty with linguistic, cognitive, and academic measures at age 12.5. Children with comprehension problems had scores within the normal range but had difficulty with expressive and receptive language and pragmatics. Children in the poor-articulation group were impaired in the area of articulation but scored within the normal range in all other tests. Children in the high overall group had high performance on all speech/language tests. The proportion of children in each group who required special education was 64% in the low overall group, 50% in the poor-comprehension group, 46.3% in the poor-articulation group, and 0% in the high overall group.

Conclusion.—Results of childhood speech/language competence assessed at 5 years of age are correlated with demographic characteristics, linguistic skills, IQ, visual-motor skills, and academic achievement at 12.5 years of age. The best group scores in descending order were high overall, poor articulation, poor comprehension, and low overall. The pattern of results was observed across language, cognitive, developmental, and academic measures. These findings underscore the urgent need for early intervention in children with pervasive speech/language impairment.

▶ This study is important in 2 ways. Too seldom do we have longitudinal follow-up. Although with the virtue of longitudinal follow-ups there are necessarily questions about attrition bias and missed intervening variables (such as the quantity and quality of remedial services), the authors have addressed these methodologic problems straightforwardly. In addition, the study confirms that this specific speech/language classification and evaluation can, with beginning school-age children, provide data that will carry predictive value and thus a basis for decisions about remediation.

J.E. Schowalter, M.D.

Seven-Year Follow-up of Speech/Language Impaired and Control Children: Psychiatric Outcome

Beitchman JH, Brownlie EB, Inglis A, et al (Clarke Inst of Psychiatry, Toronto; Mount Sinai Hosp, Toronto; Algonquin College, Ottawa, Canada)

J Child Psychol Psychiatry 37:961–970, 1996 2–14

Introduction.—Previous studies have examined the outcome and natural history of childhood speech and language (S/L) impairment. However, there are few data on the course of the associated psychiatric disorder present in so many of these children. This 7-year follow-up study looked at the psychiatric outcomes of children with S/L impairment.

Methods.—Two hundred two children from a community sample were assessed at ages 5 and 12.5 years. There were 105 children with S/L impairment (73 boys and 32 girls) and 97 normal children (62 boys and 35 girls). At both ages, the children underwent S/L testing and psychiatric assessment. The time courses of S/L and psychiatric impairment were compared.

Results.—At follow-up, psychiatric diagnoses were recorded for 37% of the children with S/L impairment and 24% of the control children. The difference was nonsignificant. Fifty-seven percent of children with both a speech and a language impairment had a psychiatric diagnosis, compared with 42% of those with a language-only disorder and 26% of those with a speech-only disorder. Children with S/L impairment were more likely than controls to have a psychiatric diagnosis at follow-up. This was so even if the S/L impairment improved, and even after controlling for concurrent psychiatric disorders. About one third of the children with S/L impairment who had no psychiatric disorder at baseline had one by follow-up.

Conclusion.—Children with early S/L impairment are at elevated risk of psychiatric problems later on, even if their S/L problem improves. As these children near adolescence, they are more likely to have a psychiatric disorder if they have a language disorder than if they have a speech disorder. More research is needed to identify other factors that may contribute to the continued risk of psychiatric disorder, and to find out which aspects of S/L impairment are associated with different rates of psychiatric risk.

► This follow-up study raises more questions than it answers. Language is a key differentiator between higher and lower functioning mammals, and between modern humans and our prehistoric progenitors. We are only at the surface of our learning regarding the neural causes of S/L disorders and regarding the pathogenic feedback loop from these disorders into disordered behavior. These linkages are 1 of the intriguing frontiers of developmental psychopathology.

J.E. Schowalter, M.D.

3 Child and Adolescent Psychiatry

Introduction

I have been a co-editor for the YEAR BOOK for 10 years. A decade of choosing the "best" articles and providing personal commentaries on them has been most enjoyable and stimulating. I have also decided that this is a good time for me to stop and allow a new eye to select what is "best" and a fresh pen to explain why. You are very fortunate that these skills will be provided in the future by a truly eminent child and adolescent psychiatrist, Peter Jensen.

What has struck me over my tenure and my review of more than 10,000 articles is the improvement in the methodology in child and adolescent psychiatry research. It has become much easier to know what we know and to know what we do not know, although this is a never-finished quest. On the clinical side, that work-in-progress called for-profit managed care in a relatively few years has forced an unprecedented re-evaluation of our therapies and has threatened our values concerning the best interest of children. My prediction is that the time for administrators' almost complete control of managed care organizations (MCOs) has peaked, and the influence of physicians on MCOs will now steadily increase. Time will be my judge.

A personal hobby-horse during my tenure as a YEAR BOOK editor has been teenage violence. The American Medical Association,[1] the World Health Organization,[2] and the Centers for Disease Control have all become strong advocates for medicalizing and studying adolescent violence as a major health problem. A Centers for Disease Control analysis of the most recent data for the United States and 25 industrialized countries on firearm-related deaths is striking.[3] It was found that the homicide rate was more than 5 times higher for the U.S. than for children in all of the other 25 countries combined. For non–firearm-related homicides, the U.S. was less than 4 times higher; and for non–firearm-related suicides, the U.S. was similar to the children's death rates in the other countries combined. The initial report from the National Longitudinal Study of Adolescent Health (Add Health) demonstrates statistically the "parent-family connectedness" (the adolescent's perception of parental love and caring) and parental expectations for good school work and delayed sexual activity are powerful forces for the reduction of adolescents' risk behaviors and emotional distress.[4] Although these and the additional findings that poor parental connectedness and the home availability of guns, alcohol, and other drugs increase the likelihood of risk factors are not surprising, they re-emphasize the importance of public policy initiative to strengthen the family. The daunting fact that adolescent violence is multi-dimensional and requires attention from home, school, and judiciary, as well as individual perspectives, must not discourage us. The price of our youths' self carnage has become just too high.

Probably the most important thing in life is to choose one's parents wisely. None of us has this option, so it is wise to remember that being born lucky or smart is dumb luck.

John E. Schowalter, M.D.

References

1. American Medical Association: Guidelines for Adolescent Preventive Services. Chicago: American Medical Association, 1994.
2. World Health Assembly: Prevention of violence: public health priority. Geneva, Switzerland: World Health Organization, Resolution WHA49.25, 1996.
3. Centers for Disease Control: Rates of homicide, suicide, and firearm-related death among children—26 industrialized countries. *MMWR Morb Mortal Wkly Rep* 46:101–105, 1997.
4. Resnick MD, Bearman PS, Blum RW, et al: Protecting adolescents from harm. *JAMA* 278:823–832, 1997.

Potpourri

► This subsection includes topic areas that only include one or two articles. You will not find any trends here, but there is much of interest and to provoke thought.

John E. Schowalter, M.D.

Psychopathology in Infancy

Zeanah CH (Brown Univ, Providence, RI; Johns Hopkins Univ, Baltimore, Md)
J Child Psychol Psychiatry 38:81–99, 1997 3–1

Purpose.—There is growing interest in the topic of infant psychopathology. Two emerging areas of research into this area are developmental psychopathology, which seeks to identify individuals who are diverging from the path of normal development; and the diagnosis of psychiatric disorders in infancy. Both approaches try to understand the origins of psychiatric disorders that appear more clearly later in development. A selective review of the developmental psychopathology of early childhood is presented.

Context for Psychopathology.—Several factors influence our concepts of psychopathology during infancy. One approach is to study groups at risk for psychopathology to identify predictors of disorders or symptom patterns. Although this has been a productive strategy, there are few specific links between risk factors and outcomes. A high number of risk factors may predict many outcomes. It is even more difficult to measure psychopathology in infants than in adults—reliance on caregiver reports opens the way to several types of reporting bias. The rapid developmental changes of infancy mean that the indicators of disturbance may change over time. Recent years have seen an appreciation of the importance of context in infant psychopathology, i.e., the infant-caregiver relationship, suggesting that symptoms during infancy may be relationship specific.

Disorders of Infancy.—Aside from the pervasive developmental disorders, there have been few studies of psychiatric disorders in infancy. The research done to date shows no clear advantage of a dimensional or categorical approach to the psychopathology of infancy—both probably have merit for research purposes. To overcome the limitations of standard nosologies, some alternative systems for the classification of disorders of infancy have been developed: the Zero to Three system and a relationship disorders approach. There have been few studies to establish the validity of most disorders of infancy. Studies to validate posttraumatic stress disorder in infancy represent a first step.

Regulation of Emotion.—Several studies have sought to examine psychopathologic variants of emotional regulation. Infants of depressed mothers are at risk for later developmental problems. This risk apparently involves both social interactive and biological processes. It remains to be determined whether the mood or regulatory disorders of these symptoms are sufficient to be considered disordered. Other studies have examined infants with difficulties in the regulation of emotion. Preliminary results suggest that infants with extreme problems of this type may have problems with sensory integration, regulating attention during cognitive tasks, and behavior problems.

Attachment.—Other studies have investigated disturbances of attachment in infants. Studies of disorganized attachment suggest that it influences the development of disruptive behaviors and that models considering these effects are needed. Reactive attachment disorder is one of the few standard diagnoses that can be made in children. However, despite the many studies of attachment in the developmental literature, there have been no recent studies of clinical disorders of attachment.

Discussion.—Increased understanding of normal infant development has led to studies of infants at risk for later psychopathology and of the biological and environmental factors affecting infants at risk. In reviewing this topic, some important areas for future research are identified, including the ways in which risk factors affect outcomes, the identification of infants who would benefit from intervention, the ways in which relationship experiences become internalized and generalized, and the stability of infant characteristics. Previous studies of emotion regulation and attachment will direct the course of research into the next decade.

▶ These leaders in infant psychiatry use infants' skill in regulating emotion and the quality of the infant's attachment to a caregiver as a springboard by which to understand developmental psychopathology. The authors are careful to stay within the data, and they conclude the article with a list of methodological areas that require attention if infant psychiatry research is to continue to prosper.

J.E. Schowalter, M.D.

Are Short Normal Children at a Disadvantage? The Wessex Growth Study

Downie AB, Mulligan J, Stratford RJ, et al (Univ of Southampton, England)
BMJ 314:97–100, 1997 3–2

Objective.—Whether short children are psychosocially disadvantaged is controversial. The ongoing longitudinal Wessex growth study examined physical growth and psychological development of a cohort of short normal children and compared the results with those of a cohort of children of average stature in a second assessment in 1994–1995.

Methods.—Of the children recruited for the first study in 1986–1987 after entering primary school at ages 5 and 6 years, 106 short normal children sex-, age-, and grade-matched with 119 normal-stature children, were reassessed at ages 11–13. Cognitive development and attainment, locus of control, behavior, self-esteem, and self-perception were evaluated. Body image was measured, as was parents' perception. Data were compared using the Mann-Whitney U test.

Results.—Short children had significantly lower intelligence quotient scores, lower measures of reading and number skills attainment, and less internalization of control. However, they did not differ from control children in measures of self-esteem, self-perception, parents' perception, or behavior. Short children were less satisfied with their height. Children from higher social classes scored higher on all measures. Short children were significantly more likely to come from working class homes.

Conclusion.—Social class appears to be a better predictor of disadvantage than height in children aged 11–13 years.

▶ My unscientific observation over the years has been that height, like wealth, means very little, unless you do not have it.

J.E. Schowalter, M.D.

Bullying, Physical Disability and the Paediatric Patient
Dawkins JL (St George's Hosp, London)
Dev Med Child Neurol 38:603–612, 1996 3–3

Background.—Bullying—the intentional, unprovoked abuse of power by 1 or more children to repeatedly cause pain or distress to another child—has traditionally been unrecognized or dismissed as a part of growing up. However, bullying can be conceptualized as a form of abuse. It is a common phenomenon, especially in junior–middle schools. The victims of this abuse are usually anxious, insecure children who are cautious, sensitive, and quiet. These children have been characterized as having low self-esteem and feelings of being stupid, ashamed, and unattractive. When asked why they are bullied, children often refer to physical attributes. Rates of bullying in children with and without visible abnormalities were investigated.

Methods and Findings.—Forty-six boys and girls with visible abnormalities and 57 with no such abnormalities were included. Most children in the former group had cerebral palsy. All children anonymously filled out Olweus' self-report bullying questionnaire. Logistic regression analysis indicated that the most important factors increasing the chance of being bullied were having fewer friends, being alone at playtime, being male, and needing extra help in school. Although significantly more children with visible abnormalities were bullied than those without, the former were not more likely to be bullied after these 4 factors were taken into consideration.

Conclusions.—Children with cerebral palsy and similar conditions affecting their appearance, gait, and mobility are more likely than children with no visible abnormalities to be bullied by their peers. Such children require special support and protection at school.

► Bullies bully those whom they believe they can dominate, and bullies take pleasure in causing distress. Not surprisingly, this study shows that bullies prey most on those disabled schoolmates who are most isolated. Caregivers should become aware that prevention of bullying is a possible and worthwhile objective.

J.E. Schowalter, M.D.

Effects of Self-induced Mental Imagery on Autonomic Reactivity in Children
Lee LH, Olness KN (Case Western Reserve Univ, Cleveland, Ohio; Rainbow Babies and Children's Hosp, Cleveland, Ohio)
J Dev Behav Pediatr 17:323–327, 1996 3–4

Background.—In adults, mental processing changes are associated with changes in cardiovascular responses. However, the extent of this phenomenon has not been well documented in children. The effects of mental imagery on cardiac rate, skin temperature, or electrodermal activity in children were investigated, and the relation of such changes to age, sex, and other variables was determined.

Methods.—Thirty-eight girls and 38 boys, aged 5 to 15 years, were included in the study. The children were in good health, had no learning disabilities, and had no previous experience with hypnosis or biofeedback training. Autonomic reactivity was measured during baseline and mental processing periods. The children were asked to think about being in a quiet, pleasant place for 120 sec, then, after a resting period, about an exciting activity, such as a sport, for another 120 sec. The children were asked to describe what they had been thinking about during the 2 monitoring periods.

Findings.—Pulse rates in all children significantly declined during quiet and relaxing imagery and significantly increased during active imagery. Skin temperatures rose significantly during both quiet and active imagery. Electrodermal activity declined during active imagery. Changes in these parameters were unrelated to age or sex.

Conclusions.—The deliberate change of mental imagery produces immediate autonomic changes in children. These findings raise the questions of whether average daily thinking processes produce autonomic changes over long periods and whether such changes have clinical significance.

► It is instructional to periodically remind ourselves of just how suggestible we are as human beings. Suggestion is ever so much more powerful than we would like to believe.

J.E. Schowalter, M.D.

Anxiety Disorders in Children and Adolescents: A Review of the Past 10 Years

Bernstein GA, Borchardt CM, Perwien AR (Univ of Minnesota, Minneapolis; Univ of Florida, Gainesville)

J Am Acad Child Adolesc Psychiatry 35:1110–1119, 1996 3–5

Purpose.—The current state of knowledge of the anxiety disorders of childhood and adolescence was reviewed, with a focus on the literature of the past 10 years.

Anxiety.—Behavioral inhibition to the unfamiliar, a temperamental characteristic defined as the tendency to be shy or show fear and withdrawal in novel situations, appears to be an enduring trait that is linked to anxiety. Avoidant disorder, separation anxiety disorder, and agoraphobia were significantly more prevalent in young children with behavioral inhibition. Insecure attachment to parents also appears to be a risk factor for the development of childhood anxiety disorders. In middle childhood, the most common anxiety disorders are separation anxiety disorder, overanxious disorder, and specific phobias. Isolated subclinical anxiety disorder symptoms have also been found to be common. In adolescence, the most commonly self-reported symptoms are fear of heights and public speaking, blushing, excessive worry about past behavior, and self-consciousness. Panic disorder is uncommon in childhood and begins to increase in frequency with sexual maturity. Adolescence is the peak period for the onset of this disorder.

Assessment of Anxiety.—Assessment should include onset, development, context, medical history, school history, and social history. A family psychiatric history should be obtained. Structured psychiatric interviews, clinical rating scales, self-report instruments, and parent report measurements are all useful in the assessment of anxiety.

Treatment of Anxiety.—As there appears to be an association between an insecure parent-child bond and anxiety, treatment to improve parent-child interactions may be useful in the preschool years. Older children can be treated with education, consultation with caregivers and health providers, cognitive-behavioral interventions, psychodynamic psychotherapy, family therapy, and pharmacotherapy. There are also specific interventions for some specific anxiety disorders. Very little information exists on pharmacologic interventions for the anxiety disorders of childhood. Medications that may be commonly considered for these conditions include tricyclic antidepressants, benzodiazepines, serotonin reuptake inhibitors, beta-blockers, buspirone, and monoamine oxidase inhibitors.

Conclusions.—This review article examined the research of the last 10 years on anxiety disorders in children and adolescents. Important areas for future research include the neurologic basis of anxiety disorders, longitudinal studies of the course of these disorders through childhood, and investigation of optimal treatment modalities.

► As a child and adolescent psychiatrist, I am frequently pressed by parents, schools, and others to prescribe "antianxiety" medications. The wish for a pill-cure, and my answer that there is none, frequently elicit a reaction that I am not much of a clinician.

J.E. Schowalter, M.D.

School Phobia With Separation Anxiety Disorder: A Comparative 20- to 29-Year Follow-up Study of 35 School Refusers

Flakierska-Praquin N, Lindström M, Gillberg C (Univ of Göteborg, Sweden)
Compr Psychiatry 38:17–22, 1997 3–6

Introduction.—In an earlier study, 35 individuals who were seen in a psychiatric clinic because of school phobia were followed up. Study subjects were aged 7–12 years when seen at the clinic and 24–29 years at the time of the first follow-up; in this new follow-up, all were older than 30. It was hypothesized that school phobia case patients would have persisting psychiatric problems and fewer social contacts than comparison groups, but would function better than nonschool refusal psychiatric patients.

Methods.—The school phobia group included 19 girls and 16 boys; 21 had received outpatient treatment only and 14 were treated as inpatients. All were of normal intelligence and had no indications of major social or family dysfunction. All 35 cases met *Diagnostic and Statistical Manual of Mental Disorders,* ed 3, revised, criteria for separation anxiety disorder. Only 2 children did not live with both parents. Comparison groups were 35 child psychiatric patients and 35 normal children matched for age and sex; all were similar in social class and amount of schooling. Follow-up data were obtained from case records, adult psychiatric clinic records, national health insurance records, demographic registers, and police registers.

Results.—The percentage of those taking more than 45 sick-leave days during a 3-year period was greater in the nonschool refusal psychiatric group (58%) than in the normal (24%) or school phobia (21%) groups. The national police register listed 9 (21%) of those in the nonschool refusal psychiatric group vs. 6% each for the other 2 groups. In addition to a higher rate of criminality, the nonschool refusal psychiatric group had poorer psychological adjustment than the others. School phobia cases had more psychiatric consultation and lived with their parents more often than those in the general population group and had fewer children than both comparison groups.

Discussion.—In one of the few studies of school refusers to employ strict diagnostic criteria and lengthy follow-up, investigators report some long-term effects of a childhood diagnosis of school phobia in association with separation anxiety disorder. Individuals treated for school phobia as children continue to apply for psychiatric help and appear to have a limited sphere of social relationships. Their outcome is closer, however, to that of "normal" children than to that of children who were not school refusers but were treated for other psychiatric problems.

► The authors' hypotheses were confirmed, albeit with a small sample size. The outcomes suggest that the original diagnoses were correct. The diagnoses of school phobia and truancy are at times confused. Shyness and social phobia tend to be protective factors for conduct problems, whereas truancy is a risk factor.

J.E. Schowalter, M.D.

Obsessive-Compulsive Disorder in Children and Adolescents: A Review of the Past 10 Years

March JS, Leonard HL (Duke Univ, Durham, NC; Brown Univ, Providence, RI)
J Am Acad Child Adolesc Psychiatry 35:1265–1273, 1996 3–7

Introduction.—Although 1 in 200 adolescents is reported to have obsessive-compulsive disorder (OCD), few receive a correct diagnosis or appropriate treatment. Drawing on the clinical and research literatures and the authors' own clinical experience, pediatric OCD was reviewed from the standpoint of basic knowledge expected for American Board of Psychiatry and Neurology recertification in child and adolescent psychiatry.

Epidemiology and Diagnosis.—In up to one half of affected adults, OCD developed during childhood. Only 4 of 18 children with OCD, however, are identified and receive professional care. Health care providers may be unfamiliar with the disorder or unwilling to use proven treatments. To merit a diagnosis of OCD, either obsessions or compulsions must be present and the symptoms must be distressing and time-consuming. Affected individuals must see the compulsions as excessive and recognize at some point that the obsessions originate in the mind, although this requirement is waived for children.

Phenomenology.—Common obsessions include harm to self or others; sexual, aggressive, and contamination themes; symmetry urges; and the need to tell, ask, or confess. Typical compulsions include washing, checking, counting, ordering/arranging, and hoarding. Boys are more likely to have prepubertal onset, and girls are more likely to have OCD start during adolescence. Children with a variety of psychiatric disorders may have these behaviors, and children with OCD may have additional diagnoses—particularly tic, attention-deficit, anxiety, and affective disorders.

Treatment.—Cognitive-behavioral therapy has proved to be an effective and durable treatment for OCD. Treatment relies primarily on repeated exposure and response prevention, typically implemented in a gradual fashion. Medication trials show the benefits of serotonin re-uptake inhibitors (SRIs), particularly clomipramine; also effective are the selective SRIs, including fluvoxamine. At least 10 weeks of treatment should be completed before response can be assessed, and about one third of patients will not respond to monotherapy. As in adults, OCD appears to be a chronic, waxing-and-waning illness in many children. The disorder may be improved by a calm, supportive family and exacerbated by a family with high "expressed emotion."

Conclusions.—A great deal of information is now available on OCD in the pediatric population, and ongoing research offers promise for improvements in diagnosis and treatment. With a combination of an SRI and OCD-specific cognitive-behavioral therapy, most children now can be successfully treated.

► This is one of the *Journal of the American Academy of Child Adolescent Psychiatry's* special articles chosen to review an area in anticipation of the first American Board of Psychiatry and Neurology's recertification examination in child and adolescent psychiatry. When I began practice thirtysomething years ago, OCD was considered an extremely rare disorder in children. Maybe etiologic factors have intensified over the years, but more likely we did not see what we did not look for. One wonders whether in 35 years some commentator will make the same remark about something we are missing now.

J.E. Schowalter, M.D.

Does PTSD Transcend Cultural Barriers?: A Study From the Khmer Adolescent Refugee Project

Sack WH, Seeley JR, Clarke GN (Oregon Health Sciences Univ, Portland; Oregon Research Inst, Eugene)

J Am Acad Child Adolesc Psychiatry 36:49–54, 1997 3–8

Objective.—Whether young Cambodian survivors of war have signs of posttraumatic stress disorder (PTSD) similar to those of white and black combat survivors and rape survivors was studied.

Methods.—Interviews were conducted in the United States with 209 Cambodian adolescents and young adults, aged 13 to 25 years. During the Pol Pot War in Cambodia (1975 to 1979), many of these individuals were separated from their parents, had malnutrition, or witnessed executions of family members or other atrocities. Questions included the Diagnostic Interview for Children and Adolescents, which contains 17 items about PTSD. A parent or guardian was interviewed separately.

Results.—Fifteen participants reported no history of trauma, so the reference sample was 194 participants. Factor analysis identified 17 symptoms of PTSD in the sample, grouped into 4 categories: (1) arousal (hypervigilance, sleep disturbances, irritability, concentration difficulties, sense of foreshortened future, avoidance of situational reminders of trauma); (2) avoidance (physiologic reactivity, excessive startle response, avoidance of thoughts of trauma, no memory of trauma); (3) intrusion (emotional reactivity, intrusive thoughts, nightmares, flashbacks); and (4) numbing (loss of interest in daily activities, detachment, restricted affect). These results were confirmed by the interviews with parents and guardians. Logistic regression analysis showed that in predicting a diagnosis of PTSD, the 4 most salient symptoms are avoidance of situational reminders of the trauma, no memory of traumas, detachment, and increased irritability.

Conclusions.—The profile of PTSD in Cambodian war survivors is similar to that in traumatized white and black adults. Despite cultural differences, this diagnosis appears to be appropriate, when indicated, for refugee populations.

▶ This is a very thoughtful study and discussion. Ernst Kris differentiated "shock" from "strain" trauma more than 40 years ago.[1] Researchers now debate the differences and similarities of "single blow" or "protracted" trauma. What is striking to me is how "neurophysiologic" severe emotional trauma can be. It is as though the mind and brain have been dealt a damaging blow and this effect ranges across geographic and ethnic boundaries.

J.E. Schowalter, M.D.

Reference

1. Kris E: The recovery of childhood memories in psychoanalysis. *Psychoanal Study Child* 11:54–88, 1956.

Traumatic Brain Injury in Children and Adolescents: Psychiatric Disorders in the First Three Months

Max JE, Smith WL Jr, Sato Y, et al (Univ of Iowa, Iowa City; Univ of Montana, Missoula; Cedar Centre Psychiatric Group, Cedar Rapids, Iowa)

J Am Acad Child Adolesc Psychiatry 36:94–102, 1997 3–9

Introduction.—Previous studies of children and adolescents who sustain traumatic brain injury (TBI) found that behavioral changes and psychiatric disorders often develop after the injury, particularly among those with more severe TBI. Other variables related to psychiatric disorder were the child's preinjury behavior, early postinjury intellectual level, and psychosocial circumstances. These and other variables were assessed as predictors of psychiatric outcome in the first 3 months after TBI in a prospective follow-up study.

Methods.—Eligible for participation were consecutively admitted TBI patients aged 6–14 years at the time of injury and who had a CT scan on admission. Excluded were patients with penetrating TBI, posttraumatic amnesia of 3 months or more duration, a history of child abuse or mental retardation, and pre-existing acute or chronic serious illness. The 50 patients enrolled in the study were assessed for severity of injury and results of neuroimaging. Information was also gathered on preinjury psychiatric, behavioral, adaptive, and family functioning and on the family's psychiatric history.

Results.—The 50 children and young adolescents had a mean age of 10.30 years; 64% were boys and 98% were white. The TBI was considered mild in 52%, moderate in 18%, and severe in 30%. At 3-month follow-up, 37 of the children were available for re-assessment. New psychiatric disorders developed in 17 of those 37 patients within the 3-month period. The most frequent diagnoses were organic personality disorder in 10 (resolved in 4), major depression in 5 (all resolved), attention-deficit hyperactivity disorder in 6, oppositional defiant disorder in 3, posttraumatic stress disorder in 2 (both resolved), and separation anxiety disorder in 2 (1 resolved). Significant predictors of development of a "novel" psychiatric disorder in the first 3 months after TBI were increasing severity of injury, the presence of a lifetime psychiatric disorder, family psychiatric history, family dysfunction, and lower socioeconomic class/preinjury intellectual function.

Conclusion.—During the first 3 months after TBI, many children and adolescents are given diagnoses of a new psychiatric disorder. The significant risk factors reported here can help to identify and treat those with an increased likelihood of posttraumatic changes.

► Most of us know that TBI is associated with an increased likelihood of psychiatric disorders, but this study emphasizes that behavioral problems often occur within the ensuing 3 months. These data emphasize how important it is to have a child psychiatrist available to and used by emergency department and neurosurgical staff. This is currently done in some medical centers, but not in many.

J.E. Schowalter, M.D.

Tourette Disorder: A Cross-cultural Review

Staley D, Wand R, Shady G (St Boniface Gen Hosp, Winnipeg, Manitoba, Canada)

Compr Psychiatry 38:6–16, 1997 3–10

Background.—Tourette's disorder (TD), a complex disorder of chronic motor and vocal tics, appears in childhood or adolescence and can cause significant functional impairment. The disorder is much more common in males than in females. Many patients also have obsessive-compulsive disorder and/or attention deficit hyperactivity disorder, together with various inappropriate behaviors. Treatment with dopamine antagonists is usually effective in reducing motor and vocal symptoms, and psychotherapy is a useful adjunct modality. Whereas many studies of TD have been published in Europe and North America, less is known about the manifestations of TD in other cultures. A review of case reports and clinical studies was undertaken to ascertain the cross-cultural similarities and differences in the etiologic factors, prevalence, clinical characteristics, and treatment outcome of TD.

> *Case Reports.*—The first report of TD outside Europe or North America appeared in 1963 (a 15-year-old Chinese boy from Hong Kong). Since then, a substantial number of case reports of TD have come from a wide range of countries and geographic regions. Most of the 39 cases listed in this study occurred in males (72%). At the time of treatment, their mean age was 20.1 years; mean duration of the disorder was 12 years. Vocal tics were the most common clinical feature, and echolalia and coprolalia were frequently noted (31% and 74% of cases, respectively). Symptoms often fluctuated, and stress increased their intensity. Comorbid conditions reported frequently included depression (31%) and obsessive-compulsive disorder (26%). Pharmacologic treatment was reported in 79% of the case studies. Symptom relief was noted in 77% of reports, and the most successful agent was haloperidol.

Clinical Investigations.—Cross-cultural clinical studies of TD have come from Japan, Hong Kong, China, Russia, Korea, and New Zealand. Findings have been similar to those of western studies. Many of the clinical investigations note psychobehavioral problems, including aggression and sleep difficulties. The 3 cross-cultural studies that employed electroencephalographic examinations all found a high incidence of electroencephalographic abnormality. Dopamine antagonists successfully treated symptoms, and the dosage was gradually increased until an effective dose was established.

Discussion.—Tourette's disorder appears throughout the world with similar characteristics. There is a strong male predominance, and symptoms—commonly motor tics—start to appear in childhood. The major effect of culture appears to be the vocal phenomena associated with TD, especially coprolalia. A uniformity of response to medication suggests that TD has a common biological basis independent of culture or geography.

► Tourette's disorder (TD) has become a very important entity, not only in its own right but by providing theoretical hints as it hovers between psychiatry and neurology and overlaps with more benign tics, obsessive-compulsive disorder, attention deficit disorder, intelligence, etc. It is also a personal favorite of mine because, in the early 1960s, I correctly made the diagnosis during a pediatric consultation. Tourette's disorder was not well known then, and my diagnosis gave me a stature in the Peds Department that felt very good indeed.

J.E. Schowalter, M.D.

Weight Modification Efforts Reported by Black and White Preadolescent Girls: National Heart, Lung, and Blood Institute Growth and Health Study

Schreiber GB, Robins M, Striegel-Moore R, et al (Westat, Inc, Rockville, Md; Wesleyan Univ, Middletown, Conn; Natl Heart, Lung and Blood Inst, Bethesda, Md; et al)

Pediatrics 98:63–70, 1996 3–11

Background.—The percentage of American adolescent girls who are overweight has risen markedly between 1978 and 1990. Research has shown that being overweight is significantly more common among black women than white women. Although genetic predisposition and socioeconomic status are major determinants of obesity, these factors alone do not explain the racial differences observed. Compared with white women, black women appear to accept a larger body size, have greater body satisfaction, and are less likely to diet to lose weight. Attempts to modify weight among white and black pre-adolescent girls were investigated.

Methods and Findings.—Data were obtained on 1,213 black and 1,166 white girls, aged 9 and 10 years. Compared with white girls, black girls were taller and heavier and showed earlier signs of puberty. However, the white girls were more dissatisfied with their weight, body shape, and body parts. About 40% of the girls said they were trying to lose weight. About 75% of those in the fourth quartile of body mass index (BMI) were trying to lose weight. After adjustment for BMI, there were no significant between-group differences in the prevalence of those trying to lose weight. However, significantly more black girls were trying to gain weight. In a multiple logistic regression analysis, the major factors associated with attempted weight loss were a high BMI, the mother telling the daughter she was too fat, and body dissatisfaction. Chronic dieting was associated only with a high BMI and the mother telling the daughter she was too fat. Attempts to gain weight were predicted by being black, having a low BMI, and the mother telling the daughter she was too thin.

Conclusions.—Attempts to lose weight and chronic dieting did not differ between white and black pre-adolescent girls in this study. Attempts to gain weight are much more common among black girls. Mothers' opinions of their daughters' weight play an important role in the girls' efforts to lose or gain weight.

► One need only look at the female form as painted by past masters or to check out the weights of Playboy Bunnies over the decades to learn that cultural norms for the female form change. What seems less clear is whether these changes come more from what men want or from what mothers want, or even whether these 2 are related.

J.E. Schowalter, M.D.

A Participant's Observations: Preparing DSM-IV

Shaffer D (Columbia Univ, New York; New York State Psychiatric Inst)

Can J Psychiatry 41:325–329, 1996 3–12

Purpose.—Personal experience by a participant on the task force that created the *Diagnostic and Statistical Manual of Mental Disorders*, ed 4, (DSM-IV) is described.

Charge to the Working Group.—The working group was instructed to keep changes between DSM-III-R and DSM-IV to a minimum, only making changes to correct widely recognized mistakes or those that were justified by empirical evidence. A transparent process was designed. The working groups had autonomy and were drawn from many groups. Suggestions and advice were actively sought from outside the working groups. Empirical data were used to set thresholds, frequencies, and durations. If such data were not available, less precise terminology was used. The DSM-IV was to be made more compatible with the International Classification of Diseases system.

Results.—Development of DSM-IV was primarily based on designed field trials and secondary data analyses. Commissioned literature reviews were less useful.

Conclusions.—Nosology is inherently difficult. The DSM-IV development process was carefully planned and the profession is indebted to the American Psychiatric Association for its effort in producing this system. As the field is evolving rapidly, more changes can be expected by the time a task force begins work on DSM-V.

► This is a fascinating personal "diary" of an insider author of what is our bible for the next half-dozen or so years. Dr. Shaffer is to be thanked for allowing the rest of us, albeit belatedly, to be insiders too.

J.E. Schowalter, M.D.

Regulatory Issues in Pediatric Psychopharmacology

Laughren TP (Food and Drug Administration, Rockville, Md)

J Am Acad Child Adolesc Psychiatry 35:1276–1282, 1996 3–13

Background.—Labeling information on the use of psychotropic agents in children and adolescents has been inadequate, mainly because of the lack of valid research data relevant to such use. The many obstacles to research in pediatric psychopharmacology have included some of a regulatory nature. Recently, a regulation with the potential to stimulate research interest and activity in this area was finalized.

Regulatory Issues in Pediatric Psychopharmacology.—The Food and Drug Administration (FDA) has made several efforts to encourage more informative labeling of drugs for use in children. A recent labeling initiative stresses the possibility of extrapolating efficacy data from adult studies to pediatric populations under certain conditions. This regulation requires pharmaceutical sponsors to reassess existing data on their drugs to determine whether there is a basis for modifying labeling for pediatric use. The new regulation includes a reminder that, in certain situations, the FDA may require new pediatric studies.

Conclusions.—The FDA has renewed its long-standing commitment to better labeling for the use of pharmacologic agents in children. Investigators and sponsors must understand the basic regulatory requirements for obtaining new claims. Preclinical and clinical approaches for evaluating the possible effects of these drugs on growth and development also should be re-examined.

► Although not an article endorsed by the FDA, Dr. Laughren's discussion of the FDA's direction is illuminating. Psychopharmacologic agents seldom are as effective with children as they are with adults. Developmental considerations, such as liver functioning, need to be much better understood, but at the same time pharmaceutical firms must not be allowed the easy option of not researching a medication's effectiveness only on the basis of unlikely remunerativity. I believe that if an agent works for adults, testing for children should be strongly encouraged, barring some obvious danger.

J.E. Schowalter, M.D.

Impact of Medicaid Managed Care on Child and Adolescent Emergency Mental Health Screening in Massachusetts

Nicholson J, Young SD, Simon L, et al (Univ of Massachusetts, Worcester; Northeastern Univ, Boston)

Psychiatric Serv 47:1344–1350, 1996 3–14

Objective.—How the change to managed care for Medicaid benefits in Massachusetts has affected emergency mental health screening of children and adolescents was investigated.

Methods.—At a university medical center, records were reviewed for all emergency screening episodes for children and adolescents during 2 periods: for the 12 months before implementation of managed care (period A), and for 12 months after implementation, beginning in the seventh month after implementation so that the staff had time to adjust (period B). Two types of data were collected: patient attributes (sex, age, problem when first seen, diagnosis, and hospitalization history) and system attributes (payer, referral source, and disposition).

Results.—The number of emergency screening episodes was significantly higher in period B than in period A, 393 vs. 297. This was expected because the managed care company requires screening before hospitalization. In period B, among Medicaid-covered episodes, significantly fewer problems when first seen were labeled "threatening behavior" (suicidal ideation or attempts, self-abusive behavior, or assaultive or homicidal behavior) than in period A, and significantly more were given the milder label of "problem behavior" (destructive behavior, substance abuse). This may reflect the pressure on staff to keep youths out of inpatient care. The percentage of inpatient admissions significantly decreased in period B, as did the percentage of discharges to home. There, decreases were balanced almost exactly by a significant increase in the percentage of referrals to short-term residential treatment and to other programs that had contracts with the managed care company.

Conclusions.—The managed care company met its goals of reduced hospital admissions and shorter lengths of stay. However, it remains to be seen whether these outcomes will reduce costs in the long term. Studies of recidivism and quality of care are in order.

▶ Massachusetts was earlier than most states in converting patients receiving Medicaid from fee-for-service to managed care. Although all in all their initial mental health effort worked quite well for adults, it underserved children.

Perhaps it is my age, but I still cringe whenever I hear or read about a patient referred to as a "client." I am also sure in my heart that I will never accept being called a "provider." It is comforting to look at my diploma and see that it still reads "Medical School," not "Provider School." This is, of course, linguistic warfare. Managed care wants to run as a business, not as a source of medical care. To lower the 2,000+ year-old honored title of "physician" to "provider" helps underline that the care of patients' bodies and illnesses is really no more personal than producing ball bearings.

J.E. Schowalter, M.D.

The Great Smoky Mountains Study of Youth: Functional Impairment and Serious Emotional Disturbance

Costello EJ, Angold A, Burns BJ, et al (Duke Univ, Durham, NC)

Arch Gen Psychiatry 53:1137–1143, 1996 3–15

Background.—The United States Alcohol, Drug Abuse, and Mental Health Administration defines severe emotional disturbance (SED) in children as a *Diagnostic and Statistical Manual of Mental Disorders*, ed 3, revised (*DSM-III-R*) diagnosis plus functional impairment. In turn, functional impairment is defined as "difficulties that substantially interfere with or limit role functioning in 1 or more major life activities."

Objective.—The rates and correlates of SED in children were investigated.

Methods.—Highly trained lay interviewers visited homes to interview 804 randomly selected children, aged 9, 11, and 13 years. A parent of each child was interviewed separately. The interviewers used the third edition of the Child and Adolescent Psychiatry Assessment, which generates *DSM-III-R* diagnoses and measures of impairment, and the Child and Adolescent Functional Assessment Scale. Later they completed the Children's Global Assessment Scale, based on the results of the interview.

Results.—Rates of SED varied with functional impairment score and with the assessment instrument used. The Child and Adolescent Psychiatry Assessment and the Child and Adolescent Functional Assessment Scale gave similar maximum rates of SED: 6.8% and 7.6%, respectively. The Children's Global Assessment Scale identified a maximum rate of 4.2%. Functional impairment and *DSM-III-R* diagnosis were independently correlated with mental health service use by children with SED. Ignoring functional impairment, the percentage of children with a *DSM-III-R* diagnosis was 20.3%. Children living below the federal poverty line were at significantly greater risk of SED. Three of 5 (60%) children with SED had not recently received mental health care in any setting, and 4 of 5 (80%) had not recently received professional mental health care.

Conclusions.—There is clearly a need to improve access to mental health services for children with severe problems. Defining SED as functional impairment plus a *DSM-III-R* diagnosis will reduce the number of children who are eligible for care and help identify those with greater need. More work is needed to define what constitutes "substantial interference" with a child's functioning.

► For those of us who are clinicians, mental health managed care directors, or managers (Medicaid, Medicare, or commercial), these types of data are needed desperately. It is appalling how difficult it is to confirm how much the

State, the Feds, indemnity, or managed care payers pay or have paid for mental health care. What percentage of per member per month premiums should be expected? Is it 2%, 6%, 10%, or what? Should it be $2, $6, $10 per member per month? Each of these numbers is used in some part of the country, but what is, objectively, the reasonable rate or range of rates? This is most often settled now by shouting, pounding the table, relying on friendships, using blackmail, or whatever leverage you have at hand. We must get data to do this better.

J.E. Schowalter, M.D.

The Impact of Legislation to Improve Coordination of Services to Children With Serious Emotional Disturbance

Petti TA, Phillips JR, Williams JD, et al (Indiana Univ, Indianapolis; Indiana Family and Social Services Administration; Indiana Youth Services Assoc; et al)

Psychiatric Serv 47:1239–1243, 1996 3–16

Background.—State legislation in Indiana has mandated the establishment of local coordinating committees to prevent inappropriate removal of children and adolescents with serious emotional disturbance from the home and to facilitate the development of community-based initiatives. The impact of this legislation was evaluated.

Methods.—A survey was first sent to the directors of mental health, welfare, education, and probation agencies of each county to estimate how well the mandated structures and processes had been established. Then, the directors of key agencies in 7 representative counties underwent a structured interview.

Findings.—A total of 310 completed surveys were received from all 92 counties in Indiana. Seventy-three counties had functioning committees. Committee success was most often attributed to improved coordination among providers. Half the survey respondents believed that the existence of the committee improved services. More than half the respondents said that there were too few service options available. Other problems were rigid funding opportunities, which limited options, and lack of staff time to properly prepare for and attend meetings. During the structured interviews, agency directors reported that the committee too often formalized decisions already made, that consideration of individual cases came too late in the process, and that less restrictive options had often already been attempted without success. The directors also said that the committee process had not attained the major objective of pooling resources to address the needs of particular children.

Conclusion.—The extent to which a state mandate can effect broad change without additional resources needs further study. Sufficient funding and a fiscal strategy to support coordination and staffing of local coordinating committees are essential for success.

► The mixed results in Indiana are not surprising. The importance of integrating mental health services so that they can be both efficient and appropriate is matched by the turf issues that make this so difficult to accomplish. As managed health care budgets and social service budgets are being ratcheted downward simultaneously, success in attempting better integration becomes all the more important, while every sector becomes all the more self-possessive.

J.E. Schowalter, M.D.

Economic Evaluations and Interventions for Children and Adolescents With Mental Health Problems

Knapp M (London School of Economics and Political Science)
J Child Psychol Psychiatry 38:3–25, 1997 3–17

Objective.—There is a growing need for interventions for children and adolescents with mental health disorders. These disorders can have long-lasting consequences, yet there have been few economic evaluations of the interventions for them. The demand for economic evaluations of interventions for children and adolescents with mental disorders, along with the modes of evaluation and a discussion of past, current, and future research in this area, was reviewed.

Demand.—Discussion of the demand for economic evaluation must begin with the recognition of scarcity, which means that there are too few resources to meet the present needs or demands. Although scarcity is always present, it is compounded by the growing prevalence of mental health problems among children and adolescents, the low proportion of identified need that is treated appropriately, and the expense of effective treatments. All this is occurring against a background of economic pressures and government cutbacks. Other pressures affecting demand include broader socioeconomic changes, social and family expectations, and market forces. Demands for economic evaluation come from health care users and purchasers, managed care organizations, policy makers, marketers, and other sources.

Modes of Evaluation.—The demand for economic evaluation raises questions about how the evaluations should be conducted. Economic evaluations tend to focus on the criteria of effectiveness, economy, efficiency, and equity. The 3 major modes of economic evaluation are cost-benefit analysis, which addresses the social justification of a particular treatment; cost-effectiveness analysis, which is done to ensure that the health care resources allocated are being used to the best effect; and cost-utility analysis, which values the impact of a treatment on health-related quality of life.

Evaluative Evidence.—Economic evaluations may ask what treatment should be provided, as well as when, where, to whom, and how treatment should be provided. Much work is ongoing in many of these areas; however, this work is unlikely to meet the growing demand for economic evaluation of child and adolescent mental health care. Part of the problem is a clash between the interests of clinical and economic researchers. Future economic evaluations will have to consider the multi-agency nature of child and adolescent mental health interventions; the long persistence of many of the disorders; and the importance of external factors, such as parents and society at large. Costs and outcomes will have to be measured, and the links between costs and outcomes elucidated. Finally, there is a need to study how all of these various elements interconnect and coordinate, and which incentives can help to achieve the desired goals. Economic evaluations could help to overcome the most serious problems facing child and adolescent mental health services today: the fragmentation of service systems and the lack of coordination of their responses to needs.

Discussion.—There is a need for economic evaluations of mental health interventions for children and adolescents, as well as a need to review the modes of evaluation, the available research, and unmet research needs. For the present, scarcity of economic evaluations is one of the major problems facing the planning and provision of child and adolescent mental health services.

► This is a "must-read" article for anyone interested in the basic economics of child and adolescent psychiatry. Knapp is a professor at the London School of Economics, but he knows a surprising amount about the clinical aspects of our work. This data-rich essay will serve as a database for the rest of us to use in our negotiations and in thinking about how best to understand current and future economic constraints.

J.E. Schowalter, M.D.

Depression and Suicide

► These are the issues in child and adolescent psychiatry that probably cause the greatest amount of acute worry and long-term heartache.

John E. Schowalter, M.D.

Depression Screening in Adolescents With Somatic Complaints Presenting to the Emergency Department

Porter SC, Fein JA, Ginsburg KR (Children's Hosp of Philadelphia; Univ of Pennsylvania, Philadelphia)

Ann Emerg Med 29:141–145, 1997 3–18

Objective.—Suicide is the third most common cause of death in adolescents. Adolescents may seek medical help for somatic problems in the weeks or months preceding a suicide attempt. Because depression is associated with somatic complaints, emergency department (ED) methods were instituted to determine the frequency of depression screening for adolescents seen in the ED.

Quick screen for depression/risk of suicide.

How is school going?
How are you feeling?
Whom do you talk to when you are feeling down or sad?
Have you ever tried to hurt yourself before?
What are your plans for the future (summer, next school year, after high school)?

BOX.—Quick screen for depression/risk of suicide. (Courtesy of Porter SC, Fein JA, Ginsberg KR: Depression screening in adolescents with somatic complaints presenting to the emergency department. *Ann Emerg Med* 29:141–145, 1997.)

Methods.—Emergency department records of 408 of 2,786 patients, aged 11 to 17 years, seen in the ED for abdominal pain, chest pain, headache, hyperventilation, dizziness/fainting, and weakness/fatigue between February and June 1995 were retrospectively reviewed for documentation of a depression screen (Box).

Results.—Depression or suicidal ideation was noted on charts of 17 (4.2%) of the patients (4 males). Patients with chronic conditions were screened as frequently as patients without a history. Patients with both a somatic complaint and a nonspecific diagnosis were screened with a frequency of 7.5%. Screening prevalence was significantly higher among black than nonblack patients. Significantly more nonblack patients than black patients were described as being in fair condition rather than in good condition (26.0% vs. 9.8%). Significantly more black than nonblack patients were admitted to the hospital (33.0% vs. 13.4%).

Conclusions.—Very few adolescents with somatic complaints received depression screening, although black adolescents received such screening significantly more frequently than nonblack adolescents. There is a need to educate ED personnel to the need for depression screening for adolescents seeking medical care for somatic complaints.

▶ In my mind, depression is the most underdiagnosed disorder in psychiatry. Given its vast co-morbidity and its powerful link to suicide, we must arouse ourselves to better educate primary care clinicians to use depression screening devices in their offices, in school clinics, and in EDs. If done, a large reduction of morbidity and mortality will result from a small increase of expenditures.

J.E. Schowalter, M.D.

Childhood and Adolescent Depression: A Review of the Past 10 Years. Part II

Birmaher B, Ryan ND, Williamson DE, et al (Univ of Pittsburgh, Pa)
J Am Acad Child Adolesc Psychiatry 35:1575–1583, 1996 3–19

Background.—Patients with early-onset major depressive disorder (MDD) or dysthymic disorder (DD) require accurate diagnosis with prompt treatment and preventive interventions. A selective review of the past 10 years' literature on MDD and DD in adolescents and children was presented.

Findings.—The article reviews the assessment; treatment, including psychosocial and psychopharmacologic interventions; and prevention of early-onset MDD and DD. In terms of assessment, there are now reliable diagnostic systems and standardized interviews for early-onset MDD and DD. There have been few controlled studies of psychotherapeutic treatments for early-onset MDD. The available studies suggest that cognitive-behavioral therapy (CBT) is beneficial. One study found fluoxetine to be effective in the acute management of early-onset MDD. Recent results suggest that the selective serotonin reuptake inhibitors may constitute a useful initial treatment. Placebo-controlled studies have shown no advantage of tricyclic antidepressant therapy. However, these studies have had small sample sizes and methodologic flaws. There is evidence that CBT may have a role to play in the prevention of MDD.

A combination of treatments seems best for pediatric MDD and dysthymia, especially given the frequency of comorbidity and the psychosocial and academic effects of depression. Mental health problems are common among the parents of depressed youths, suggesting the need for concurrent treatment of children and parents.

Discussion.—Both psychosocial and pharmacologic treatments appear to be useful in these patients. Psychotherapy is a useful initial treatment, especially for CBT. For patients who do not respond, antidepressant medications may be indicated. Drug treatment should also be considered for youngsters whose depression interferes with their academic and social functioning, who have recurrent depression that does not respond to psychotherapy, or who have psychotic or bipolar depression. More study is needed of the short- and long-term effectiveness of psychotherapy and drug treatment, alone and in combination.

► Comorbidity is a bugaboo generally for psychiatric nomenclature. Until we sort out this problem better, it is going to be difficult to more specifically target our therapeutic priorities.

J.E. Schowalter, M.D.

Discriminating Depression and Anxiety in Youth: A Role for Diagnostic Criteria

Gurley D, Cohen P, Pine DS, et al (Univ of Colorado, Denver; Columbia Univ, NY; New York State Psychiatric Inst; et al)

J Affect Disord 39:191–200, 1996 3–20

Objective.—To address the controversy about symptoms of anxiety and depression in adolescence, these questions were studied: Do such symptoms reflect an underlying emotional disorder, or are they distinguishable?

Methods.—The data were taken from a large, ongoing community-based study of pathopsychology in 976 youth living in upstate New York. The study began in 1975, when the index respondents were 1 to 10 years old. Separate interviews were conducted of children and parents using the Diagnostic Interview Schedule for Children, modified to incorporate *Diagnostic and Statistical Manual of Mental Disorders,* ed 3, revised criteria. Most of the youth, along with newly recruited youth, were re-interviewed in 1983 (when they were aged 9 to 18 years) and from 1985 to 1986 (when they were aged 11 to 20 years). The original sample was 91% white and about equally divided between girls and boys. Maternal education averaged 12.6 years. Socioeconomic status varied widely.

Results.—Across age groups, there was considerable co-morbidity of depression and anxiety. The association was strongest in youth who did not have an emotional disorder (major depression, simple phobia, social phobia, separation anxiety, or obsessive-compulsive disorder). Symptoms of anxiety and depression were more discriminable among youths who had at least 1 emotional disorder than among those without.

Conclusions.—As has been suggested for adults, it appears that some youths have a mixture of impairing symptoms of anxiety and depression even though they do not meet *Diagnostic and Statistical Manual of Mental Disorders,* ed 3, revised criteria for an emotional disorder. These youths may most often be seen in primary care or community settings.

► When I was in my training close to 40 years ago, anxiety and depression were taught as 2 hermetically sealed compartments. I knew for myself and for some of my patients that 1 mood often brought forth the other and vice versa in a reverberating circuit. These current findings are reassuring to me, in retrospect, that my psychopathology was not that severe.

J.E. Schowalter, M.D.

Response of Families to Two Preventive Intervention Strategies: Long-term Differences in Behavior and Attitude Change

Beardslee WR, Wright E, Rothberg PC, et al (Children's Hosp, Boston)

J Am Acad Child Adolesc Psychiatry 35:774–782, 1996 3–21

Background.—Empirical data have shown that the children of parents with affective disorders are at risk for poor outcomes. The long-term effects of 2 types of preventive interventions designed to reduce this risk in children with 1 or 2 affected parents were studied.

Methods.—Fifty-four parents in 28 families were included. All had had an episode of affective disorder in the preceding year. After assessment, the parents were randomly assigned to a clinician-facilitated, manual-based, psychoeducational preventive intervention or to a standardized lecture-group discussion including similar educational material. Standard diagnostic interviews, child behavior scales, and semi-structured interviews with parents about the effects of the intervention were used.

Findings.—Neither intervention was associated with harmful effects. In both groups, ratings of degree of upset about reported concerns declined over time. More behavior and attitude changes occurred in the families receiving the clinician-facilitated intervention than in the lecture group after the intervention. This between-group difference persisted at further follow-up assessment.

Conclusions.—Although both interventions resulted in behavior and attitude changes, the clinician-facilitated intervention was more beneficial. The hypothesis that linking cognitive information to the family's life experience leads to long-term changes is supported.

► Psychotherapy research is difficult to do, and at a time when managed care often seems to want to prescribe first and talk later, such studies are particularly welcome. This study won the American Academy of Child and Adolescent Psychiatry's 1996 Psychotherapy Research Award.

J.E. Schowalter, M.D.

Presentation and Course of Major Depressive Disorder During Childhood and Later Years of the Life Span

Kovacs M (Univ of Pittsburgh, Pa)

J Am Acad Child Adolesc Psychiatry 35:705–715, 1996 3–22

Introduction.—Major depressive disorder (MDD) among children and adolescents is well recognized. Questions remain regarding similarities/differences in the psychopathology of the diagnosis of MDD in youths and adults. Six phenomenologic aspects of MDD were evaluated to determine whether the features of MDD vary across the age span.

Methods.—Operational psychiatric diagnostic criteria and systematic evaluations were given preference in a review of relevant literature. Six phenomenologic features of MDD were evaluated in this review of inpatient and outpatient literature: episode number, symptom constellation, psychiatric comorbidity, recovery from the index episode of MDD, recurrence of MDD, and switch from unipolar MDD to bipolar affective illness. Patients ranged in age from 6 to over 80 years.

Results.—In clinical settings, juveniles with MDD were almost entirely first-episode probands. Reports indicate that the cardinal symptoms of MDD are similar in both age groups. Comorbidity is well documented in the juvenile and adult age groups but entails different combinations and sequencing of specific disorders by age. Attention-deficit disorders or enuresis-encopresis are specific disorders of youth. Panic disorders are more likely to be observed in adults. Regardless of age, the majority of depressed patients have comorbid disorders. Anxiety is the most prevalent diagnosis observed in conjunction with depression in all age groups. Youths seem to recover somewhat faster from their index episode of depression than do adults. The recurrence rate of depression is similar for both age groups. The risk of bipolar switch may be as much as 3-fold for juveniles as compared with adults.

Conclusion.—Symptoms and recurrence rates of juvenile-onset depression are similar to depression symptoms and rates in adults. An early onset of depression is predictive of a particularly serious form of affective illness. The treatment and management of juveniles with MDD require long-term monitoring, clinical care, and patient education.

► There are no chronic psychiatric disorders to my knowledge for which early onset does not in general also indicate greater severity and poorer prognosis. An interesting study would be to determine whether depressed young people are more or less able, when compared with depressed adults, to know that something is wrong with their mood. We know from epidemiologic surveys that parents are less aware than their adolescent offspring of the child's depression. We also know that with adults, depression is woefully underdiagnosed.

J.E. Schowalter, M.D.

Cardiovascular Effects of Therapeutic Doses of Tricyclic Antidepressants in Children and Adolescents

Wilens TE, Biederman J, Baldessarini RJ, et al (Harvard Med School, Boston; Washington Univ, St Louis; Univ of Pittsburgh, Pa)

J Am Acad Child Adolesc Psychiatry 35:1491–1501, 1996 3–23

Background.—For 3 decades, tricyclic antidepressants (TCAs) have played an important role in the pharmacotherapy of psychiatric disorders in children. However, sudden death has been associated with their use, raising concerns about possible cardiovascular risk. The evidence on TCA-associated cardiovascular effects in children and adolescents was reviewed.

Methods and Findings.—The literature from 1967 to 1996 was reviewed, and relevant studies were identified. Twenty-four studies of imipramine, amitriptyline, desipramine, or nortriptyline were reviewed. Seven hundred thirty children were included. Tricyclic antidepressant therapy was associated with minor increases in blood pressure, heart rate, and the ECG conduction parameters PR, QRS, and QT_c. Minor treatment effects were found on Holter ECG monitoring and exercise testing. Some ECG changes were related to specific agents. There were few age-related ECG

TABLE 2.—Suggested Guidelines for Monitoring ECGs and Vital Signs of Children and Adolescents Receiving Tricyclic Antidepressants

Parameter	Children	Adolescents
Vital signs		
Heart rate	≤110–130 beats/min*	≤110–120 beats/min*
Blood pressure	<120/80 mm Hg	<140/90 mm Hg
Electrocardiogram		
PR interval	<200 msec	<200 msec
QRS interval	≤120 msec ± >30% over baseline	±120 msec
QT_c interval	≤460–480 msec	≤460–480 msec

*For 2 consecutive weeks.
(Courtesy of Wilens TE, Biederman J, Baldessarini RJ, et al: Cardiovascular effects of therapeutic doses of tricyclic antidepressants in children and adolescence. *J Am Acad Child Adolesc Psychiatry* 35(11):1491–1501, 1996.)

differences among TCA-treated children, adolescents, or adults. Relatively higher serum TCA levels were associated with ECG abnormalities.

Conclusions.—Cardiovascular changes of uncertain but probably minor clinical significance are associated with TCA in children, as in adults. More information is needed. Guidelines exist for TCA use in children and adolescents (Table 2).

► The shift by child and adolescent psychiatrists to use selective serotonin reuptake inhibitors as first-choice antidepressants in part results from the wish not to have to deal with the uncertainties inherent in TCAs' impact on the cardiovascular system.

J.E. Schowalter, M.D.

Arguments for and Against Teaching Suicide Prevention in Schools

Hazell P, King R (Univ of Newcastle, Callaghan, Australia)
Aust N Z J Psychiatry 30:633–642, 1996 3–24

Background.—Because of the increasing incidence of suicide among youths, school-based suicide prevention programs have been proposed. The arguments for and against teaching such a curriculum were summarized.

The Arguments.—The 2 authors developed their arguments independently after reviewing the available literature on school-based programs before debating the issue at an Australian conference on suicide prevention. In support of school-based programs, 1 author argues that the school has the responsibility, that problems that interfere with education may be resolved through such a program, and that suicide prevention can be considered part of health education. Such programs would acknowledge a duty of care to parents and the community, as well as the students. Primary prevention programs in schools are directed at potential "helpers"—the peers that provide a primary support for troubled adolescents—rather than at-risk students. The goal of increasing teenagers' tendency to approach adults for help appears to be attainable through school-based programs, as evidenced by data in the literature. The other author argues that the evaluation research does not support the inclusion of suicide prevention programs in schools. The evidence from this literature indicates that such programs are not effective or efficient, not universally acceptable, and not necessarily safe.

Conclusions.—Arguments for and against teaching suicide prevention in schools can be made on the basis of existing literature. Those persuaded by the argument for such programs will want to see secondary schools adopt them. Those persuaded by the argument against such programs will want to see suicide prevention resources allocated in other ways.

► My approach to suicide prevention for a general middle or upper school population is to stress the importance of alerting a trusted adult when youths or one of their friends feels suicidal. Often students mention their suicidality to a friend but say that the friend must not tell anyone. I give a few anecdotes in which this wish was honored, the child died, and the friend then felt guilty forever. Most students do not know that suicidal wishes are usually transient and, if the individual lives through them, will go away.

J.E. Schowalter, M.D.

PATHOS: A Screening Instrument for Adolescent Overdose: A Research Note

Kingsbury S (Dept of Child and Adolescent Psychiatry, Health Centre, Hoddesdon, England)

J Child Psychol Psychiatry 37:609–611, 1996 3–25

Background.—A 5-question screening instrument has been developed to identify adolescents at high risk for suicide among those taking a drug overdose. The concurrent validity of this instrument was tested.

Methods.—The questionnaire is designed to assess depression, hopelessness, premeditation, and suicidal intent. The instrument acronym—PATHOS—refers to key words in the 5 questions: Have you had **P**roblems for longer than 1 month? Were you **A**lone in the house at the time? Did you plan the overdose for longer than **T**hree hours? Are you feeling **HO**peless about the future? Were you feeling **S**ad for most of the time before the overdose? This instrument, along with the validating instruments, was administered to 45 adolescents admitted to 1 center for overdose.

Findings.—The PATHOS was strongly correlated with other measures of psychiatric state, including the Beck Hopelessness Inventory, the Beck Depression Inventory, and the Beck Suicide Intent Scale. The PATHOS also predicted all high-risk patients and missed none; all miscalculations were positives.

Conclusion.—This instrument may be useful as an aid for nonpsychiatric staff involved in the management of adolescent overdose. Additional research is needed to explore this possibility and to determine the questionnaire's predictive validity in the short or long term.

▶ Although PATHOS seems to me to reach rather far to find an acronym, it does seem a worthy screening technique for primary care clinicians. What is so needed is to give screeners an easy, unforgettable tool, and PATHOS does this with only a little bathos.

J.E. Schowalter, M.D.

Suicidal Adolescents After Hospitalization: Parent and Family Impacts on Treatment Follow-through

King CA, Hovey JD, Brand E, et al (Univ of Michigan, Ann Arbor; Henry Ford Wyandotte Hosp, Mich)

J Am Acad Child Adolesc Psychiatry 36:85–93, 1997 3–26

Introduction.—Adolescents who make known suicide attempts usually receive inpatient stabilization and comprehensive evaluation, but little is known about predictors of posthospitalization follow-through with recommended drug treatment, individual therapy, and family therapy interventions. A group of 66 suicidal adolescents participated in a study designed to help determine optimal follow-through strategies.

Methods.—Study participants ranged in age from 13 to 17 years and had been hospitalized with significant suicidal thoughts, intents, or behaviors. The 44 girls and 22 boys had a mean age of 15.0 years; 86.4% were Caucasian. Most had mood disorders, primarily major depressive disorder (72.7%). Other frequently noted disorders were alcohol use (18.2%), other substance use (15.2%), conduct disorder (24.2%), and social phobia (15.2%). Baseline evaluations were completed during the first week of hospitalization and telephone follow-up interviews conducted at a mean of 30.5 weeks after hospital discharge.

Results.—Nineteen of the 66 adolescents had made serious suicide attempts, 12 had made mild suicide attempts or gestures, 22 had serious suicidal intent, and 13 expressed significant suicidal ideation. Psychoactive medications were recommended for 51 patients, two thirds of whom reported complete follow-through. The 61 patients for whom individual psychotherapy was recommended attended a mean of 15.2 sessions. A mean of 6.61 sessions were attended by the 62 patients with a recommendation of parent guidance/family therapy. Follow-through was significantly better for medication (66.7%) and for individual therapy (50.8%) than for parent guidance/family therapy (33.3%). The poorest follow-through in parent guidance/family therapy was found in the most dysfunctional families and in those with the least involved/affectionate father-adolescent relationships. There were associations between less medication follow-up and mothers' hostility and between less individual therapy/family therapy and mothers' depressive and paranoid symptoms.

Conclusion.—Many suicidal adolescents fail to obtain continuing treatment after hospitalization. Compliance was best for medication recommendations and poorest for parent guidance/family therapy. Because parents have a strong impact on maintenance of treatment, parent psychiatric evaluations may be essential for successful follow-through.

▶ Many divisions worry about this common problem of maintaining children's treatment after suicidal behavior. As managed care makes hospitalization less available, follow-up is now more often devised under the difficult constraints imposed by an emergency department visit. One approach Yale now uses when concern is high is to provide an in-home service. This intensive outpatient treatment is cheaper than hospitalization, relatively close observation can be provided based on the frequency of visits, and work with parental figures is more likely to occur.

J.E. Schowalter, M.D.

Child Survivors of Suicide: Psychosocial Characteristics

Pfeffer CR, Martins P, Mann J, et al (Cornell Univ, White Plains, NY; New York Hosp; New York Hosp, White Plains; et al)

J Am Acad Child Adolesc Psychiatry 36:65–74, 1997 3–27

Background.—Children and adolescents who experience the suicidal death of a family member or friend are known to have an increased likelihood of mood disorders, which in turn increases their risk for a variety of adverse events. A group of children and young adolescents who recently experienced the suicidal death of a relative was evaluated for psychiatric symptoms and social adjustment. It was hypothesized that these survivors of suicide would have clinically significant symptoms of depression, anxiety, and poor social adjustment.

Methods.—The children were recruited from the community and ranged in age from 5 to 14 years. Research interviews with children and parents were conducted by psychiatrists, psychologists, social workers, and nurse practitioners. A number of standard research instruments were used to assess the children's psychiatric symptoms and social adjustment. The strongest predictors of outcome were identified by multiple linear regression models.

Results.—The study group included 16 families with 22 children, 12 boys and 10 girls. Twelve families were white and 4 were African American or Hispanic. The 17 surviving caretakers were 11 mothers, 4 fathers, 1 grandmother, and 1 aunt (all were biologically related). Eight suicide victims were fathers, 4 were mothers, 3 were brothers, and 1 was a sister. The mean age of the child at the time of death was 8.58 years; mean time between the death and study entry was 1.05 years. No child witnessed the suicide or saw the body of the victim at the time of death. In all but 4 of the 16 families, the children had been told immediately that the death was a suicide.

Compared with a standard community sample, child survivors of suicide had a higher rate of internalizing symptoms and poorer school adjustment. Six families had at least 1 child who reported recent assaultive behavior and 5 had at least 1 child who reported recent suicidal ideation. Half of the surviving caretakers had clinically significant levels of depression, and 25% of families had children who reported clinically significant symptoms of depression. Children with at least moderate symptoms of posttraumatic stress were reported by approximately 40% of families. Psychosocial features of the children were significantly associated with parental psychiatric symptoms and stressful life events.

Discussion.—Child survivors of suicide have higher rates of psychosocial problems than children who have not experienced the suicide of a relative. Symptoms of posttraumatic stress were common, as were symptoms of depression and anxiety, and the children's caretakers were similarly affected. Preventive interventions should address the needs of both the child survivors and their caretakers.

▶ There are no surprises here. Life is not fair, and risk factors tend to cluster. For these children, their traumatic event is added usually to problematic genetic loading and to problematic life circumstances that have just become worse. I hope the investigators continue to follow this cohort to find out which interventions help, which do not help, and what the longer term outcomes will be.

J.E. Schowalter, M.D.

Psychosocial Risk Factors of Child and Adolescent Completed Suicide
Gould MS, Fisher P, Parides M, et al (Columbia Univ, New York)
Arch Gen Psychiatry 53:1155–1162, 1996 3–28

Background.—The psychosocial risk factors for adolescent and childhood suicide have not been well studied. The socioenvironmental characteristics of children and adolescents who committed suicide between June 1984 and May 1986 in the New York area were assessed, and these children were compared with a matched control group.

Study Design.—Psychological autopsies were performed on 120 suicides completed by a person younger than 20 years of age in the New York area. The study area included rural, urban, and suburban districts, with diverse ethnic and socioeconomic characteristics. A random comparison sample of 147 children, stratified on the age, ethnic, and sex distribution of the study group, was identified from the study area. Information on the completed suicides was obtained from an adult member of their household, a sibling or friend, and at least 1 teacher. The interval between suicide and assessment was 28–976 days. The demographic variables included composition of household, socioeconomic status, parental education, parental occupation, marital status, and the school or work status of the suicides. The parent-child relationship, physical punishment, parental psychopathologic characteristics, family history of suicidal behavior, stressful life events, school or work problems, and psychiatric diagnoses were all evaluated.

Findings.—The suicide victims were older, more likely to be boys, and less likely to be African-American than the general youth population. The male-to-female ratio increased with age among the suicide population. The suicide victims were significantly more likely to live with a nonintact family of origin than the community controls. Suicide victims had less frequent and less satisfying communication with both parents. Suicide victims were significantly more likely to have had a mother with a history of mood disorder symptoms, a father with a history of trouble with the police, and a family history of suicidal behavior. Suicide victims had experienced more negative stressful life events, such as school suspension, appearance in juvenile court, recent separation of parents, or break-up with girlfriend or boyfriend. Significant suicide risk was also associated with difficulties in school, neither working nor being in school, and not attending college. Experiencing an interpersonal loss increased the risk of suicide only for boys. Hispanic youth were not affected by disciplinary crises. Failing a grade was a risk factor only for white youths. Poor communication with the father was a significant suicide risk only for those older than 16 years. These factors were independent of psychopathology in their contribution to suicide risk.

Conclusions.—The socioenvironmental factors discussed in this paper significantly increase the risk of suicide in a child or adolescent. The size of this effect is equivalent to that for psychiatric diagnostic factors. In addition to diagnostic profiles, the psychosocial characteristics are a necessary component of suicide risk assessment in young people.

▶ I like this study very much. The authors were very careful with the methodology and they persuasively outline quite specific psychosocial risk factors for teenagers' suicides. I look forward to others' attempts at replication.

J.E. Schowalter, M.D.

Attention Disorders

▶ Biederman's articles must make us wonder about our diagnostic system. If everything overlaps, are we left with anything specific? It has not come to this yet, but disturbing questions are raised that require much debate before the proposed *DSM IV-R* is published.

John E. Schowalter, M.D.

Increased Methylphenidate Usage for Attention Deficit Disorder in the 1990s

Safer DJ, Zito JM, Fine EM (Johns Hopkins Univ, Baltimore, Md; Univ of Maryland, Baltimore)

Pediatrics 98:1084–1088, 1996 3–29

Objective.—Use of methylphenidate (Ritalin) for attention deficit disorder (ADD) has increased steadily since 1971, with some increase estimates as high as 6-fold. The extent and reasons for the increased use of the drug were reviewed.

Description of the Methylphenidate Data Sources Reviewed.—The Baltimore County Health Department biennial survey of public school students receiving treatment for ADD, the Maryland Medicaid database, the Automated Reports Consolidated Orders System Database, National Prescription Audit, the Scott-Levin National Physician's Drug and Diagnosis Audit, the Rhode Island Division of Drug Control, State of Michigan triplicate prescription survey, New York State Health Department prescription survey, and the Northwest Region Kaiser Permanente HMO dataset were used to track the use of methylphenidate from 1990 through 1995.

Results.—These data showed that between 1990 and 1995 use of methylphenidate for treating ADD has increased 2.5 times. Reasons for increasing use of the drug included an increasing number of students being treated, more students continuing medication into their teens, more students with ADD without hyperactivity being given medication, increased use in girls, and a more positive perspective for medicating children with ADD. Approximately 50% to 60% of children with ADD with hyperactivity in Baltimore County are being medicated. About 1.3–1.5 million children are estimated to be receiving methylphenidate as of mid-1995, twice the number receiving medication in 1987.

Conclusion.—There is a 2.5–fold, not a 6-fold, increase in the number of children being treated with methylphenidate for ADD as a result of longer duration of treatment, treatment of more girls and more children with ADD without hyperactivity. The findings do not address the appropriateness of treatment.

► It is helpful to have these figures. Safer has for decades been a good chronicler of ADD diagnosis and treatment statistics. It is still somewhat appalling to me how this condition and its treatment are so American. Are we alarmists or is the rest of the world blind to the obvious? I also wonder what it will mean for methylphenidate consumption that in 1997 Abbott Laboratories had to add to its product labeling a boxed warning for pemoline (Cylert) that it is associated with life-threatening hepatic failure and should not be considered as a first-line medication for ADD?

J.E. Schowalter, M.D.

Attention Problems Versus Conduct Problems as Six-Year Predictors of Problem Scores in a National Sample

MacDonald VM, Achenbach TM (Univ of Vermont, Burlington)

J Am Acad Child Adolesc Psychiatry 35:1237–1246, 1996 3–30

Background.—Follow-up studies of attention-deficit hyperactivity disorder (ADHD) show that this disorder frequently persists into adolescence and young adulthood and is correlated with an increased risk of academic problems, conduct disorders, and criminal involvement. However, because of the frequent co-occurrence of ADHD and conduct disorder or oppositional defiant disorder and the stability of aggressive behavior, researchers have questioned whether the continuation of early co-morbid conduct problems accounts for the unfavorable outcomes associated with ADHD. The extent to which attention problems, the continuation of early co-morbid conduct problems, and overall initial problems are responsible for poor outcome scores on the Child Behavior Checklist and related measures 3 and 6 years after initial evaluation was determined.

Methods.—A nationally representative sample of girls and boys aged 4 through 16 years was studied. In 1986, 2,734 (92.1%) of the eligible children were interviewed. Follow-up interviews in 1989 and 1992 were completed with 90.7% of the 1986 group and with 96.4% of the 1989 group, respectively. Standardized ratings of attention, conduct, and other problems, using sex-specific scores to define deviance, were obtained.

Findings.—Children found to be deviant in both attention and conduct scored significantly higher on behavior problems than children deviant only in attention or conduct at outcome. Initial attention problems contributed minimally to later conduct problems after adjustment for initial conduct problems. Predictive patterns were comparable across sex and age groups.

Conclusions.—Subsequent conduct problems associated with attention problems are best explained by the continuation of early co-morbid conduct problems and perhaps by the overall level of initial psychopathology. Pure attention problems did not appear to have specific effects relative to other types of deviance.

Is Childhood Oppositional Defiant Disorder a Precursor to Adolescent Conduct Disorder?: Findings From a Four-Year Follow-up Study of Children With ADHD

Biederman J, Faraone SV, Milberger S, et al (Massachusetts Gen Hosp, Boston; Harvard Med School, Boston; Massachusetts Health Ctr, Boston; et al)

J Am Acad Child Adolesc Psychiatry 35:1193–1204, 1996 3–31

Background.—Studies have found a high rate of overlap among attention-deficit hyperactivity disorder (ADHD), oppositional defiant disorder (ODD), and conduct disorder (CD). Compared with the data on ADHD

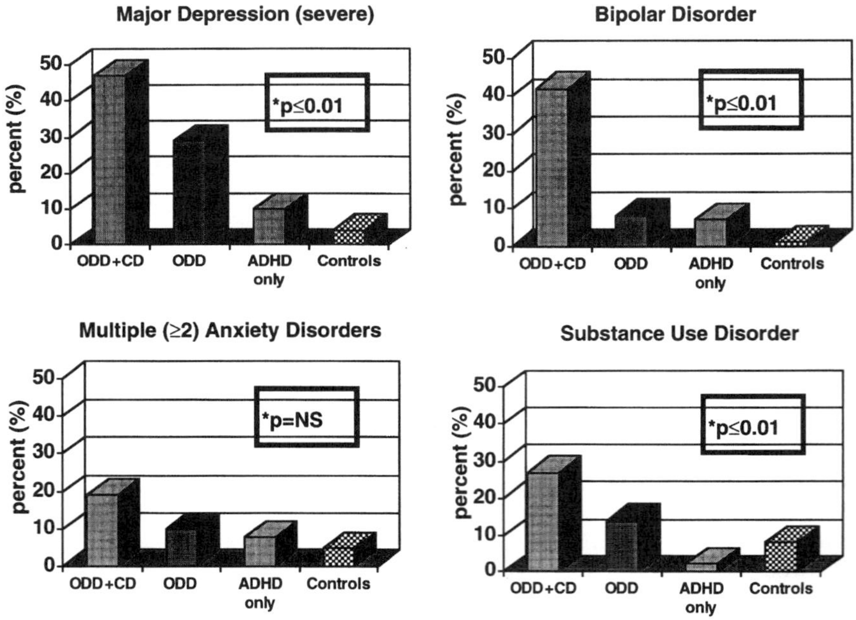

FIGURE 4.—Incidence of co-morbid psychiatric disorders at follow-up. *Abbreviations: ODD*, oppositional defiant disorder; *CD*, conduct disorder; *ADHD*, attention-deficit hyperactivity disorder. *Omnibus tests include ADHD probands only. (Courtesy of Biederman J, Faraone SV, Milberger S, et al: Is childhood oppositional defiant disorder a precursor to adolescent conduct disorder?: Findings from a four-year follow-up study of children with ADHD. *J Am Acad Child Adolesc Psychiatry* 35(9):1193–1204, September, 1996.)

and CD overlap, relatively little is known about the overlap between ADHD and ODD.

Methods and Findings.—One hundred forty children with ADHD and 120 healthy children were assessed on multiple domains at study enrollment and again 4 years later. Sixty-five percent of the children with ADHD at baseline had co-morbid ODD, and 22% had co-morbid CD. Thirty-two percent of those with ODD had co-morbid CD. In all but 1 child with CD, ODD was also present, preceding CD onset by several years. Children with ODD and CD had more severe symptoms of ODD, more co-morbid psychiatric disorders, lower Global Assessment of Functioning Scale scores, more bipolar disorder, and more abnormal Child Behavior Checklist clinical scale scores than children with ADHD and non-CD ODD and children without ODD or CD. The findings of ODD without CD at baseline did not increase the risk of CD at the 4-year assessment at mid-adolescence (Fig 4).

Conclusions.—Two subtypes of ODD associated with ADHD were identified in this study: 1 prodromal to CD and 1 subsyndromal to CD not likely to progress to CD in later years. The correlates, courses, and outcomes of these subtypes differ.

► These 2 articles (Abstracts 3–30 and 3–31) reinforce the clinical finding that children who have a quite pure strain of ADHD do not have the long-term poor social outcome that is routinely found in patients who are co-morbid with ADHD and CD. As a consultant over the years to many schools, I always ask teachers how disruptive is the behavior of the child in question. Children with pure ADHD can roam the room far and wide without attracting attention. A child with ODD or budding CD will have the ability to only drop his pencil and bend over to pick it up to have part or all of the class in an uproar.

J.E. Schowalter, M.D.

Attention-deficit Hyperactivity Disorder and Juvenile Mania: An Overlooked Comorbidity?

Biederman J, Faraone S, Mick E, et al (Massachusetts Gen Hosp, Boston; Harvard Med School, Boston; Harvard School of Public Health, Boston)

J Am Acad Child Adolesc Psychiatry 35:997–1008, 1996 3–32

Introduction.—The pediatric and adult literature report co-occurrence of attention-deficit hyperactivity disorder (ADHD) and bipolar disorder (BPD). However, there has been little systematic investigation regarding these possible comorbid conditions. The psychiatric, cognitive, and functional correlates of ADHD with and without comorbid BPD in children were evaluated by using data from a 4-year family history and follow-up investigation of ADHD.

Methods.—A total of 140 children with ADHD and 120 normal controls underwent *Diagnostic and Statistical Manual of Mental Disorders,* ed 3, revised, structured diagnostic interviews at baseline and at 4 years. Research subjects were evaluated for cognitive, academic, social, school, and family functioning.

Results.—At the 4-year follow-up, 91% of the children with ADHD and 91% of the normal controls were available. At baseline, 11% of the children with ADHD also had a diagnosis of BPD. An additional 12% of the children had a diagnosis of both ADHD and BPD at the 4-year follow-up. When compared with controls, children with ADHD had significantly higher rates of mania at baseline and at the 4-year follow-up. Children with ADHD and comorbid BPD were significantly more likely to have additional psychopathology, psychiatric hospitalization, and severely impaired pyschosocial functioning than other children with ADHD. The clinical picture of mania in children with ADHD was mostly irritable and mixed with rapid cycles and increased activity. Children with ADHD and a new diagnosis of BPD at the 4-year follow-up had higher initial rates of comorbidity, more symptoms of ADHD, worse scores on the Child Behavior Checklist (Fig 1), and a more severe family history of mood disorder than did children with ADHD and no BPD.

Conclusion.—Children with ADHD are at increased risk for BPD and its associated severe morbidity, dysfunction, and incapacitation. The clin-

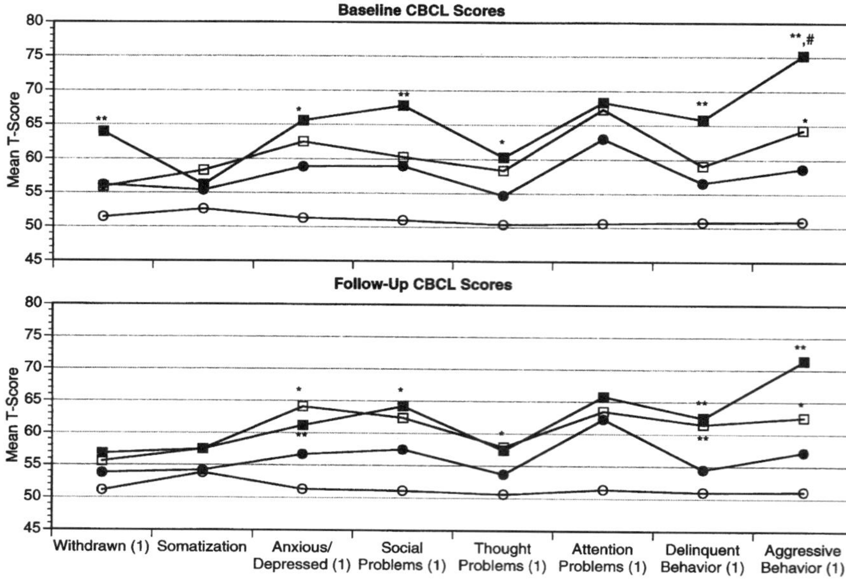

FIGURE 1.—Child Behavior Checklist (*CBCL* scores for the baseline bipolar disorder (*BPD*) group (*black boxes*), follow-up BPD group (*white boxes*), non-BPD attention-deficit hyperactivity disorder (*ADHD*) group (*black circles*), and normal controls. (*white circles*). ***P* <0.01. **P* <0.05 vs. the non-BPD group. #P < 0.05 vs. the follow-up BPD group. (1) *P* < 0.01 vs. controls for all ADHD groups. (Courtesy of Biederman J, Faraone S, Mick E: Attention-deficit hyperactivity disorder and juvenile mania: An overlooked comorbidity? *J Am Acad Child Adolesc Psychiatry* 35(8):997–1008, 1996.)

ical picture is typified by severe irritability, a mixture of symptoms of depression and mania, and multiple episodes.

► This paper sparked controversy within the child and adolescent psychiatry community. The reaction stems largely from the question of what is the meaning of the diagnosis of ADHD. Its frequency (in this country) of diagnosis is almost matched by its vast array of comorbidity. To add bipolar disorder to the already overflowing ADHD comorbidity bin caused some people to believe that Biederman had finally thrown the comorbidity net too far. Controversy is fun, but only future research will confirm or disconfirm what ADHD is and isn't.

J.E. Schowalter, M.D.

Child Behavior Checklist Findings Further Support Comorbidity Between ADHD and Major Depression in a Referred Sample

Biederman J, Faraone S, Mick E, et al (Massachusetts Gen Hosp, Boston; McLean Hosp, Belmont, Mass; Harvard Med School, Boston)

J Am Acad Child Adolesc Psychiatry 35:734–742, 1996 3–33

Background.—Continuing research on depressive disorders in children has identified high levels of psychiatric co-morbidity among patients with

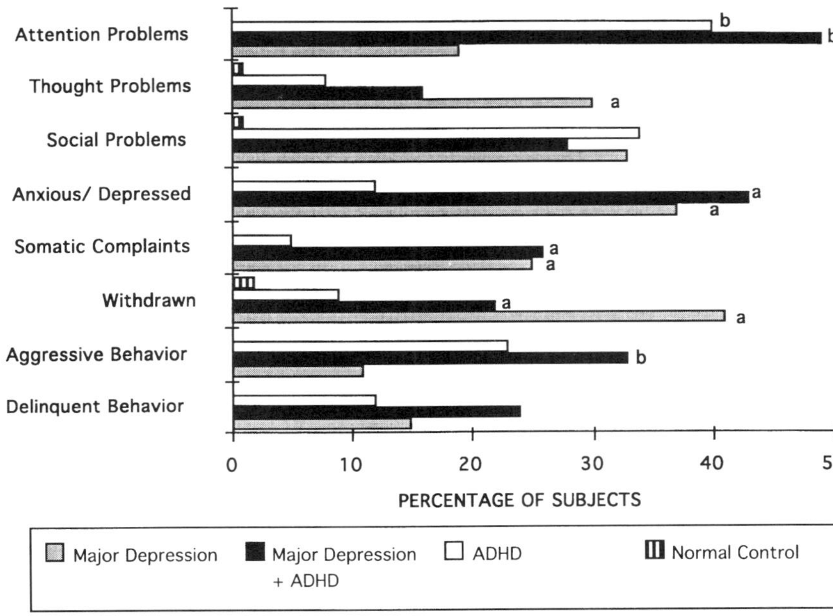

FIGURE 2.—Frequency of abnormal elevations of scores on clinical scales of the Child Behavior Checklist. All scales were significantly lower in normal controls when compared with all 3 psychopathologic groups. [a]$P \leq 0.05$ vs. ADHD; [b]$P < 0.05$ vs. major depression. *Abbreviation: ADHD*, attention-deficit hyperactivity disorder. (Courtesy of Biederman J, Faraone S, Mick E, et al: Child behavior checklist findings further support comorbidity between ADHD and major depression in a referred sample. *J Am Acad Child Adolesc Psychiatry* 35:734–742, 1996.)

a diagnosis of major depression. Using the Child Behavior Checklist (CBCL), the co-morbidity between attention-deficit hyperactivity disorder (ADHD) and depression was studied. Whereas co-morbidity between juvenile major depression and anxiety and conduct disorders is relatively well accepted, some authors suggest that co-morbidity between ADHD and depression is an artifact of overlapping symptoms.

Methods.—From a sample of 424 children and adolescents referred for major psychopathology, 136 received a diagnosis of nonbipolar major depression and 152 received a diagnosis of ADHD. The final sample for analysis consisted of 67 children with major depression plus ADHD, 27 with major depression only, and 97 with ADHD only; also studied were 115 normal control children. Structured diagnostic interviews were administered, and the diagnoses considered positive if *Diagnostic and Statistical Manual of Mental Disorders-III-R* criteria were unequivocally met. The CBCL was completed by the mother. Total predictive value and the odds ratio were used to evaluate the convergence of CBCL scales with the structured interview-derived diagnoses.

Results.—Because sociodemographic characteristics differed significantly among the 4 groups, analyses were corrected by age, sex, and family intactness. The CBCL clinical scales revealed significant differences within psychopathologic groups and between these groups and controls (Fig 2). Irrespective of co-morbidity with ADHD, the CBCL Anxious/Depressed scale discriminated between depressed and nondepressed children; the Attention Problems scale discriminated ADHD from non-ADHD children, irrespective of co-morbidity with major depression. Among children with both major depression and ADHD, CBCL correlates of both disorders were present.

Discussion.—Previous reports of a high overlap between major depression in children and ADHD do not appear to reflect rater or assessment biases. Various scales of the CBCL—an empirically derived taxonomic system—were able to discriminate children with and without major depression and children with and without ADHD, irrespective of co-morbidity with ADHD and major depression.

▶ Many clinicians note the co-morbidity of ADHD and major depression in some of their patients. An interesting study for the future will be to attempt to measure whether depression occurs more frequently in those patients who are more bothered by their ADHD symptoms. I am struck that some patients accept ADHD symptoms as *just the way I am*, whereas others experience the symptoms as dystonic and shameful.

J.E. Schowalter, M.D.

Motor Vehicle Driving Competencies and Risks in Teens and Young Adults With Attention Deficit Hyperactivity Disorder

Barkley RA, Murphy KR, Kwasnik D (Univ of Massachusetts, Worcester)
Pediatrics 98:1089–1095, 1996 3–34

Background.—Attention deficit hyperactivity disorder (ADHD) is a behavioral disorder that begins in childhood and consists of poor sustained attention, impulsiveness, and excessive activity relative to peers. Some research has suggested that those with ADHD are more likely to be involved in motor vehicle crashes. To examine this issue, the driving knowledge, skills, and negative outcomes of older teens and young adults with ADHD were compared with those of a control group without ADHD.

Study Design.—The study group consisted of 25 young adults who met the *Diagnostic and Statistical Manual of Mental Disorders*, ed 4 criteria for ADHD and 23 age-, gender-, and education-matched controls from the same community. The 4 ADHD participants who were taking stimulants were asked to refrain from medication for the 24 hours before testing. Testing consisted of a structured interview concerning psychiatric disorders, education, work, drug use, criminal history, and driving history. A videotape test of driving knowledge was then administered, followed by a computer-simulation driving test. Official driving records were obtained from the state.

Findings.—The ADHD young adults were cited more frequently for speeding, were more likely to have suspended licenses, were involved in more and more serious crashes, and were self-rated and rated by others as having poorer driving habits. There was no difference between the 2 groups in driving knowledge. During the computer-simulated driving test, the ADHD participants had more erratic steering, as well as more crashes and scrapes than the control participants.

Conclusions.—The results of this study of young drivers with and without ADHD demonstrated that ADHD is associated with a greater risk of erratic and unlawful driving behaviors that result in more traffic citations, license suspensions, and motor vehicle crashes. The problems of the ADHD drivers were not in driving knowledge, but in the actual performance of motor vehicle operation. Attempts to lower the driving risk associated with ADHD should not focus on knowledge but on self-regulation during driving.

► The take-home point of this article is not that these findings are surprising or counterintuitive, but that they are not better ensconced in clinicians' consciousness. As clinicians we worry much about a young person's ADHD symptoms in regard to school or job success, but too seldom do we worry about the effect of these symptoms on life and limb.

J.E. Schowalter, M.D.

Autism

Autism: Towards an Integration of Clinical, Genetic, Neuropsychological, and Neurobiological Perspectives

Bailey A, Phillips W, Rutter M (Inst of Psychiatry, London)

J Child Psychol Psychiatry 37:89–126, 1996 3–35

Introduction.—Systematic research over the last 2 decades has provided useful information about autism that needs to be integrated. The current state of knowledge on genetic, neuropsychological, and neurobiological findings related to autism was reviewed.

Genetic Factors.—The possibility of genetic causes of autism was initially ignored because the incidence of more than 1 child with autism was so rare. The discovery of the fragile X anomaly in children with autism prompted major research interest in other chromosomal anomalies possibly related to autism. There may be a correlation between autism and tuberous sclerosis, untreated phenylketonuria, and an increase in the rate of other chromosomal anomalies. The genetic component in autism may make it an obvious candidate for molecular genetic strategies, but there are no strong candidate genes available to undergo the rigors of molecular analysis.

Neuropsychological Approaches.—In the 1950s and 1960s, it was thought that the psychological abilities of children with autism were not able to be measured. Clearly, focused research has shown that the cognitive deficits of children with autism are not a result of impaired social development. Autism is a complex syndrome, a constellation of features that cluster together such as sensory-perceptual abnormalities, mental retardation, language impairment, and mind hypothesis. Questions now need to focus on why these features cluster together.

Neurobiology.—Functional analyses of autism are fraught with methodologic problems that have poor reproducibility. Neuroanatomical, neuroimaging, postmortem, neurophysiological, and neurochemical studies have revealed subtle abnormalities that are hard to offer as empirical truth. One finding that deserves further investigation is that of increased brain size in patients with autism.

Conclusion.—Integration of the many levels of research findings is needed to help give a full understanding of autism, point out limitations, and stimulate future investigation. What has been done thus far has revolutionized concepts of autism over the last 3 decades. A concerted attack on autism can be made by integrating conceptual and technological advances from the various areas of expertise.

► Do not bother to crack open even your latest textbook. If you want the best critique of current understanding of autism, read this superb synthesis. Autism is the most fascinating neurodevelopmental disorder of all. Its basis, or I should say bases, flirt with what makes us human, as conventionally defined. This beginning at integrating a broad array of studies may well provoke readers' disagreement with this statement or that conclusion, but the authors have provided the reader with some 360 references, so you can chase primary sources for yourself.

J.E. Schowalter, M.D.

The Neuropsychology of Autism

Happé F, Frith U (Univ College, London)
Brain 119:1377–1400, 1996 3–36

Introduction.—Cognitive neuropsychology has offered some promising advances in linking brain abnormality and symptoms in autism. Major trends in autism were reviewed at the biological, behavioral, and cognitive levels.

Biology.—People with autism rarely have children, but there is evidence of genetic factors and family clustering in this biologically based disorder. Autism is characterized as a disorder without physical stigmata, but physical and brain tissue anomalies have been identified that may provide clues to the timing of this developmental abnormality.

Behavior.—Autism is diagnosed on the basis of behavior, not biology. The core behavioral elements of autism are social, communication, and imagination impairments and restricted, repetitive activities.

Cognition.—Autism as a disorder of social insight is a significant cognitive theory but does not explain the total disease manifestation. Other major cognitive theories include mentalizing impairment, executive dysfunction, and weak central coherence. The overlap and correlation between theories is not understood. The nonsocial impairments observed in autism deserve further investigation.

Conclusion.—Current and upcoming findings in the biological, behavioral, and cognitive levels of autism research are promising and may offer the field of neuropsychology its first understanding of a developmental disorder.

► This invited review with over 300 references offers possible points of integration between biological, behavioral, and cognitive influences. What is most different, and would therefore be most enlightening for YEAR BOOK readers, is the focus on major cognitive theories.

J.E. Schowalter, M.D.

Executive Function in Parents of Children With Autism

Hughes C, Leboyer M, Bouvard M (Univ of Cambridge, England; INSERM U 155, Paris; Hôpital Robert Debré, Paris)

Psychol Med 27:209–220, 1997 3–37

Purpose.—Previous studies have shown impairment of executive function in patients with autism. Studies disagree as to whether the parents of autistic children have social abnormalities, although there is strong evidence for a genetic component to autism. If executive dysfunction is a major feature of autistic children, their parents may have a similar but subtler impairment. The executive function of parents of autistic children was studied.

Methods.—Three groups of adults performed computerized tests of executive function: 40 parents of autistic children, 40 parents of children with learning disabilities, and 36 adults from families with no history of psychiatric disorders or learning disability. The study included tests of attentional-shifting skills, visuospatial planning, and working memory. For control purposes, a computerized test of spatial memory span was administered. Interviewers' pretest impressions of the subjects in each group were recorded as well.

Results.—Many of the parents of autistic children showed impaired executive function, most commonly the fathers. There were no differences between groups on the test of spatial memory span, nor on other "nonexecutive" measures. Thus, the parents in the autism group seemed to be just as attentive and motivated as those in the other groups. The finding of executive dysfunction was correlated with the interviewers' impression of social abnormality among the parents in the autistic group.

Conclusion.—A significant proportion of the parents of autistic children appear to have executive dysfunction. Although they have normal memory, their planning skills and attentional flexibility may be lacking. More research is needed to see whether this represents some inherent familial trait or is related to the problems of caring for an autistic child. Executive function may be involved not only in the stereotypes of autism but also in the entire behavioral phenotype.

▶ Back to the future. Kanner[1] originally believed that autistic children had "refrigerated parents." His review was soon afterward dismissed, because many of the children in his study had fathers who were Johns Hopkins faculty members. Everyone knew that professors tend to be icy types, so Kanner's parental findings were considered to be the result of selection bias.

J.E. Schowalter, M.D.

Reference

1. Kanner L: Autistic disturbances of affective contact. *Nervous Children* 2:217–250, 1943.

Childhood Schizophrenia

Childhood-onset Schizophrenia

Kumra S, Frazier JA, Jacobsen LK, et al (Natl Inst of Mental Health, Bethesda, Md; Harvard Univ, Boston; Northwestern Univ, Chicago; et al)
Arch Gen Psychiatry 53:1090–1097, 1996 3–38

Introduction.—Childhood-onset schizophrenia is frequently treatment refractory. There are no known controlled trials of atypical neuroleptics in children or adolescents with schizophrenia. Findings of the first double-blind investigation of clozapine in children with early-onset schizophrenia who were treatment refractory were reported.

Methods.—Twenty-one children and adolescents aged 6–18 years were randomized to a 6-week double-blind, parallel comparison of clozapine or haloperidol. Weekly behavioral ratings were performed on each child by a psychiatrist. During the weekly visits, children were evaluated for side effects. Patients underwent baseline and 6-week blood tests, encephalograms, and electrocardiograms.

Results.—Clozapine was significantly superior to haloperidol on all measures of psychosis. There was also significant improvement in positive and negative signs of schizophrenia in children who received clozapine, compared with those who received haloperidol. The 2 drugs were similar in minor side effects. Drowsiness and salivation were more pronounced in the clozapine group and insomnia was more prevalent in the haloperidol group. Of 10 patients receiving clozapine, 5 had a drop in the absolute neutrophil count below 1,500 mm, 5 had clinically significant seizure activity, and 1 had a clinically significant elevation in hepatic enzymes.

Conclusion.—Clozapine was superior to haloperidol in reducing positive and negative symptoms in children with early-onset schizophrenia. Children and adolescents with schizophrenia who are treated with clozapine must be carefully monitored for side effects.

► Clozapine has proven that a better neuroleptic can be found. As its younger wannabees enter long-term trials, we will see whether there is a way to maintain such stellar efficacy while taming that too-high-a-price side effect profile.

J.E. Schowalter, M.D.

Childhood-onset Schizophrenia: Biological Markers in Relation to Clinical Characteristics

Alaghband-Rad J, Hamburger SD, Giedd JN, et al (Natl Inst of Mental Health, Bethesda, Md)

Am J Psychiatry 154:64–68, 1997 3–39

Background.—Two previous studies have shown a significant correlation between negative (deficit) symptoms in schizophrenia and decreased total cerebral volume. These findings have received little attention, but they may be important. Other research suggests that negative symptoms are the core manifestations of developmental abnormalities in schizophrenia and that they are associated with earlier age of onset.

Objective.—The relation between cerebral volume and clinical measures were investigated in patients with childhood-onset schizophrenia.

Methods.—From 600 patients with schizophrenia who were referred and 138 who were screened in person, 29 met the *Diagnostic and Statistical Manual of Mental Disorders,* ed 3, revised criteria for schizophrenia

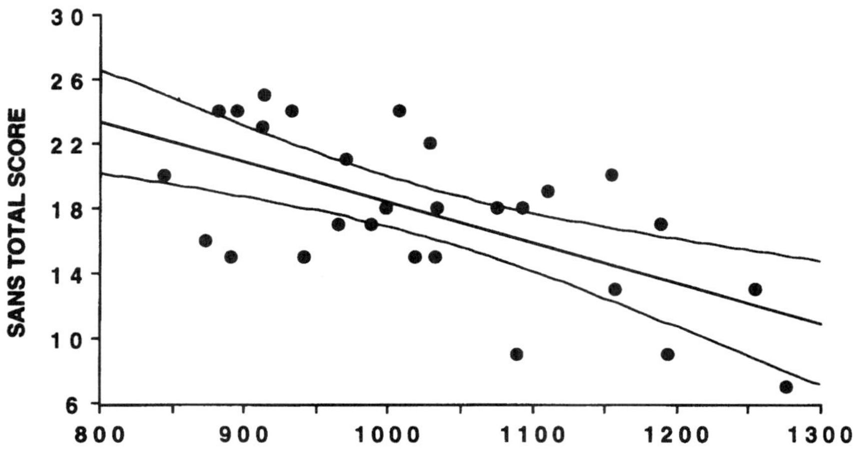

FIGURE 1.—Correlation between total cerebral volume and total negative symptoms (Scale for the Assessment of Negative Symptoms) of participants with childhood-onset schizophrenia. The *middle line* represents the regression, and the *top and bottom lines* represent the 95% confidence interval. The correlation between total cerebral volume and Scale for the Assessment of Negative Symptoms score was significant ($r = -0.65$, $N = 28$, $P < 0.001$). (Courtesy of Alaghband-Rad J, Hamburger SD, Giedd JN, et al: Childhood-onset schizophrenia: Biological markers in relation to clinical characteristics. *Am J Psychiatry* 154:64–68, 1997. Copyright 1997, the American Psychiatric Association. Reprinted by permission.)

and had had onset at or before age 12 years (age range, 10 to 19 years; mean age at onset, 10.2 years). All had had an IQ score of 70 or above before the onset of psychosis. Chart review and interviews were used to study the patients' language development and symptoms of autism, the mother's obstetric complications, and type of onset. Type of onset was rated as subacute (6 months or less elapsed between the first nonspecific symptoms and the first psychotic symptoms) or insidious (more than 6 months elapsed). Brain MRI was used to determine total cerebral volume and lateral ventricular volumes. Participants also were rated on the Brief Psychiatric Rating Scale), the Scale for the Assessment of Negative Symptoms (SANS), and the Scale for the Assessment of Positive Symptoms.

Results.—For the entire group, there was a significant negative correlation between SANS score and total cerebral volume (Fig 1). Four other relationships were significant for boys: smaller cerebral volume was significantly associated with SANS score, Scale for the Assessment of Positive Symptoms score, Brief Psychiatric Rating Scale score, and the presence of language disorders. In addition, boys were more likely than girls to have had insidious onset of schizophrenia.

Conclusions.—These patients seem to have a general pattern of brain maldevelopment. Compared with the later-onset disorder, childhood-onset schizophrenia may have a more homogeneous or more potent neurobiological basis.

► Although it has limitations because of the small sample size and ever-present possibilites for a selection bias, this study is important in pointing out a strong association between smaller cerebral volume and negative symptoms, IQ notwithstanding. Negative symptoms have always been more difficult to understand and to treat than positive symptoms. Studies such as this are helping us to better put negative symptoms into a biophysiologic context.

J.E. Schowalter, M.D.

Prenatal Growth Markers in Schizophrenia: A Monozygotic Co-twin Control Study

Davis JO, Bracha HS (Southwest Missouri State Univ, Springfield; Univ of Arkansas, Little Rock; VA Med and Regional Office Ctr, Honolulu, Hawaii)

Am J Psychiatry 153:1166–1172, 1996 3–40

Introduction.—Earlier investigations have reported that dermatoglyphics may help determine the timing of a prenatal dysgenesis in schizophrenia. Monozygotic twins who were discordant for schizophrenia were analyzed for evidence of prenatal growth differences between the affected and well co-twins.

Methods.—Twenty-six monozygotic twin pairs discordant for schizophrenia, 13 monozygotic twin pairs concordant for schizophrenia, and several normal monozygotic twin samples were evaluated for 4 dermato-

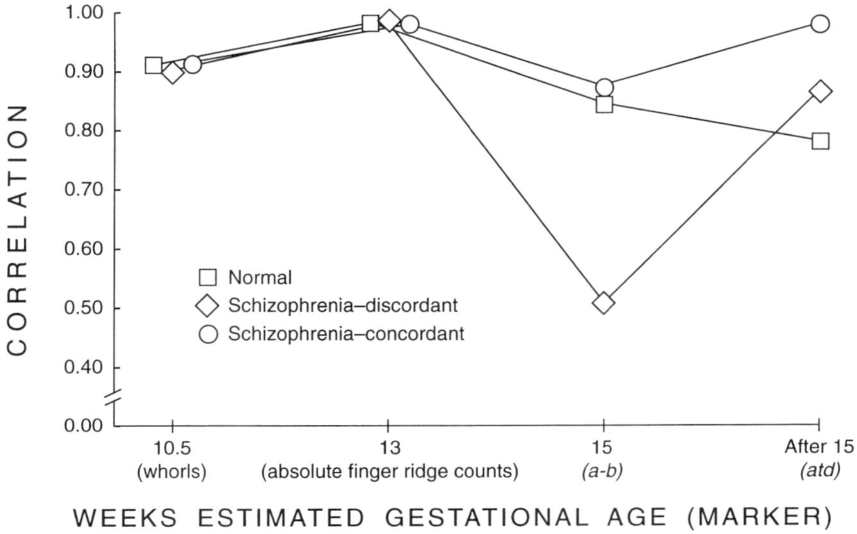

Number of Twin Pairs:				
Normal	7	136	142	527
Schizophrenia–concordant	13	13	13	9
Schizophrenia–discordant	26	26	19	12

FIGURE 3.—Intraclass correlations for dermatoglyphic similarity of monozygotic twins discordant and concordant for schizophrenia and normal monozygotic twins. (Courtesy of Davis JO, Bracha HS: Prenatal growth markers in schizophrenia: A monozygotic co-twin control study. *Am J Psychiatry* 153:1166–1172, copyright 1996, the American Psychiatric Association. Reprinted by permission.)

glyphic markers of prenatal growth: finger patterns, finger ridges, *a-b* ridges, and *atd* angles. Intraclass correlations of the 4 dermatoglyphic chronomarkers were used to create dermatoglyphic profiles to show the developmental trends for all twin groups (Fig 3).

Results.—There were more *a-b* ridge count differences between the affected and well co-twins, compared with concordant and normal monozygotic twin pairs. In the affected twins in discordant pairs, fewer epidermal ridges developed in the *a-b* interdigital area of their right palms, compared with their normal co-twin. No significant differences were detected between the affected twin and their normal co-twin on markers associated with fetal development before 13 weeks' or after 15 weeks' gestational age.

Conclusion.—Findings show that developmental differences occurred in the period between 13 and 15 weeks' gestational age. This evidence for a time-specific and time-limited embryopathy in patients with schizophrenia suggests that it would be helpful to evaluate other organs that develop at the same time as the CNS. These efforts could help define the timing and nature of what could be preventable, nongenetic influences in the development of severe psychiatric disorders.

► This is an exciting finding that pinpoints the 13- to 15-week gestational age as possibly critical in the developmental differentiation between at least some schizophrenia-discordant monozygotic twins. These dermatoglyphic findings fit nicely with the neurologic findings (also from surface ectoderm) which have earlier been traced to this gestational period. It is fascinating to watch how these embryonic studies are beginning to complement one another.

J.E. Schowalter, M.D.

Adolescence

► Birth to age 3 is a crucial time for development in regard to how children are treated. In the next most crucial developmental period, adolescence, we are confronted with how many ways, often negative, that children treat themselves and others. The following articles, related to each other mainly by covering a specific age-range, address some aspects of this mosaic of teenage development.

John E. Schowalter, M.D.

Prevalence and Impact of Exposure to Interpersonal Violence Among Suburban and Urban Middle School Students

Campbell C, Schwarz DF (Univ of Pennsylvania, Philadelphia)
Pediatrics 98:396–402, 1996 3–41

Background.—Many studies have shown that a high percentage of children are exposed to violence in some way. However, most previous studies have included relatively small numbers of children and focused mostly on low-income, black children in inner-city neighborhoods. The prevalence of exposure to violence in preadolescent children in communities varying by family income was investigated.

Methods.—The participants were 228 sixth-graders in a suburban middle school (school A) and 209 sixth-graders in an urban middle school (school B) in Philadelphia. The students completed a questionnaire anonymously.

Findings.—Eighty-nine percent of the students from school A and 96% from school B reported knowing someone who had been robbed, beaten, stabbed, shot, or murdered. Fifty-seven percent from school A and 88% from school B had witnessed a robbing, beating, stabbing, shooting, or murder. Forty percent and 67%, respectively, had personally been robbed, beaten up, stabbed, shot, or caught in gun cross fire. Fifty-nine percent of the school A children and 73% of the school B children reported hearing gunfire in their neighborhood. At least 1 positive response in all 3 categories of knowing a victim, witnessing violence, and being a victim of

TABLE 1.—Topics Covered in the Questionnaire Survey

Witness of violent events
Personal victimization
Victimization of friends and acquaintances
Patterns of communication in reaction to violent events
Patterns of conflict resolution
Television and other media viewing habits
Physical symptoms
Demographic information

(Courtesy of Campbell C, Schwarz DF: Prevalence and impact of exposure to interpersonal violence among suburban and urban middle school students. Reproduced by permission of *Pediatrics*, Vol. 98, pages 396–402, Copyright 1996.)

violence was reported by 82% of the students in school A and 97% in school B. Children in school had significantly more symptoms of somatization syndromes, depression, and posttraumatic stress disorder. Only 1% to 8% of the students had been seen by a medical or mental health professional for such problems (Table 1).

Conclusions.—A substantial proportion of children in urban and suburban schools are exposed to violence. Children in the urban school, whose exposures were greater, had a higher incidence of symptoms that sometimes occur after traumatic stress. Although most of the children talked with someone about their experience, they rarely consulted a health professional.

► I have to believe that violence in general and violence to children in particular are slowly but surely becoming intolerable to a larger segment of the population, suburban and urban. The 1996 congressional elections went almost unanimously against candidates backed by the National Rifle Association. There is a God!

J.E. Schowalter, M.D.

Adolescent Resiliency to Family Adversity

Fergusson DM, Lynskey MT (Christchurch Hosp, New Zealand)
J Child Psychol Psychiatry 37:281–292, 1996 3–42

Introduction.—Children whose families experience an accumulation of difficulties, such as poverty, abuse, conflict, and change, are at increased risk for behavioral and mental health problems. Teenagers with multiple problems rarely come from families with a lack of adversity during childhood, yet many children reared under adverse circumstances make a satisfactory adjustment. To identify factors associated with adolescent resiliency to childhood disadvantages, data collected during a 16-year longitudinal study of a birth cohort of New Zealand children were reviewed.

Methods.—The 1,265 children enrolled in the Christchurch Health and Development Study were born during mid-1977 and have been studied at birth, 4 months, 1 year, and at annual intervals until age 16 years. Children were grouped according to level of family adversity: 54.5% were in the lowest adversity group and 5.4% in the highest adversity group. The rate of multiple-problem teenagers was 21.6% in the highest adversity group but only 0.2% in the lowest adversity group. Measures of risk included conduct/oppositional defiant disorders; self-report offending; police contact; frequent truancy; school dropout; and the use of cannabis, cigarettes, and alcohol. Fifteen factors associated with resiliency also were included in the analyses: among these were intelligence, self-esteem, interest in sport, novelty seeking, parental bonding, and the nature of the home environment. A total of 940 cases of adolescents from the original sample were available for analysis.

Results.—Of the 171 teenagers in the high-risk group, 63 (36.8%) were without externalizing behaviors such as delinquency, substance use, and school problems. These resilient adolescents differed from their peers by having higher intelligence and self-esteem and lower levels of novelty seeking, early-onset attention-deficit behaviors, and conduct behavior disorders. Those who were resilient were more likely to enjoy school and had fewer affiliations with delinquent peers. In logistic regression analysis, predictors of resiliency were less exposure to family adversity, having higher IQ scores at age 8 years, and having lower affiliations with delinquent peers and lower reported rates of novelty seeking at age 16 years.

Discussion.—Resilience to a high level of family adversity is probably the result of several factors acting together, rather than a single factor. In general, teenagers from high-risk family backgrounds who achieve a satisfactory adjustment have at least average intelligence and show low tendencies to novelty seeking and to association with delinquent peers.

► New Zealand is the home of some of child psychiatry's most significant longitudinal studies. This one comes up with 3 resiliency factors, which make intuitive sense for avoiding externalizing problems. Nerds may be laughed at in school, but at age 30 years, nerds may be having the last laugh.

J.E. Schowalter, M.D.

Maternal Correlates of Adolescent Sexual and Contraceptive Behavior

Jaccard J, Dittus PJ, Gordon VV (State Univ of New York; Univ at Albany)

Fam Plann Perspect 28:159–165,185, 1996 3–43

Introduction.—Certain family variables have been identified as predictors of adolescent sexual behavior. Some studies, for example, find a relation between low parental levels of supervision over dating activities and high-risk sexual behavior by adolescents. A survey of 751 black youths focused on 3 variables likely to influence adolescent sexual behavior: maternal disapproval of premarital sex, maternal discussion of birth control, and the quality of the parent-child relationship.

Methods.—Potential study participants, identified through a random sampling of households, were living in the inner city of Philadelphia. Those eligible were aged 14 to 17 years at the time of the study, were unmarried, had a biological mother who was black, and had a mother or female caregiver living in the home. The adolescents and their mothers were interviewed separately at home and with the assurance that responses were confidential. Eighty-four percent of those invited agreed to participate.

Results.—The mean age of the adolescent boys and girls was 15 years and the mean age of the adult women was 40 years. Eighty-five percent of adolescents lived with their biological mother and 94% were in school. The most frequently reported religious affiliation was Baptist (44%). The median family income was approximately $16,000. More than half of the adolescents reported engaging in sexual intercourse (65% of males and 50% of females), and many who were sexually active used no contraceptive method at first intercourse (68% of males and 47% of females). Whereas 66% of mothers did not think their child had engaged in sexual intercourse, this was true for only 42%. Most mothers expressed disapproval of this behavior, but 25% were ambivalent or had a positive attitude toward sexual intercourse by adolescents. Youths who were less likely to engage in sexual intercourse had a more satisfying parent-child relationship and felt that their mothers encouraged abstinence. Increased discussions about birth control predicted a greater likelihood that the adolescent had initiated intercourse and were associated with increased contraceptive use by males, but not by females.

Discussion.—Maternal variables were confirmed to have an influence on adolescent sexual behavior. The overall quality of an adolescent's relationship with his or her mother was related to the initiation and frequency of sexual intercourse and the consistency with which birth control was used. Family-based interventions may help to reduce unintended pregnancies in adolescents.

► It is safe to say that mothers know much more about infants as responsibilities than adolescents do, and this knowledge seems able to modify adolescents' fantasies that infants are trophies or will be supportive companions. Conversely, there are some data that teenaged boys who spend much time talking about sex with their fathers are on average more promiscuous.

J.E. Showalter, M.D.

Relationship Between Cigarette Smoking and Health Risk and Problem Behaviors Among US Adolescents

Escobedo LG, Reddy M, DuRant RH (Ctrs for Disease Control and Prevention, Atlanta, Ga; Harvard Med School, Boston)

Arch Pediatr Adolesc Med 151:66–71, 1997 3–44

Background.—Rates of smoking among adolescents remain high and may have increased in certain groups during recent years. Many factors are known to affect teen smoking, including high school dropout status, socioeconomic status, and school performance. However, there are few data on how smoking is affected by the health risk and problem behaviors common among adolescents. The effects of these health- and behavior-related factors on smoking by adolescents were evaluated.

Methods.—The study included a national probability sample of 10,645 United States youths aged 12–21 years. The response rate was 74%, with oversampling of black and Hispanic subjects. The subjects were questioned privately about cigarette smoking and other health risk and problem behaviors that are common among adolescents.

Results.—Factors associated with a greater likelihood of smoking included white race, older age, high school education, and living in the Northeastern United States. The prevalence of smoking was adjusted for sociodemographic behaviors and health risk and problem behaviors. For white male adolescents, smoking was significantly linked to marijuana use (odds ratio [OR], 3.7), binge drinking (OR, 2.1), and fighting (OR, 1.4). The same factors were also related to smoking for white females and for black and Hispanic youths of both sexes. For whites, smoking was also linked to using smokeless tobacco, having multiple sex partners, and not wearing a bicycle helmet. Among Hispanic youths, smoking was related to having multiple sex partners for females and to carrying weapons for males.

Conclusion.—Factors associated with cigarette smoking among United States adolescents included marijuana use, binge drinking, and fighting. The precise pattern of associations varies by race and sex. However, the factors may cluster to form a syndrome of related risk behaviors. The results suggest the need for effective interventions to keep adolescents from starting smoking and to help them quit.

► We currently have the most powerful set of government forces ever assembled against teenage smoking. Smoking's multiple correlations with other health risks are obvious, but society should be aware that to paint any behavior as ultra-dangerous is likely to increase its popularity within the most vulnerable segment of the adolescent population.

J.E. Schowalter, M.D.

Nicotine Patch Therapy in Adolescent Smokers

Smith TA, House RF Jr, Croghan IT, et al (Mayo Clinic, Mayo Found, Rochester, Minn)

Pediatrics 98:659–667, 1996 3–45

Background.—Tobacco use is the largest cause of preventable death in the United States. Most lifetime smoking behavior begins during adolescence, but little information is available on effective smoking cessation programs for teenagers. Nicotine patch therapy has been very successful as an adult smoking cessation program. A nonrandomized, open-label clinical trial of nicotine patch therapy was performed in smokers younger than 18 years.

Study Design.—Twenty-two smokers aged 13–17 years, who smoked more than 20 cigarettes per day and were attempting to quit smoking, were recruited from 5 public high schools in Rochester, Minnesota. The participants received daily nicotine patch therapy for 8 weeks, with weekly individual behavioral counseling and group support for 8 weeks. Follow-up visits were conducted at 3 and 6 months and a survey was mailed after 1 year. Smoking abstinence was self-reported and verified by expired air carbon monoxide.

Results.—At entry to this study, participants smoked more than 20 cigarettes per day and had smoked for more than 2 years. Their average age was 16 years and 68% were girls. Of the 22 participants, 19 completed patch therapy, 3 had biochemically validated smoking cessation at week 8 and continued to be smoke free at 6 months' follow-up. There was a significant decrease in nicotine withdrawal scores after patch initiation. The most common adverse event was skin reactions to the patch. Other reported adverse events were headaches, nausea and vomiting, tiredness, dizziness, and arm pain. None of the adverse events were considered serious or led to discontinuation of the patch. Adolescents had lower blood cotinine levels than adults with comparable smoking rates.

Conclusions.—Nicotine patch therapy appeared to be safe and well tolerated in this small group of adolescent smokers. Placebo-controlled trials will be necessary to establish the efficacy of nicotine patch therapy in the adolescent smoker population.

► I believe most of the medical world in this country has been surprised by the degree of success that is being published about nicotine patch therapy for adult smokers. Success rates for teenagers are not yet available. Safety, however, is a start, and if a teenager can reach age 20 nonsmoking, the odds are that he or she will stay nonsmoking.

J.E. Schowalter, M.D.

Young Adult Drug Use and Delinquency: Childhood Antecedents and Adolescent Mediators

Brook JS, Whiteman M, Finch SJ, et al (Mount Sinai School of Medicine, New York; State Univ of New York, Stony Brook; Columbia Univ, New York)

J Am Acad Child Adolesc Psychiatry 35:1584–1592, 1996 3–46

Objective.—The relation between childhood aggression and young adult delinquency was investigated. Specifically, 3 hypotheses were developed (Fig 1): (a) childhood aggression correlates with drug use during early adolescence, late adolescence, and young adulthood; (b) at each stage of development, drug use has an effect on delinquency; and (c) childhood aggression affects young adult delinquency via continued drug use during adolescence, or continued delinquency.

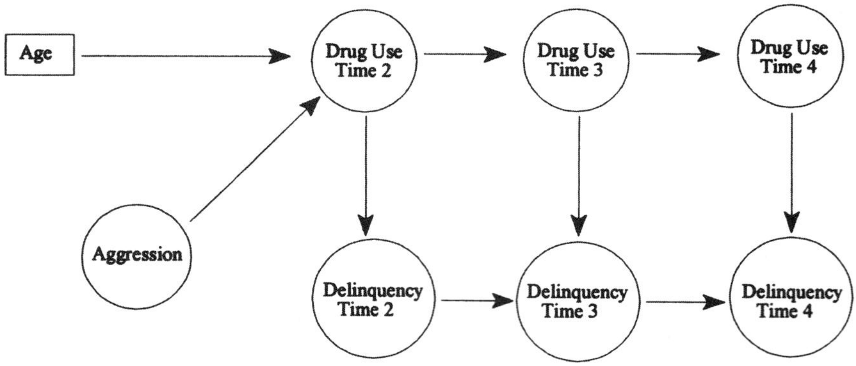

FIGURE 1.—Hypothesized model for interrelation of aggression, drug use, and delinquency. *Circles* represent latent constructs; *1-headed arrows* represent paths of influence between variables. (Courtesy of Brook JS, Whiteman M, Finch SJ, et al: Young adult drug use and delinquency: Childhood antecedents and adolescent mediators. *J Am Acad Child Adolesc Psychiatry* 35(12):1584–1592, 1996.)

Methods.—In this long-range study, a representative sample of children and their mothers were interviewed in their homes 4 times: when the child was aged 5 to 10 years (T1), when the child was 13 to 18 years (T2), when the child was 16 to 21 years (T3), and when the child was 22 to 27 years (T4). Questions concerned the child's personality, behavior, and development, as well as family structure, family health, and demographic factors. At T2 to T4, the mothers and the adolescents/young adults were interviewed separately, and the adolescents/young adults also completed a questionnaire about their personality, behavior, mental health, and drug use. The original number of children was 500, but this article reports only on the 358 young adults for whom there are complete data (163 men, 195 women). At T4, the sample was 91% white, the mean family income was $37,500, and mothers and fathers both had a mean of 12.7 years of schooling.

Results.—In males, childhood aggression was significantly correlated with drug use and delinquency at T2 and T3. There was strong continuity of both drug use and delinquency from T2 to T3 and from T3 to T4. Significant relations were found between drug use at T2 and drug use at T3 and T4, and between drug use at T2 and delinquency at T3 and T4. In females, childhood aggression was significantly correlated with drug use and delinquency at T2, T3, and T4.

Conclusions.—Adolescent drug use and delinquency should not be dismissed with a "kids will be kids" attitude, because these behaviors tend to persist into adulthood. Decreases in childhood aggression should decrease drug use by adolescents and young adults. At any stage of development, if drug use decreases, decreases in delinquent behavior can be expected.

▶ This article extends in age previous reports of the potency that early childhood aggressive behavior has as a risk factor for both later delinquency and drug use. Females and males suffer this link equally. The authors also do an excellent job of discussing the multiple possible reasons for such a strong linkage.

J.E. Schowalter, M.D.

Phenomenology of Adolescent and Adult Mania in Hospitalized Patients With Bipolar Disorder

McElroy SL, Strakowski SM, West SA, et al (Univ of Cincinnati, Ohio; Florida Hosp, Orlando)

Am J Psychiatry 154:44–49, 1997 3–47

Background.—Evidence suggests that bipolar disorder usually begins in adolescence. However, it has often been underrecognized and misdiagnosed in this age group. This may be partly because adolescent mania is phenomenologically different from adult mania. This hypothesis was tested in a cohort of adolescents hospitalized for acute mania and compared with a cohort of hospitalized acutely manic adults.

Methods and Findings.—Forty adolescents, aged 12 to 18 years, and 88 adults, aged 18 to 45 years, comprised the study population. Compared with the adult patients, the teenagers had a higher rate of mixed bipolar disorder and a significantly lower rate of psychotic features. The adolescents also had higher ratings for many depressive symptoms, including suicidality and depressed mood, and lower ratings for thought disorder and delusions. In addition, the rate of substance abuse was significantly lower in the adolescent group, and the rates of familial mood disorder and drug abuse or dependence were significantly higher.

Conclusions.—Adolescent mania appears to be phenomenologically different from mania in adults. A possible explanation for this finding is that teenagers and adults differ in familial loading for mood or substance use disorders or in developmental or maturational stage.

▶ In general, the earlier in an individual's life the onset of a severe disorder occurs, the poorer the prognosis. This prospective study shows that generalities also can sometimes hide complexities. I wonder, is the greater presence of depression in the younger patients 1 reason why a relatively large number of teenagers show their hypomanic side in response to antidepressant medications?

J.E. Schowalter, M.D.

Lithium Treatment of Conduct Disorders in Adolescents

Rifkin A, Karajgi B, Dicker R, et al (Elmhurst City Hosp, Queens, NY)

Am J Psychiatry 154:554–555, 1997 3–48

Introduction.—Conduct disorder is a common mental disorder in adolescents, and psychosocial treatments have not been effective. The only previous double-blind, controlled study of drug treatment for adolescents with conduct disorder found methylphenidate to be superior to placebo. A study of 33 adolescent inpatients with a diagnosis of conduct disorder examined the efficacy of lithium carbonate treatment.

Methods.—The study participants were 19 girls and 14 boys, with a mean age of 15.15 years. None had major physical disorders that might account for their behavior or a concomitant diagnosis of stereotyped movement disorder, pervasive developmental disorder, organic mental disorder, schizophrenia, or mood disorder. All had exhibited at least 3 episodes of overt aggression during the first week of hospitalization. After 1 week of placebo administration, patients were randomized to a lithium carbonate group or a matching placebo group for 2 weeks. The lithium dose was adjusted to maintain a blood level of 0.6 to 1.0 mmol/L. Clinical raters collected outcome data using the Overt Aggression Scale, Behavior Rating Scale, and Hamilton Rating Scale for Depression.

Results.—Twenty-six patients completed the study, 14 in the lithium group and 12 in the placebo group. The lithium and placebo groups showed no significant differences on various measures of clinical change. Of those who completed the study, 3 in the lithium group and 1 in the placebo group were considered responders—not a statistically significant difference. Lithium-treated patients had more side effects, but the side effects were few overall and did not lead to removal of these patients from the study. Lithium levels were not correlated with changes in score on the Overt Aggression Scale.

Conclusion.—Both lithium and placebo were ineffective in the treatment of conduct disorder in adolescents. Longer duration of treatment might prove more beneficial.

► As American society has become more violent, and violence has become accepted as a public health issue, pressure to use medicine to control violence and delinquent behaviors has risen. Unfortunately, no medication is approved by the Food and Drug Administration for delinquency or violence. As a clinical supervisor and consultant, I am worried by how often medication is used for socially unwanted behaviors. The success rate is not high.

J.E. Schowalter, M.D.

Alcohol Availability and Motor Vehicle Fatalities

Kelleher KJ, Pope SK, Kirby RS, et al (Univ of Pittsburgh, Pa; Univ of Arkansas, Little Rock)

J Adolesc Health 19:325–330, 1996 3–49

Background.—Young men comprise the population with the highest rates of drinking and problem drinking. In addition, a disproportionate number of males die in motor vehicle accidents related to drinking. The association between alcohol availability and motor vehicle fatalities among 15- to 24-year-old males was investigated.

Methods.—Data were obtained from 75 counties on alcohol availability (whether the county was wet or dry and the number of licensed on-site and off-site alcohol outlets) and on motor vehicle fatality rates among males during a 6-year period. Other variables were controlled for in computing the correlation.

Findings.—County-level motor vehicle fatality rates were unassociated with any of the alcohol availability measures examined. However, rural residence was found to be correlated with a much greater fatality rate.

Conclusion.—Ecologic models incorporating a wide range of variables explain little of the variance in motor vehicle fatality rates among young men. Thus, further legal or regulatory restrictions on alcohol outlet licensing may not have an effect on fatalities. The greater fatality rates among rural residents could not be explained by alcohol outlets.

▶ This study was included because of somewhat contrarian-seeming findings by a well-respected researcher. Everyone knows that alcohol plus young male drivers equals an enhanced chance for disability and death. High speeds make for even more mayhem. Counties seem to me to be too small to allow much differentiation. In the 1980s, when some states had an 18-year-old drinking age whereas others used age 21, teenage driving death rates were not always lower in the latter. One reason for this was that 18- to 20-year-olds drove to the next door age-18 state to buy. They then drank and drove back home. They often had to drive even faster than usual to cover the relatively greater distance to home and still make their parents' curfew. CRASH!

J.E. Schowalter, M.D.

Project Northland: Outcomes of a Communitywide Alcohol Use Prevention Program During Early Adolescence

Perry CL, Williams CL, Veblen-Mortenson S, et al (Univ of Minnesota, Minneapolis; Ctr for Health Studies, Seattle)

Am J Public Health 86:956–965, 1996 3–50

Introduction.—Alcohol use is widespread among adolescents and plays a major role in motor vehicle fatalities in this age group. Strategies to prevent alcohol use in early adolescence often use individual behavior change (demand) and environmental change (supply). A program conducted in Minnesota specifically targeted young adolescents with multilevel interventions. Results after 3 years of implementation were reported.

Methods.—Project Northland involved 24 school districts and adjacent communities in northeastern Minnesota. Residents of the area, which includes 7 American Indian reservations, are primarily of European ethnic backgrounds. The study cohort was the group of 2,351 students who were sixth graders in fall 1991. Intervention programs were implemented from 1991 to 1994 and included parent involvement/education, behavioral curricula, peer participation, and community task force activities. In each

TABLE 1.—Alcohol and Other Drug Use, Peer Influence, Self-Efficacy, and Access to Alcohol Scales: Comparison of Class of 1,998 Students in the Intervention and Reference School Districts

	All Students		Baseline Nonusers		Baseline Users	
	Intervention	Reference	Intervention	Reference	Intervention	Reference
	Tendency to use alcohol scale score,[a] mean (95% CI)					
Fall 1991	11.5 (11.0, 12.0)	11.0 (10.5, 11.5)	9.4 (9.2, 9.5)	9.5 (9.3, 9.7)	14.5 (13.8, 15.2)	13.6 (12.9, 14.4)
Spring 1992	11.7 (11.2, 12.2)	11.6 (11.1, 12.1)	10.1 (9.6, 10.6)	10.2 (9.7, 10.7)	14.3 (13.5, 15.1)	14.1 (13.2, 14.9)
Spring 1993	14.5 (13.3, 15.7)	14.9 (13.7, 16.1)	12.2 (11.2, 13.2)	13.2 (12.2, 14.2)	18.3 (16.3, 20.3)	17.8 (15.8, 19.8)
Spring 1994	16.0 (15.1, 16.8)*	17.5 (16.7, 18.5)	13.8 (13.1, 14.4)**	15.3 (14.6, 15.9)	19.7 (18.0, 21.6)	21.1 (19.3, 22.9)
	Past month alcohol use,[b] % (95% CI)					
Fall 1991	6.9 (5.0, 8.8)*	3.9 (2.0, 5.9)	0 ...	0 ...	16.6 (12.7, 20.5)*	10.6 (6.4, 14.9)
Spring 1992	7.6 (4.9, 10.4)	6.3 (3.5, 9.0)	2.4 (1.0, 3.7)	3.1 (1.7, 4.4)	15.6 (10.1, 21.1)	11.6 (5.9, 17.3)
Spring 1993	14.9 (10.3, 19.4)	17.5 (13.0, 22.0)	8.3 (5.1, 11.9)	11.8 (8.7, 15.3)	25.5 (17.1, 33.5)	27.9 (19.5, 36.4)
Spring 1994	23.6 (20.1, 27.1)*	29.2 (25.6, 32.8)	15.3 (11.7, 18.9)*	21.2 (17.7, 24.8)	36.9 (29.5, 44.2)	43.1 (35.2, 51.0)
	Past week alcohol use,[b] % (95% CI)					
Fall 1991	3.8 (2.6, 5.0)*	2.0 (1.0, 3.2)	0 ...	0 ...	9.1 (6.3, 11.9)	5.3 (2.2, 8.4)
Spring 1992	3.4 (1.4, 5.5)	3.4 (1.4, 5.4)	1.0 (0, 2.2)	1.5 (0.4, 2.7)	7.1 (2.6, 11.7)	6.7 (2.1, 11.4)
Spring 1993	7.4 (4.0, 10.8)	8.4 (5.1, 11.8)	5.0 (2.5, 8.1)	6.1 (3.6, 9.0)	11.1 (5.4, 16.7)	13.2 (7.2, 19.0)
Spring 1994	10.5 (8.0, 13.0)*	14.8 (12.2, 17.4)	5.3 (3.0, 7.6)**	9.8 (7.5, 12.1)	18.4 (12.4, 24.5)	23.6 (17.0, 30.1)
	Cigarette use,[c] % (95% CI)					
Fall 1991	6.9 (4.9, 8.9)*	4.7 (2.6, 6.7)	1.5 (0.6, 2.3)	0.9 (0, 1.7)	13.8 (8.9, 18.6)	11.5 (6.4, 16.6)
Spring 1992	8.4 (6.1, 10.6)	8.8 (6.5, 11.0)	3.1 (1.5, 4.7)	2.8 (1.2, 4.4)	15.9 (12.0, 19.8)	18.5 (14.3, 22.7)
Spring 1993	17.8 (13.5, 22.1)	19.4 (15.2, 23.7)	9.8 (5.7, 13.8)	14.3 (10.3, 18.2)	29.8 (23.4, 36.1)	29.4 (22.7, 36.1)
Spring 1994	24.8 (20.2, 29.5)	30.7 (26.0, 35.4)	15.5 (10.3, 20.7)*	24.6 (19.6, 29.7)	39.1 (32.8, 45.4)	42.7 (35.7, 49.6)
	Smokeless tobacco use,[c] % (95% CI)					
Fall 1991	1.5 (0.4, 2.5)	1.5 (0.5, 2.6)	0 ...	0 ...	3.1 (0.8, 5.3)	4.0 (1.6, 6.4)
Spring 1992	3.2 (22, 4.3)	3.4 (2.3, 4.5)	1.2 (0, 2.4)	1.3 (0, 2.5)	6.6 (4.5, 8.7)	6.8 (4.4, 9.2)
Spring 1993	7.8 (4.7, 11.0)	9.4 (6.2, 12.5)	4.0 (1.7, 6.4)	6.8 (4.5, 9.1)	14.1 (8.3, 19.9)	14.2 (8.2, 20.3)
Spring 1994	13.5 (10.2, 16.8)	16.3 (13.0, 19.7)	7.4 (3.7, 11.1)	12.3 (8.7, 16.0)	23.4 (18.9, 27.8)	23.8 (18.7, 28.9)
	Marijuana use,[d] % (95% CI)					
Fall 1991	0.7 (0, 1.3)	0.4 (0, 1.0)	0 ...	0 ...	1.7 (0, 3.4)	5.8 (0, 2.3)
Spring 1992	0.6 (0, 1.2)	1.2 (0, 1.8)	0 ...	0 ...	1.1 (0, 2.4)	2.2 (0.1, 3.6)
Spring 1993	3.5 (0.9, 6.1)	3.2 (0.6, 5.8)	1.7 (0.4, 3.1)	2.6 (1.3, 3.9)	4.4 (1.2, 7.7)	5.12 (1.7, 8.6)
Spring 1994	7.4 (4.4, 10.4)	8.6 (5.5, 11.6)	3.1 (1.3, 4.9)*	6.2 (4.4, 8.0)	14.3 (8.1, 20.5)	13.2 (6.6, 19.8)

			Peer influence scale score,[c] mean (95% CI)			
Fall 1991	19.4 (18.8, 20.1)	18.6 (18.0, 19.3)	18.2 (17.7, 18.7)	17.7 (17.2, 18.2)	21.0 (20.0, 22.0)	20.2 (19.2, 21.3)
Spring 1992	19.0 (18.5, 19.5)	19.1 (18.6, 19.6)	18.1 (17.6, 18.5)	18.0 (17.6, 18.5)	20.5 (20.0, 21.0)	20.6 (20.1, 21.2)
Spring 1993	21.9 (20.4, 23.4)	23.0 (21.5, 24.5)	20.5 (19.3, 21.8)	21.8 (20.6, 23.1)	23.9 (22.0, 25.9)	24.9 (23.0, 26.9)
Spring 1994	24.6 (23.3, 26.0)*	27.0 (25.7, 28.4)	22.8 (21.5, 24.1)*	25.4 (24.1, 26.7)	27.7 (25.83, 29.6)	29.9 (27.9, 31.8)
			Self-efficacy scale score,[f] mean (95% CI)			
Fall 1991	21.9 (21.5, 22.2)	22.0 (21.6, 22.4)	22.9 (22.4, 23.3)	22.8 (22.4, 23.2)	20.6 (20.1, 21.1)	20.5 (20.0, 21.1)
Spring 1992	21.9 (21.6, 22.3)	21.8 (21.4, 22.1)	22.9 (22.6, 23.1)	22.5 (22.2, 22.8)	20.4 (19.8, 21.1)	20.5 (19.8, 21.2)
Spring 1993	20.4 (19.4, 21.4)	20.4 (19.4, 21.4)	21.5 (20.7, 22.3)	21.2 (20.4, 22.0)	19.0 (17.7, 20.2)	19.0 (17.8, 20.3)
Spring 1994	20.2 (19.7, 20.8)	19.6 (19.0, 20.2)	21.6 (21.1, 22.0)*	20.4 (20.0, 20.9)	18.2 (17.2, 19.1)	18.4 (17.3, 19.4)
			Perceived access scale score,[g] mean (95% CI)			
Fall 1991	14.7 (14.2, 15.2)	14.7 (14.2, 15.2)	14.0 (13.4, 14.6)	14.3 (13.7, 14.9)	15.8 (15.4, 16.2)	15.6 (15.1, 16.1)
Spring 1992	15.3 (14.7, 15.9)	15.1 (14.5, 15.7)	14.5 (13.8, 15.2)	14.6 (13.9, 15.3)	16.5 (16.1, 17.0)	16.1 (15.6, 16.6)
Spring 1993	17.7 (17.0, 18.5)	18.1 (17.3, 18.8)	17.1 (16.3, 18.0)	17.7 (16.9, 18.5)	18.6 (17.8, 19.4)	18.7 (17.9, 19.5)
Spring 1994	19.2 (18.6, 19.9)	19.7 (19.1, 20.4)	18.8 (17.9, 19.7)	19.4 (18.5, 20.2)	20.0 (19.6, 20.5)	20.4 (19.9, 20.9)

Note: Values were adjusted for race and baseline measures. All-student sample sizes for all analyses were as follows: fall 1991, n = 2,351; spring 1992, n = 2,191; spring 1993, n = 2,060; spring 1994, n = 1,901. Baseline nonusers sample sizes were as follows: fall 1991, n = 1,443; spring 1992, n = 1,353; spring 1993, n = 1,273; spring 1994, n = 1,176. Finally, baseline user sample sizes were as follows: fall 1991, n = 881; spring 1992, n = 816; spring 1993, n = 766; spring 1994, n = 712.

Abbreviation: CI, confidence interval.

[a]The score range was 8 (no tendency to use alcohol) to 48 (high levels of use and intentions).

[b]At least 1 occasion.

[c]More than 1 or 2 occasions (occasionally or regularly).

[d]At least 1 occasion in the past year.

[e]The score range was 15 (no influence) to 71 (high peer influence).

[f]The score range was 5 (not being able to refuse alcohol) to 25 (being able to refuse).

[g]The score range was 6 (very difficult to obtain alcohol) to 30 (easy to obtain).

*$P < 0.05$ (differences between conditions based on F statistic).

**$P < 0.01$ (differences between conditions based on F statistic).

(Courtesy of Perry CL, Williams CL, Veblen-Mortenson S, et al: Project Northland: Outcomes of a communitywide alcohol use prevention program during early adolescence. *Am J Public Health* 86:956–965, 1996. Copyright American Public Health Association.)

year of the program, specific curricula were designed to provide students with skills to affect their social environment. Collaboration was sought with existing community organizations to create as many linkages as possible with local groups directly influencing underage drinking. The students were surveyed at baseline and at 3 follow-up periods to measure use of alcohol, tobacco, and other drugs and to evaluate their social environment, communication with parents, and perceptions about alcohol use and availability.

Results.—Four of the smaller school districts were combined with larger districts. Ten of the 20 combined districts were randomly assigned to the intervention condition and 10 to a reference condition. Most of the students in the reference districts had taken part in Project DARE. Project Northland achieved widespread participation in the after-class and community activities. By the end of eighth grade, students in the intervention program reported less onset and prevalence of alcohol use than those in the reference districts (Table 1). The percentage of cigarette users was 19% lower in the intervention group, and among baseline nonusers the percentages of students reporting cigarette use and marijuana use was significantly lower than that of the reference group. Project Northland was also successful in reducing peer norms and peer influence to use, introducing skills to resist peer influence, and increasing parent-child communication about the consequences of drinking.

Conclusion.—Project Northland, with its home-team approach and peer-led social influences curricula, delayed alcohol use onset and prevented alcohol use among sixth- through eighth-grade students living in an area of Minnesota that rated at the top of the state in terms of alcohol-related problems.

► Project Northland is to my knowledge the most impressive of many previous approaches to alcohol prevention. The key is the engagement of the community. Without that there can be no program, and probably little chance for satisfying success. What is needed now is for replication studies from other supportive communities. If I were in the gateway drug prevention seat, this replication would be at the top of my *to-do* list.

J.E. Schowalter, M.D.

4 Psychotherapy

Introduction

It is hard to believe that another year has gone by, but the appearance of this volume in print is concrete testimony to that fact. While the economic environment in support of psychotherapy has not really improved, the body of literature supporting a variety of psychotherapies as important and effective clinical modalities continues to expand. This year's selections span a wide variety of areas of investigation into psychotherapy. I am pleased to see that more individuals are beginning to study psychodynamic psychotherapy in a formal way. I have no doubt that this will allow dynamic therapies to regain some of the luster lost in the multitude of formal clinical studies of cognitive behavioral approaches. There are also a number of interesting papers this year about group and family therapy. It is unfortunate that our present educational and economic climate de-emphasizes both of these important modalities. There is no doubt that psychiatric residency programs underemphasize group and family approaches in comparison to individual interventions. This seems paradoxical since group and family interventions might be quite efficient approaches. The integration of psychopharmacologic and psychotherapeutic approaches remains one of the important frontiers of psychiatric research in clinical practice. Not much crossed my desk in this area this year, but I thought several papers were worth including to highlight this area for future work.

With all of the focus on cost effectiveness, the importance of treating individuals with serious long-term disorders has not been in the forefront. The group of articles that discusses both personality disorders and psychoses is important to reinforce the essential role of psychotherapeutic interventions in both of these groups of patients. It's too bad that the managed care companies are too focused on their profit margins to give much attention to these issues. As I have said in previous volumes, the role of psychotherapies in patients with medical illness is just being explored. I expect that we will see a continued elucidation of the value of psychotherapy in this patient population.

As has been my practice, I have also included a number of articles that focus on educational and research issues. I include these not only for the benefit of educators or researchers who read this volume but to illustrate for clinicians the exciting opportunities for further research and training in psychotherapy. I hope that you are stimulated to read some of the articles abstracted here. I have no doubt that you would find these very enjoyable reading and that your skills as a therapist, educator, or researcher would be enhanced.

Allan Tasman, M.D.

Psychodynamic and Interpersonal Psychotherapy

Which Depressed Patients Will Respond to Interpersonal Psychotherapy? The Role of Abnormal EEG Sleep Profiles

Thase ME, Buysse DJ, Frank E, et al (Univ of Pittsburgh, Pa)

Am J Psychiatry 154:502–509, 1997 4–1

Purpose.—Although it has long been suggested that patients with mild depression can be treated with psychotherapy, there has been very little clinical research data to support this impression. Previous studies have suggested that a reduced rapid eye movement (REM) sleep latency in the electroencephalographic (EEG) sleep profile in a depressed patient—along with other more state-dependent factors—may indicate the need for pharmacotherapy rather than psychotherapy alone. The possible link between EEG sleep profile and response to interpersonal psychotherapy in patients with recurrent major depressive disorder was analyzed.

Methods.—The study included 91 outpatients with a diagnosis of recurrent major depressive disorder, unipolar or bipolar II. All diagnoses were made by the Research Diagnostic Criteria, based on an interview with the Schedule for Affective Disorders and Schizophrenia. Data on EEG sleep variables monitored over 2 nights—sleep efficiency, REM latency, and REM density—were used to classify 50 patients as having a normal sleep profile and 41 as having abnormal sleep profiles. These 2 groups were compared by chi-square tests and life table and random effects model analyses for their responses to short-term interpersonal psychotherapy. Responses to pharmacotherapy for patients who did not respond to psychotherapy were analyzed as well.

Results.—Clinical outcomes were worse in patients with abnormal sleep profiles. There were significant differences between groups in terms of symptom ratings, attrition rates, and remission rates. The remission rate in response to psychotherapy was 58% in patients with normal sleep profiles, compared to 37% in those with abnormal sleep profiles. Of patients who did not respond to interpersonal psychotherapy, 75% had remissions in response to pharmacotherapy.

Conclusions.—Among patients with recurrent major depressive disorder, those with an abnormal EEG sleep profile appear less likely to respond to interpersonal psychotherapy than those with a normal sleep profile. The relationship between sleep profile and treatment response may reflect a neurobiological "boundary" that limits the effectiveness of psychotherapy in depression. It may be possible to clarify this boundary through concomitant studies of hypothalamic-pituitary-adrenocortical axis activity.

► This study is a follow-up and replication of a previous study done by the same investigators. Once again they have found evidence that an abnormal biological finding has predictive significance regarding response to interpersonal psychotherapy. Further, those patients with the EEG abnormality who did not respond to therapy had a very good response to pharmacotherapy when it was tried subsequently. We continue to need more studies like this that will help us further define predictive variables. This would allow more rational prescription of psychotherapy or pharmacotherapy, not just in depression but in a wide variety of disorders.

A. Tasman, M.D.

Does Brief Dynamic Psychotherapy Reduce the Relapse Rate of Panic Disorder?

Wiborg IM, Dahl AA (Univ of Oslo, Norway)

Arch Gen Psychiatry 53:689–694, 1996 4–2

Background.—Drug treatments—antidepressants and certain benzodiazepines—are effective therapy for patients with panic disorder (PD), with and without agoraphobia. However, many patients will have a full or partial relapse after the end of drug therapy. There have been few studies of the efficacy of combined drug and psychotherapy approaches for PD. Whether the addition of brief dynamic psychotherapy could reduce the relapse rate of PD after the end of drug treatment was investigated.

Methods.—The randomized trial included 40 patients with PD, as defined by the DSM-III-R. All received 9 months of treatment with clomipramine—alone or with 15 weekly sessions of brief dynamic psychotherapy. The psychotherapy focused on the psychosocial vulnerability of patients with PD, with the goal of helping them to achieve more adaptive patterns in their interpersonal relationships. Assessments of anxiety and depression were performed at baseline and follow-up. The patients were interviewed in blinded fashion at 6, 12, and 18 months after the start of treatment.

Results.—Within 6 months, all patients in both groups were free of panic attacks. At the 18-month follow-up, the relapse rate was 75% in the patients receiving clomipramine only vs. 20% in those receiving clomipramine plus psychotherapy. At 9 months, there was evidence of reduced anxiety in the clomipramine plus psychotherapy group.

Conclusions.—Adding brief dynamic psychotherapy to clomipramine treatment appears to reduce the rate of relapse after drug treatment. The psychotherapy intervention used in this study may work by reducing the psychosocial vulnerability associated with PD. Psychotherapy appears to improve many different outcome measures, including not only panic attacks but also anticipatory anxiety, avoidance behavior, and disability.

► Once again, we have a study indicating that there may a synergistic effect when both medication and psychotherapy are prescribed at the same time.

This is one of the few studies of this nature to use brief dynamic psychotherapy rather than cognitive behavioral therapy. Although the mechanism of action of the reduced relapse rate is not known, this issue certainly warrants further study. Another interesting aspect of this issue is whether treatment provided by 1 individual has a different effectiveness rate than when the therapy is split between 2 individuals.

A. Tasman, M.D.

Varieties of Transference Patterns in Psychotherapy

Connolly MB, Crits-Christoph P, Demorest A, et al (Univ of Pennsylvania, Philadelphia; Amherst College, Mass)

J Consult Clin Psychol 64:1213–1221, 1996 4–3

Introduction.—The concept of transference is key to current theories of clinical psychotherapy. However, there has been little research into the nature of the construct of transference. The quantitative assessment of interpersonal themes method was used to examine the nature of transference of interpersonal patterns in patients' psychotherapy narratives.

Methods.—The analysis included patients participating in a study of psychotherapy for opiate addiction. It examined the association between interpersonal patterns with significant others in a patient's life and the pattern with the therapist early in the course of treatment. By cluster analysis, similar relationships were categorized for 35 patients.

Results.—The data suggest that most patients had a main pattern that was more pervasive than other patterns. However, it was not always the pattern that was most apparent in the relationship with the therapist. When the patients narrated an episode about the therapist early in treatment, transference of interpersonal patterns to the therapist was a fairly common finding. In this group, the main and single-object cluster profiles were significantly correlated with the therapist profiles. About 60% of narratives about the therapist early in treatment described a pattern in the patient-therapist relationship that was similar to a theme evident in narratives about at least 1 other person. The transferred pattern was sometimes a less pervasive one, or sometimes one that was apparent in just 1 other relationship. Furthermore, for 40% of patients, there was no evidence of transference to the therapist at an early stage of the relationship. The number of interpersonal patterns and the objects of the most pervasive patterns were not significantly different for patients receiving cognitive therapy vs. dynamically oriented therapy.

Conclusions.—The repetitive interpersonal patterns patients display with other people in their lives are often expressed in their relationship with a psychotherapist, the results suggest. The findings do not describe the full complexity implicit in theories of transference. Patients participating in different kinds of therapy tell narratives about their relationships with others that include patterns; these similarities are not simply encouraged by dynamically oriented therapy.

► The understanding in use of the transference and psychodynamic psychotherapy has been a matter of significant debate for decades. Some have argued that transference is an artifact of the artificiality of the patient-therapist relationship within a very constrained and artificial situation. This study reveals that patients do tend to exhibit a characteristic set of interpersonal relationship patterns of response in their lives and that there may be a typical interpersonal pattern within the therapeutic relationship that may be related to other relationships in the patient's life. This study provides a response to critics of dynamic psychotherapy's reliance on an understanding of the transference, in that it demonstrated that, even in cognitive therapy, patients tend to exhibit a characteristic interpersonal pattern that has similarities to those which exist outside the therapy. These findings, although preliminary, lend support to use of the transference as a means for gaining greater understanding of a patient's interpersonal relationship styles.

A. Tasman, M.D.

Techniques to Accelerate Dynamic Psychotherapy

Fosha D, Slowiaczek ML (New York Univ)

Am J Psychother 51:229–251, 1997 4–4

Background.—Approaches to short-term dynamic psychotherapy seek to accelerate personality change through focus on emotional experiences during sessions, high level of therapist involvement, patient collaboration, and attention to time limits. Recent approaches have examined the experience of deep affect as a route to therapeutic change. Accelerated experiential/dynamic psychotherapy (AEDP) emphasizes affective rather than defended relating in the patient-therapist relationship, as well as affect-focused strategies that counteract the patients' defenses. This affect-centered model of relational dynamics was presented, along with specific techniques for therapeutic action.

Conceptual Framework.—The developmental theory behind AEDP places affect in the context of an emotional relationship. Accelerated experiential/dynamic psychotherapy tries to support creative rather than defensive motivational tendencies. The therapist tries to minimize iatrogenic contributions to the defensive repetition of stereotypic patient response through support, affirmation, and emotional engagement. A goals of AEDP is to help the patient experience emotions that were previously unbearable, including core affects, self-experiences, and relational experiences; emotional pain; healing-associated affects; and positive breakthrough feelings. These expressive experiences must be differentiated from communications related to defensiveness or avoidance. The therapist must be able to quickly distinguish between defensiveness or relational repetition and genuine emotions or attempts at genuine relating.

Therapeutic Techniques.—The techniques of AEDP can be grouped into relational, restructuring, and experiential/affective interventions. Relational interventions try to activate the patient's potential for open relating in the relative safety of therapy. These interventions foster and focus on the relationship between the patient and therapist. The therapist affirms that any feelings that come up in the interaction can and should be discussed openly. The therapist systematically expresses empathy and support and uses affective self-disclosure to create an environment of openness and intimacy. Work with patients is collaborative, encouraging patients to understand the depths of their resources.

The restructuring interventions help the therapist rapidly process the clinical interactions and encourage the patients to recognize their patterns of experiential and relational responses. This is the most cognitive category of interventions, and includes monitoring fluctuations in openness vs. defensiveness and in positive vs. negative emotional experiences; working with defensive responses; working with anxiety, shame, and guilt responses; working with relational patterns; and linking dynamic patterns with interpersonal environments. The third group is experiential/affective interventions, which can be used to bypass defenses and prime affective experiences, or, once affect has been elicited, to deepen affect and work through the accompanying psychodynamic factors. These interventions include facilitating genuine affective experience; naming and acknowledging affective experience; striving for specificity and detail; examining physical sensations associated with emotional reactions; using portrayal to explore the dynamic/experiential correlates of imagined interactions; and facilitating the mourning process. These techniques were described in detail, including illustrative clinical vignettes.

Discussion.—These AEDP interventions can deepen the patient's affective experience in the emotionally close patient/therapist relationship. Used effectively, they enhance the patient/therapist bond, increase the patient's self-esteem, reduce defensiveness and anxiety, and promote emotional healing. The AEDP techniques promote adaptive over defensive reactions, encourage emotional engagement rather than neutrality and abstinence, and emphasize health and change over pathology and stasis.

► These authors are pursuing an issue that has been raised since the days of Sigmund Freud, that is, can psychotherapy be shortened without diminishing its effectiveness? These investigators focused on methods for intensifying affect and found that this enhances the therapeutic relationship and therapeutic change. This approach clearly needs more study. It is worth cautioning that any approach that intensifies affect through techniques and manipulations can be easily misused by an inexperienced therapist.

A. Tasman, M.D.

Cognitive and Behavioral Psychotherapy

Cognitive Therapy With Inpatients

Stuart S, Wright JH, Thase ME, et al (Univ of Iowa, Iowa City; Univ of Louisville, Ky; Western Psychiatric Inst & Clinic, Pittsburgh, Pa)
Gen Hosp Psychiatry 19:42–50, 1997 4–5

Introduction.—Even with the current emphasis on cost control, many psychiatric inpatient units continue to rely heavily on psychotherapy, particularly in the treatment of depression. Patients routinely participate in group and individual psychotherapy, which are intended not only to be primary therapy but also to increase compliance with drug therapy. Several units started using cognitive therapy (CT) principles as the organizing theories for their therapy programs. There is evidence that CT improves continuity of care after hospital discharge. The principles and types of inpatient CT were reviewed.

Inpatient Cognitive Therapy.—Treatment settings use a wide range of CT models, including primary therapist, staff, "add-on," comprehensive, and flexible models. Modifications of CT for inpatient use include increased frequency of patient contact, greater structure, more intensive use of psychoeducational tools, early behavioral emphasis, and chances to learn CT skills while in the "therapeutic milieu." Although some inpatient programs are based on individual CT, most apply cognitively oriented group therapy, family therapy, and adjunctive approaches such as occupational and recreational therapy. Few research data are available so far; however, the results suggest that CT can have an additive effect when used with drug therapy for some patients with depression. Other studies suggest that CT alone—even without biological therapies—can be an effective treatment for severe depression. However, there is still a need for randomized, controlled trials of fully implemented inpatient CT programs.

Discussion.—The use of CT for depression in inpatients has been attracting interest. More experience with this approach should stimulate further research into the benefits and cost-effectiveness of inpatient psychotherapy. It should also spur development of specific forms of psychotherapy for the many disorders that require inpatient treatment.

▶ As hospital lengths of stay have decreased, less and less attention has been paid to the therapeutic milieu on an inpatient unit. This is in part because of the diminished emphasis on a psychodynamic way of understanding milieu processes, which required a certain amount of stability and length of time to develop. These authors describe an innovative approach to structuring a program around CT parameters and suggest that this may be a helpful approach, especially in an environment in which lengths of stay are fairly brief.

A. Tasman, M.D.

Cognitive Behavior Therapy for Chronic Fatigue Syndrome: A Randomized Controlled Trial

Deale A, Chalder T, Marks I, et al (King's College Hosp and Inst of Psychiatry, London)

Am J Psychiatry 154:408–414, 1997 4–6

Objective.—There is still no established cause or treatment for chronic fatigue syndrome. Cognitive behavioral therapy has been used for patients with chronic fatigue syndrome, but there have been few randomized, controlled trials of this approach. Cognitive behavior therapy was compared with relaxation for patients with chronic fatigue syndrome.

Methods.—The randomized trial included 60 patients with chronic fatigue syndrome, diagnosed according to British and American case definitions. The patients were randomly assigned to undergo 13 sessions of either cognitive behavior therapy or relaxation during a 4- to 6-month period. The cognitive behavior therapy was aimed at a graded approach to increasing activity, along with cognitive restructuring. Before, during, and after treatment, the patients were assessed on measures of functional impairment, fatigue, mood, and global improvement.

Results.—Seven patients discontinued treatment. Of those who completed therapy, the cognitive behavior therapy group showed greater improvements in functional impairment and fatigue. At last follow-up, a substantial improvement in physical functioning was achieved in 70% of patients who completed cognitive behavior therapy, compared with 19% of those who completed relaxation therapy.

Conclusions.—For patients with chronic fatigue syndrome, cognitive behavior therapy is more effective than a control relaxation intervention. The benefits of cognitive behavior therapy are sustained over follow-up. Given the variability of chronic fatigue syndrome, a flexible range of behavioral and cognitive techniques individualized to the patient is probably the most effective approach to therapy.

▶ During the last few years, there have been reports on the utility of cognitive behavioral therapy in a variety of syndromes in which there is both an emotional and physical impairment. This study of the benefits of cognitive behavioral therapy in patients with chronic fatigue syndrome showed that it was very useful in this difficult-to-treat group. More important, the improvements were sustained for at least 6 months after the cessation of treatment. Whether the cognitive behavioral therapy specifically treated the depression that many patients with chronic fatigue syndrome are reported to have is unclear, but this approach certainly warrants further clinical use.

A. Tasman, M.D.

A Prospective Test of Criteria for Response, Remission, Relapse, Recovery, and Recurrence in Depressed Patients Treated With Cognitive Behavior Therapy

Riso LP, Thase ME, Howland RH, et al (Univ of Pittsburgh, Pa; Univ of Oregon, Eugene)

J Affect Disord 43:131–142, 1997 4–7

Purpose.—One study (*Arch Gen Psychiatry* 48:1053–1059, 1991.) suggested that the literature is inconsistent in its descriptions of the course and outcomes of depression. Many common definitions that describe the outcomes of depressive disorders are used inconsistently and are largely untested. Having a standardized, validated set of outcome definitions would aid research into the naturalistic course and treatment of depressive disorders. The validity was tested of 5 key definitions of outcome in major depressive disorder: response, remission, recovery, relapse, and recurrence.

Methods.—Definitions for each of the 5 outcome terms were put into operation, based largely on the Hamilton Rating Scale for Depression. They were then validated for their ability to predict the response to acute treatment and during a 3-year follow-up period. The validation sample was a group of patients with nonbipolar major depressive disorder treated by cognitive behavior therapy.

Results.—Moderate to excellent validity was demonstrated for all definitions studied, including all 7 definitions of treatment response. The study was successful in empirically differentiating between terms that are often confused in the literature: response vs. remission and relapse vs. recurrence.

Conclusions.—The outcome definitions studied predict later function and can generally be distinguished from one another. There is evidence that validity could be improved further with continued refinement of the outcome definitions.

► This study of depressed patients treated with cognitive behavior therapy attempted to develop a standardized and valid set of definitions of response, remission, relapse, recovery, and recurrence for use in further psychotherapy research. The authors found good support for their approach, which is worthy of further investigation and would facilitate psychotherapy research.

A. Tasman, M.D.

Body Dysmorphic Disorder: A Preliminary Evaluation of Treatment and Maintenance Using Exposure With Response Prevention

McKay D, Todaro J, Neziroglu F, et al (Fordham Univ, New York)

Behav Res Ther 35:67–70, 1997 4–8

Background.—Recent studies defined body dysmorphic disorder (BDD) as a chronic, debilitating psychiatric disorder with etiologic and symptomatic similarities to obsessive-compulsive disorder. Exposure with response prevention may be effective in alleviating the symptoms of BDD. The results of treatment and maintenance with exposure with response prevention in patients with BDD were reported.

Methods.—Ten patients with BDD, diagnosed according to the *Diagnostic and Statistical Manual of Mental Disorders,* ed 3, revised, were studied. Each took part in a standard behavior therapy protocol with exposure in vivo or in imagery, and with response prevention. During treatment, the patients were evaluated weekly for symptom severity, depression, anxiety, and avoidance. After treatment, the patients were randomly assigned to receive a 6-month maintenance program or not. The same assessments were performed biweekly and at 6 months' follow-up.

Results.—Exposure with response prevention was associated with significant improvement in measures of avoidance, BDD symptoms, depression, and anxiety. All patients were free of symptoms at 6 months' follow-up. Those assigned to the maintenance program had continued improvement, whereas those in the control group had increased anxiety and depression.

Conclusions.—Exposure with response prevention appears to be an effective treatment for BDD. Continued improvement can be achieved with maintenance therapy. Future studies should compare the effectiveness of exposure with response prevention with that of cognitive therapy.

► Body dysmorphic disorder is another psychiatric disorder that has not been particularly amenable to traditional psychodynamic treatment approaches. This small study showed that patients had some improved symptomatology when treated with behavioral techniques of exposure with response prevention. This appears to be a promising approach for this troublesome disorder, and the results of this study certainly indicate that further investigation is warranted.

A. Tasman, M.D.

Group and Family Psychotherapy

The Effect of Managed Mental Health Care on Group Psychotherapy: Treatment, Training, and Therapist-Morale Issues

Spitz HI (Columbia Univ, New York)

Int J Group Psychother 47:23–30, 1997 4–9

Background.—Managed care is having a major impact on the practice of group psychotherapy, posing a threat to the basic relationship between the group member and therapist. The threats to group therapy in 3 major areas posed by managed care are discussed: group treatment, therapist training, and therapist morale.

Impact on Group Treatment.—Four aspects of managed care threaten the relationship between group therapist and patient, and possibly even the formation of a therapeutic alliance. These are the therapist's fiduciary obligation to group members, the patient's role in health care decision making, access to adequate treatment, and quality of care. These may impact such issues as patient selection and confidentiality. Under managed care, patients with more severe illness may simply be prescribed psychotropic medications and assigned to social support groups, with no option for more ambitious therapy. Managed care decision makers do not appreciate the role of group therapy for patients with personality disorders or "maintenance group psychotherapy" for severely impaired psychiatric patients. Group therapists must take it upon themselves to educate managed care organizations as to the constructive uses of group therapy for various groups of patients. Clinicians and managers can find common ground in their desire to provide high-quality care in a cost-efficient, nonprejudicial, and pragmatic way. The National Registry of Certified Group Psychotherapists can help managed care organizations to identify therapists who are qualified to provide group services.

Educational Implications.—Group therapists may need additional skills to maximize the benefits of group therapy in the managed care setting. In the managed care era, psychiatric residents will likely train in a number of new venues, outside the traditional inpatient hospital and outpatient clinic or agency settings. Managed care heightens the need to define the essential information and skills needed to practice as a group therapist, and will lead to increased awareness of the theory and technique of short-term group psychotherapy. The public will also need information on the help group therapy can provide for their problems.

Impact on Therapist Morale.—Managed care can have a negative influence on the attitudes of psychotherapists, threatening their identities as care giver, collaborator, and guide to group members. As therapists are more burdened with work and lose their sense of autonomy, there is an increased risk of burnout. Group leaders must be aware of these reactions and ensure that they are not imparted to the group. Under the most optimistic scenario, group therapists will become more eclectic, incorporating new research findings into a more current treatment model. They are in a position to use their knowledge of individual and group dynamics as the basis for timely group interventions, only part of which will employ classic psychoanalytic techniques. Putting psychoanalytic principles into active clinical form should prove to be a stimulating, rather than inhibiting, experience.

Discussion.—The new emphasis on managed care promises to change the practice of group therapy in many different ways. The author urges therapists to meet the challenges posed by managed care. With time and new developments, managed care will stimulate the flexibility that group therapists have always been adept at providing.

► I have always been surprised that managed care, which purports to hold efficiency of effort in high esteem, has underutilized group psychotherapy. This is not really surprising to me, because conducting good brief group psychotherapy requires a very well-trained therapist. I know of no managed care companies that provide additional psychotherapy training to their employees beyond that which the employee brought with them to the company. Dr. Spitz makes an important argument that group therapy is a useful modality and should be given more attention, especially in an environment in which short-term treatment is highly valued.

A. Tasman, M.D.

Interpretive Psychotherapy in the Inpatient Community Meeting on a Short-Term Unit

Winer JA, Klamen DL (Univ of Ill, Chicago)

Psychiatric Serv 48:91–92, 1997 4–10

Introduction.—The authors have previously described a large-group interpretive model for community meetings in the inpatient psychiatric setting. This model is still useful even with the trend toward shorter lengths of inpatient stay. Such meetings are helpful in uncovering patients' attitudes toward staff in the here-and-now, and in examining the patients' maladaptive interpretations of staff behavior. The technique of interpretive psychotherapy in patient community meetings is reviewed, focusing on its application in the short-term unit.

Community Meetings in the Short-Term Unit Setting.—Meetings are held twice a week for 45 to 60 minutes. The staff do not introduce topics; rather, they listen for what the group is thinking and feeling but may be afraid to verbalize. The patients may bring up apparently unrelated topics, but the staff must try to detect the underlying allusions to how the patients are experiencing their relationship with the staff. The staff must identify the events that patients unconsciously select as their theme. Then the staff looks for the specific, stereotypical meaning that most of the group applies to the event. These 3 components can then be merged into an appropriate and timely group intervention.

In the short-term setting, community meetings provide an invaluable "snapshot" of the unit's milieu. They also provide a useful form of quality control, often bringing to light incidents that are well known to patients but unknown to staff. The meetings also provide a useful opportunity for feedback to the staff, sometimes identifying undesirable or nontherapeutic activities or attitudes. The meetings can offer psychodynamic insights that will be useful in improving patient compliance, identifying psychologic barriers to getting well, and planning appropriate aftercare. Meetings can also help to reduce tension on the unit. Patients who are too psychotic or agitated to sit still should be excluded from the meeting. Also, the staff should bring up any obviously important issues that are not brought up by the patients.

Discussion.—Community meetings with a large-group interpretive psychotherapy approach can be usefully implemented on short-term inpatient units. These meetings can help even severely patients to understand that their negative interpretations of staff behavior are not the only way to see things. The meetings can also help staff to understand the impact of their well-intended actions on patients.

► This article makes an interesting companion to the previous article by Stuart, Wright, et al. in this volume (Abstract 4–5). These authors remind us that even in a short-term, acute treatment inpatient setting there may still be a place for a psychodynamic psychotherapeutic approach to group therapy, particularly in an inpatient community meeting. There is no question that a dynamic approach to understanding group processes on an inpatient unit can be useful. However, it is unclear in the present training environment whether many residents will have an opportunity for learning experiences in this modality.

A. Tasman, M.D.

Family Treatment of Childhood Anxiety: A Controlled Trial

Barrett PM, Dadds MR, Rapee RM (Griffith Univ, Nathan, Australia; Macquarie Univ, Sydney, Australia)

J Consult Clin Psychol 64:333–342, 1996 4–11

Background.—Alhough anxiety is one of the most common psychological problems in children, there has been little research into the treatment of childhood anxiety disorders. Cognitive behavioral therapy (CBT) may be an effective intervention, and family involvement may be important. Cognitive behavioral therapy and family management training for the treatment of childhood anxiety disorders were studied in a randomized trial.

Methods.—Seventy-nine children, aged 7–14 years, who had anxiety disorders were included. According to structured interviews, the principal diagnosis was overanxious disorder in 30 children, separation anxiety disorder in 30, and social phobia in 19. The patients were randomly assigned to receive CBT alone, CBT plus a family management intervention, and a waiting list control. The family management intervention had 3 main components: training parents to reward courageous behavior and discourage excessive anxiety in the child, to deal with their own emotions and anxiety and to use model problem-solving skills, and to use communication and problem-solving skills. After treatment and at 6 and 12 months' follow-up, the interventions were compared for effectiveness by self-report measures and clinician ratings.

Results.—After treatment, the percentage of children who no longer met the criteria for an anxiety disorder was 70% in the intervention groups vs. 26% in the control group. At 12 months, 70% of children in the CBT-only group and 96% of those in the CBT plus family therapy group no longer met the criteria for anxiety disorder. The results of the combined intervention were better in all clinical evaluation scales assessed: clinical global impression, overall functioning, overall anxiety, avoidant behaviors, change of family disruption by the child's behavior, change in parents' perception of their ability to deal with the child's behavior, and change in the child's ability to deal with difficult situations. Younger children and girls had a better response to the combined intervention.

Conclusions.—Adding a family management intervention to CBT leads to improved outcomes in children with anxiety disorders. More study is needed to define the specificity of this effect and the effectiveness of the specific components of family treatment. Long-term follow-up would also be helpful.

▶ It should perhaps not be surprising that family therapy is a useful component of treatment of children. This study clearly demonstrates the synergistic effect between individual CBT and family therapy in children with anxiety disorders. These findings should serve as an important message to both therapists and third-party reimbursers that multi-modal treatment is often more effective, and, undoubtedly, more cost-effective in the long run than unitary approaches, which may seem less expensive in the short run.

A. Tasman, M.D.

Psychopharmacology and Psychotherapy

The Role of the Alliance in the Pharmacologic Treatment of Depression

Weiss M, Gaston L, Propst A, et al (McGill Univ, Montreal; British Columbia's Children's Hosp, Vancouver)

J Clin Psychiatry 58:196–204, 1997 4–12

Background.—The best predictor of psychotherapy outcome is the alliance between the therapist and client. The influence of this alliance on the efficacy of pharmacotherapy for depression was investigated.

Methods.—Thirty-one depressed outpatients taking antidepressants were included in the study. Therapeutic alliance was assessed by the patient and therapist versions of the California Pharmacotherapy Alliance Scale. The Hamilton Rating Scale for Depression; the Beck Depression Inventory; and the Symptom, Sign, Side-Effect Checklist were administered to determine treatment outcomes.

Findings.—The alliance measures explained 21% to 56% of the variance on the 3 outcome measures. When outcome measure scores were averaged, therapist perceptions of the alliance predicted 41% of the variance in symptom improvement, and patient perceptions predicted 25%. Patient attitude toward medication was associated with somatic manifestations but not depression scores. Therapist perception of patient hostility was associated with depression. The interactions between alliance and outcomes differed among patients, resulting in associations that could be positive or negative.

Conclusions.—The therapeutic alliance between therapist and patient is correlated with outcome in the pharmacotherapeutic treatment of depression, although interindividual variability among patients may exist. Therapist perception of alliance better predicts symptom outcomes than does patient perception in the pharmacotherapeutic management of depression; in psychotherapy, the reverse is usually found.

▶ This small study reinforces what many skilled psychiatrists have understood from years of clinical work—that psychopharmacologic treatment, especially when effective, does not occur in an interpersonal vacuum. Many have asserted that there is an important interaction between the therapeutic alliance and response to psychopharmacologic interventions. One would hope that further work in this area will reinforce these findings and lend weight to those who advocate the position that combined treatment by a single therapist produces better outcomes than split therapy.

A. Tasman, M.D.

The Efficacy of Imipramine and Psychotherapy in Early-onset Chronic Depression: A Reanalysis of the National Institute of Mental Health Treatment of Depression Collaborative Research Program

Agosti V, Ocepek-Welikson K (New York State Psychiatric Inst; Columbia Univ, New York)

J Affect Disord 43:181–186, 1997 4–13

Background.—No controlled studies seem to have addressed the efficacy of psychotherapy for early-onset chronic depression. The efficacies of cognitive behavioral therapy (CBT), interpersonal psychotherapy (IPT), imipramine clinical management (ICM), and placebo were compared in a reanalysis of the National Institute of Mental Health Treatment of Depression Collaborative Research Program.

Methods and Findings.—Data on 65 outpatients with early-onset chronic depression were interpreted. All patients completed at least 3.5 weeks of treatment. Mean patient age was 31.3 years, and mean duration of major depression was 15.9 years. Forty percent of the patients met criteria for intermittent depression. Depression scores after CBT, IPT, and ICM did not differ significantly from those in the placebo group. The duration of major depression was not associated with response to a specific mode of treatment.

Conclusions.—Neither ICM, IPT, nor CBT are significantly better than a placebo condition in the treatment of early-onset chronic depression. Alhough patients were generally improved from baseline, they were still significantly depressed at the end of treatment.

▶ This analysis of results from the National Institute of Mental Health Treatment of Depression Collaborative Research Program showed that neither brief psychotherapy nor pharmacologic interventions were effective in persons with chronic depression. This finding reinforces long-held clinical wisdom that effective treatment for patients with this type of long-term mood disorder requires long-term intervention. As managed care approaches cover more and more of the population, these findings should be particularly noted because this study, even though limited by its small size, suggests that limited interventions are unlikely to be effective in severe disorders.

A. Tasman, M.D.

Personality Disorders

Psychotherapy for Histrionic Personality Disorder

Horowitz MJ (Univ of California, San Francisco)
J Psychother Prac Res 6:93–104, 1997 4–14

Introduction.—Patients with histrionic personality disorder have an excessive, symptomatic, and maladaptive style of dramatic self-presentation, typified by demanding and socially inappropriate emotional displays to get attention. The patient repeats this pattern despite the often destructive personal consequences. Configurational analysis is a dynamic approach to psychopathology that emphasizes states of mind, defensiveness, and person schemas. A 3-phase approach to the psychotherapy of histrionic personality disorder was described with configurational analysis.

Treatment Phases.—The first phase of treatment focuses on stabilizing the patient's mental state. By taking a dynamic rather than a static approach, the clinician recognizes that symptoms and behavioral problems differ in different states of minds. This phase of treatment focuses on the emotionality, rationality, and apparent self-regulation of each important state of mind. Patients with histrionic personality disorder are prone to intensely negative emotions and impulsive relationship behaviors, underscoring the need for control of mental states. The next phase aims to clarify verbal communication and modify defensive controls. In patients with histrionic personality disorder, inhibition of ideation may lead to a cloudy communication style, which can make it difficult to select a topic for psychotherapeutic focus. Once the safety of the psychotherapeutic relationship is established and the patients' excessive distortions and inhibitions have been addressed, issues of conflict and concern can be identified and addressed.

The third phase addresses person schema, in which the goal is to change irrational and conflicted structures of belief. Mental states—particularly maladaptive state cycles—are explained in terms of configurations of role-relationship models. In patients with histrionic personality disorder, these models may be segregated, dissociated, distorted, and contradictory. The patient's mental state may shift explosively when the model underlying nonconscious mental processing suddenly shifts. Therapy must address the patient's irrational, conflicted self-views and views of others. Therapy should address the patient's fears of being abandoned and belief in the inability to manage basic life tasks; define excessive dependence on and idealization of unreliable people; clarify irrational and negative self-beliefs; and support realistic, positive, and competent self-concepts in opportunity-appropriate role-relationship models. Adaptive recognition of the patient's personal skills may be a useful complement to the clarification of dysfunctional beliefs in self-concepts.

Discussion.—This approach permits identification of individual states of mind, definition of specific defensive maneuvers, and gradual formation of distinctive role-relationship models. The suggested treatment phases can serve as a useful guideline for clinicians and a teaching document for trainees.

► All personality disorders are difficult to treat, in part because specific treatment approaches for different personality disorders have not been well delineated. This article is an important step in the treatment process for a personality disorder that receives little attention these days. One hopes that this promising construct might be investigated more formally to assess its utility.

A. Tasman, M.D.

Tailoring the Psychotherapy to the Borderline Patient
Howitz L, Gabbard GO, Allen JG, et al (Menninger Clinic, Topeka, Kan)
J Psychother Prac Res 5:287–306, 1996 4–15

Objective.—Patients with borderline personality disorder pose a psychotherapeutic challenge. There is disagreement as to the best form of therapy; some authors suggest psychoanalysis or exploratory psychotherapy, whereas others suggest an explicitly supportive approach designed to strengthen the patient's adaptive defenses. However, the diagnosis of borderline personality disorder encompasses a broad range of functional levels, from close to the neurotic border to close to the psychotic border. The literature was reviewed and some new research was done, with the suggestion that psychotherapy for patients with borderline personality disorder should be tailored to the individual's level of functioning.

Psychotherapeutic Approach.—When considering psychotherapy for borderline patients, most authors use a "lumping" strategy. That is, they suggest 1 approach for the "average" patient, while allowing that some patients outside the majority require different treatment. The current authors propose that the most appropriate approach for a particular patient should be based on clearer diagnostic differentiation, taking into account the developmental considerations, ego functions, and relationship patterns for that patient. Patients' patterns of closeness and distance and the appropriateness of expressive psychotherapy should be assessed. Patients at either extreme are not well suited for interpretation. Uncovering work is more likely to be successful in patients who alternate between the 2 extremes. In addition, patients who demonstrate flexibility in their response patterns are more likely to be able to accept the intimacy and separateness involved in transference interpretation. The differentiation between pathologic and healthy interpretation is another important consideration. Patients whose oscillations show greater integration between good and bad internal representations are more likely to be ready for transference exploration.

► Those who spend significant parts of their clinical lives treating patients with borderline personality disorder are well aware that there is no unified way of understanding all such patients, or even an individual patient, at all phases of treatment. The approach described in this article argues for flexibility of understanding and a categorization of patients who may have a general diagnosis of borderline personality disorder but represent particular subtypes within that diagnosis. This approach, too, should be studied in more formal research protocols to elucidate its utility.

A. Tasman, M.D.

A Review of Inpatient Group Therapy for Borderline Personality Disorder

Springer T, Silk KR (Univ of Michigan, Ann Arbor)

Harvard Rev Psychiatry 3:268–278, 1996 4–16

Background.—Lengths of stay for psychiatric inpatients have been decreasing steadily. Consequently, the demand has grown for effective inpatient treatments for severely disturbed patients with personality disorder, particularly borderline personality disorder (BPD). Group forms of therapy are frequently used on inpatient units, yet there have been few published reports of this approach. The literature on inpatient group therapy for patients with BPD was reviewed.

Inpatient Group Therapy for BPD.—Studies of inpatient group therapy have had conflicting results. Some studies suggested that psychoanalytic or insight-oriented group therapy is not helpful or can even cause deterioration. However, other studies suggested that problem-solving group therapy can be helpful in the inpatient setting. The results seem better when patients with personality disorder are analyzed separately. A notable finding is that patients with personality disorders—especially those with BPD—perceive group therapy as very helpful, even during a brief hospitalization. Most of the studies cited are older and have some methodological flaws. This questions their applicability to the present situation, in which hospital stays are very brief and patients are more severely and acutely ill.

Dialectical Behavior Therapy.—The value of psychodynamic and psychoanalytic group therapy has been questioned, particularly for inpatients. Good results were reported with outpatient Dialectical Behavior Therapy (DBT),[1] leading to interest in the possibility of DBT for patients with BPD. However, there have been few empirical studies of inpatient DBT. Although 1 study of DBT on a medium-stay unit gave encouraging results, the results were not as good on a short-stay unit. Pending further research, clinicians should carefully consider the advantages and disadvantages of DBT before deciding to try it. The natural enthusiasm for any potentially effective treatment for patients with personality disorder must be tempered with the understanding that what works in an intensive outpatient treatment setting may not apply in the short-term inpatient setting. Future studies should compare DBT with other types of group therapy, modified for inpatient use, and with a no-group control condition.

► It is well known that hospitalized patients with BPD are notoriously difficult to treat. These authors critically review the use of Linehan's DBT[1] in a group model in a short-term inpatient setting for patients with BPD. Although they conclude that there are pros and cons to the approach, a number of clinicians have found that this can be an effective aspect of a multi-modal treatment intervention. This approach warrants further clinical use to assess its utility.

A. Tasman, M.D.

Reference

1. Linehan MM: *Cognitive-Behavioral Treatment of Borderline Personality Disorder.* New York, Guilford, 1993.

Techniques for Reducing Therapy-interfering Behavior in Patients With Borderline Personality Disorder: Similiarities in Four Diverse Treatment Paradigms

Allen DM (Univ of Tennessee, Memphis)

J Psychother Prac Res 6:25–35, 1997 4–17

Introduction.—Patients with borderline personality disorder (BPD) are very difficult to deal with in psychotherapy. A key to success is the management of patient behaviors that elicit a strongly negative response from the therapist and interfere with the psychotherapeutic process. Strategies for dealing with these provocative behaviors—were examined, and striking similarities were noted. A theoretical model to explain the effectiveness of these approaches was proposed.

Theoretical Model.—All 4 interventions interrupt the process by which the patient with BPD tries to induce a specific reaction in the therapist. The reaction anticipated by the patient is the same as encountered in the patient's ongoing social environment. In the 4 interventions, the therapist's actions contrast with those expected by the patient. This limits and defines patient-therapist interactions so that patients tend to alter their provocative response patterns. Some key observations lead to the new model. Many of the behavior patterns of patients with BPD appear to be induced, at least partly, by the behaviors and responses of others in patients' social systems. Patients with BPD attempt to induce "what they fear and wish to confirm"[1] in their therapists. When the individuals in the patient's social environment inconsistently appease the patient, they create conditions in which the patient learns behaviors destructive to relationships.

In this new model, the patient with BPD expects that the therapist will respond in the same way that the patient's family does, while desperately hoping for a different response. Whenever the patient is unable to re-create the maladaptive aspects of the family relationship in therapy, the likelihood of additional provocative behavior decreases. From the range of possible responses to the provocative behavior, the particular reaction chosen is determined by the patient's and the caretaker's predispositions and conflicts.

The caretaker may try to find ways of helping the patient feel better quickly, or may indulge the patient's unreasonable demands. Such efforts are likely to fail; when they do, the patient may become even more negative toward the caretaker, leading to hostility on the part of the caretaker.

The described interventions seek to avoid this trap. Therapists should be comfortable with their own limitations, unafraid of the patient's anger, and unwilling to attack the patient when provoked. They do not try to "take care of" and thereby infantilize the patient. They maintain respect of the patient's suffering, abilities, and values, as well as the expectation that the patient will behave reasonably and cooperatively. Therapists admit errors when they occur, in the hope of interrupting the process whereby mistakes reinforce the patient's problematic behaviors. This approach often has a calming effect on the patient with BPD. The patient may become less difficult, less crisis oriented, more cooperative, and better able to work on the areas of their lives that can be changed through therapy.

Discussion.—Based on reported interventions, a theoretical model for dealing with provocative behavior in psychotherapy by patients with BPD was proposed. If successful in the patient-therapist relationship, this approach may lead to techniques for changing the patient's behavior in other key relationships. Future studies should be done to validate the effectiveness of the described approach and to explore ways of generalizing it to affect the patient's life outside psychotherapy.

▶ This is another formulation of how psychotherapy can be modified to deal with the provocative behavior of patients with BPD. The "proof is in the pudding," and one hopes this technique will be more widely studied to determine its effectiveness.

A. Tasman, M.D.

Schizophrenia and Psychosis

Two-Year Outcome of Social Skills Training and Group Psychotherapy for Outpatients With Schizophrenia

Marder SR, Wirshing WC, Mintz J, et al (Univ of California, Los Angeles)
Am J Psychiatry 153:1585–1592, 1996 4–18

Objective.—Social skills training and group therapy were evaluated for effectiveness in protecting against psychotic relapse and improving social adjustment of community-dwelling patients with schizophrenia.

Methods.—Eighty male outpatients with schizophrenia were randomly assigned to either social skills training or supportive group therapy 2 times weekly for 6 months and then weekly for 18 months. All received low-dose fluphenazine (5–10 mg every 14 days), with random assignment to prodromal supplementation with oral fluphenazine (5 mg 2 times daily) or placebo. Psychotic exacerbation and scores on the Social Adjustment Scale II (SAS-II) were monitored.

Results.—Social skills training provided more benefit than group therapy on 2 of the 6 SAS-II clusters. Significant interactions were seen between psychosocial and drug treatment for 3 SAS-II items. The advantage was greatest with active drug supplementation. Social skills training significantly decreased psychotic exacerbation in the placebo group.

Conclusion.—Social skills training resulted in greater improvement than group therapy in important social adjustment areas among patients assigned to active drug prodromal supplementation but not those in the placebo group. Patients not randomly assigned to supplementation (because they had no prodromal period) had relatively good SAS-II outcomes with either modality. The SAS-II difference between social skills training and group therapy was significant only among patients with early-onset schizophrenia (before the median age of 24 years). Perhaps patients with later onset received less benefit because they had already acquired mature social skills.

► Social skills training has proven to be useful in the overall management of patients with schizophrenia. This study reinforces our view of the utility of social skills training and particularly emphasizes its use as part of a multimodal intervention that includes psychopharmacologic management. Even though this study found that not all patients improved with this intervention and that even those who did had only modest benefit, social skills training remains an important part of the overall therapeutic armamentarium.

A. Tasman, M.D.

Cognitive Therapy and Recovery From Acute Psychosis, A Controlled Trial: I. Impact on Psychotic Symptoms

Drury V, Birchwood M, Cochrane R, et al (All Saints Hosp, Birmingham, England; Univ of Birmingham, England)

Br J Psychiatry 169:593–601, 1996 4–19

Background.—In the United Kingdom, cognitive therapy is currently being developed for patients with psychosis. A trial of cognitive therapy to hasten the resolution of positive symptoms and reduce residual symptoms in acute psychosis was conducted.

Methods.—Sixty-nine of 117 patients with acute nonaffective psychosis at 1 center satisfied inclusion criteria. Forty of those patients underwent stratified randomization. The experimental intervention, which involved individual and group cognitive therapy, was compared with treatment consisting of matched hours of therapist input providing structured activities and informal support. Clinicians unaware of group allocation provided routine pharmacotherapy. Weekly monitoring was done by self-report and mental state assessments during admission and in the subsequent 9 months.

Findings.—Positive symptoms declined in both groups, though this decline was more pronounced in the patients receiving cognitive therapy. Moderate or severe residual symptoms were noted at 9 months in 5% of the cognitive therapy group and in 56% of the control group.

Conclusions.—Cognitive therapy appears to be a valuable adjunct to pharmacotherapy and standard care for patients with acute psychosis. The challenging and testing of delusions in a nonconfrontational manner can be helpful for such patients.

Cognitive Therapy and Recovery From Acute Psychosis, A Controlled Trial: II. Impact on Recovery Time

Drury V, Birchwood M, Cochrane R, et al (All Saints Hosp, Birmingham, England; Univ of Birmingham, England)

Br J Psychiatry 169:602–607, 1996 4–20

Background.—In previous research, cognitive therapy had a significant impact on the rate and degree of recovery of positive symptoms in acute psychosis. Whether these effects would generalize to other characteristics of acute psychosis, such as dysphoria, insight, and "low level" psychotic thinking, was investigated in the current study.

Methods and Findings.—Dysphoria, insight, and psychotic thinking were assessed in 40 patients in the first 6 months after they were seen for acute psychosis. Survival analysis was used to determine time to recovery from psychosis using 3 increasingly stringent definitions in the cognitive therapy and control groups. Depending on the definition used, cognitive therapy was associated with a 25% to 50% decrease in recovery time.

Conclusions.—In these patients, the effects of cognitive therapy extended beyond positive symptoms and included insight, dysphoria, and "low level" psychotic thinking. However, this kind of clinical recovery required a median of 20 weeks.

► Cognitive therapy approaches have been little studied in schizophrenia, especially in patients with acute psychosis. These 2 studies (Abstracts 4–19 and 4–20) show that cognitive therapy may be worthy of further investigation in this group of patients, again as part of a multi-modal approach to treatment. Even though there are methodologic concerns that limit the conclusions that one can draw from this study, further investigation is clearly warranted.

A. Tasman, M.D.

Coping With Negative Symptoms of Schizophrenia: Patient and Family Perspectives

Mueser KT, Valentiner DP, Agresta J (Dartmouth Med School, Hanover, NH; Med College of Pennsylvania, Philadelphia; Northern Illinois Univ, DeKalb)

Schizophr Bull 23:329–339, 1997 4–21

Background.—A better understanding of how schizophrenic patients and their families cope with negative symptoms would be of value for several reasons. Such coping strategies were studied.

Methods.—Semistructured interviews were conducted separately with patients and their families to elicit coping strategies and their perceived efficacy. Coping responses were classified as behavioral-cognitive, social-nonsocial, or problem focused–emotion focused.

Findings.—Overall, the number of coping strategies was associated with perceived coping efficacy among patients and families, regardless of strategy type. The efficacy of perceived coping tended to be greatest for apathy and lowest for blunting. Efficacy of alogia, anhedonia, and inattention was intermediate. Family members with more knowledge about schizophrenia used more coping strategies and reported a greater efficacy of coping. Coping strategies were generally unrelated to patient rejection by family members and to the patient's or relatives' distress.

Conclusions.—Schizophrenic patients and their families use a wide variety of strategies to cope with negative symptoms. Additional studies are needed to determine whether families may benefit from psychoeducational approaches to teaching them how to better manage negative symptoms.

► Coping with the negative symptoms of schizophrenia is difficult for both the patient and the family. This study suggests an approach that involves looking at coping strategies that might be useful for further research. Whether the strategies used by patients and their families can be incorporated into a specific therapeutic method, however, remains unknown.

A. Tasman, M.D.

Cognitive-Behavioral Treatment of Panic Attacks in Chronic Schizophrenia

Arlow PB, Moran ME, Bermanzohn PC, et al (Long Island Jewish Med Ctr–Hillside Hosp, Glen Oaks, NY)

J Psychother Prac Res 6:145–150, 1997 4–22

Background.—Although panic attacks are thought to be relatively common among patients with schizophrenia, few studies of treatments for this disorder have been reported. Cognitive-behavioral therapy (CBT) has been shown to be effective for panic disorder in nonschizophrenic patients. Thus, use of this CBT for the treatment of panic attacks in patients with schizophrenia was studied in an open clinical trial.

Methods and Outcomes.—Eight of 11 patients meeting *Diagnostic and Statistical Manual of Medical Disorders*, 3rd ed., revised, criteria for schizophrenia and panic disorder completed a 16-week clinical trial of CBT. Ratings showed a statistically significant decrease in panic symptoms after treatment compared with baseline values. In addition, the number of panic attacks was significantly reduced.

Conclusions.—Cognitive-behavioral therapy in the integrated treatment of patients with schizophrenia and panic disorder appears promising. Further exploration of CBT in this population is warranted.

► This small study is another in an emerging body of literature investigating the utility of CBT in schizophrenia. This study in particular investigated utility in dealing with panic attacks in patients with schizophrenia and found CBT to be useful. I look forward to further investigation.

A. Tasman, M.D.

Personal Therapy: A Disorder-relevant Psychotherapy for Schizophrenia

Hogarty GE, Kornblith SJ, Greenwald D, et al (Univ of Pittsburgh, Pa)

Schizophr Bull 21:379–393, 1995 4–23

Background.—Little evidence supports empirically validated individual psychotherapy for schizophrenia. Personal therapy, a disorder-relevant psychotherapy for patients with schizophrenia, was described.

Personal Therapy.—This treatment tries to address the apparent limitations of traditional psychotherapy by modifying the "model of the person." The modification accommodates an underlying pathophysiology, minimizing potential iatrogenic effects of maintenance antipsychotic medication, controlling sources of environmental provocation, and extending treatment to a time when crisis management is reduced and stabilization is better ensured. Through graduated, internal coping strategies, personal therapy attempts to provide an increasing awareness of personal vulnerability, such as the internal cues of affect dysregulation. Foresight is increased through the accurate appraisal of emotional states, their appropriate expression, and assessment of the reciprocal response of others. Phase-specific psychoeducation and behavior therapy techniques are used to supplement these strategies. Preliminary observations of 2 patient groups—1 living with their families and the other living independently—suggest that improvement over time differs among patients treated with personal therapy.

► Long-term therapeutic relationships with schizophrenic patients often have an ad hoc quality. These authors attempt to develop a model into which a particular approach to long-term psychotherapy in such patients can be incorporated. Although this new approach to psychotherapeutic intervention has not been well studied, and although the results mentioned in this report are not as well supported as one might like, this is an interesting modification that might allow a clear conceptual framework for interventions over time to occur.

A. Tasman, M.D.

Behavioral Medicine

Reduction in Drug Requirements for Hypertension by Means of a Cognitive-Behavioral Intervention
Shapiro D, Hui KK, Oakley ME, et al (Univ of California, Los Angeles; Univ of California, Irvine)
Am J Hypertens 10:9–17, 1997 4–24

Background.—The use of relaxation and stress reduction has been used successfully as alternative or adjunctive methods of treating physical disorders. However, studies of combined drug and behavioral treatments have yielded inconclusive results. The efficacy of a cognitive-behavioral intervention as adjunctive treatment for hypertension was tested.

Methods.—Thirty-nine patients with unmedicated clinic diastolic blood pressures of 95 mm Hg or greater were randomly assigned. The patients underwent a 6-week cognitive-behavioral treatment or measurements only. After treatment, medication levels were decreased in a systematic stepdown procedure, and patients were followed up for 1 year thereafter.

Findings.—The cognitive-behavioral intervention was twice as effective as the control procedure in decreasing medication requirements. Seventy-three percent of the patients in the treatment group were at lower levels of medication at 12 months than at randomization, compared with 35% of patients in the control group. Fifty-five percent of the patients in the intervention group and 30% in the control group remained completely free of medications at 12 months. Medication reductions were associated with maintained, controlled levels of clinic, ambulatory, and home blood pressure.

Conclusions.—Adding a group-administered cognitive-behavioral intervention to the pharmacologic treatment of hypertension is beneficial for decreasing drug requirements for hypertensive patients. The costs and potential adverse effects of antihypertensive medications are thereby reduced.

► Cognitive-behavioral therapy reduced the requirements of medication for hypertension. The effects of this intervention persisted in many patients for nearly 1 year after the cessation of the psychotherapeutic intervention. Further work in this area is definitely indicated.

A. Tasman, M.D.

Stress Reduction Through Mindfulness Meditation: Effects on Psychological Symptomatology, Sense of Control, and Spiritual Experiences
Astin JA (Univ of California, Irvine)
Psychother Psychosom 66:97–106, 1997 4–25

Background.—Mindfulness meditation techniques emphasize the development of detached observation and awareness of the contents of consciousness. Previous studies suggest that a stress reduction program based on training in mindfulness meditation may be useful for decreasing stress-related symptoms and helping patients cope with chronic pain. However, such research has been limited by a lack of adequate control groups.

Methods.—Twenty-eight volunteers were assigned to an experimental or a control group. Patients in the first group underwent an 8-week stress reduction program based on mindfulness meditation training, and patients in the second group received no treatment.

Findings.—Greater changes occurred in the intervention than in the non-intervention group. Patients in the former group had greater decreases in overall psychologic symptoms, greater increases in overall domain-specific sense of control and use of an accepting or yielding mode of control in their lives, and higher scores on a measure of spiritual experiences.

Conclusions.—The techniques of mindful meditation may be a powerful cognitive-behavioral coping strategy for changing the ways in which people respond to life events. Such techniques may also be of benefit in preventing relapse in affective disorders.

► Mindfulness meditation is well known to persons working in behavioral medicine, especially those familiar with the work of John Kabat-Zinn. Mindfulness meditation has not been widely used, however, outside of behavioral medicine. It will be interesting to learn how mindfulness meditation could be used as an adjunct to other psychotherapeutic approaches in patients with psychiatric illness. One would hope that articles such as this might stimulate further research.

A. Tasman, M.D.

Impact of Psychotherapy: Does It Affect Frequency of Visits to Family Physicians?

Golden GA (Victoria Family Med Centre, London, Ont)

Can Fam Physician 43:1098–1102, 1997 4–26

Background.—Research has shown that patients with psychological disorders extensively use medical resources. The current study determined whether a course of psychotherapy with a psychologist would affect the frequency of patients' visits to their family physicians.

Methods.—Thirty-three patients completing a course of psychotherapy between 1984 and 1991 were included in the study. The patients did not pay a direct fee for psychotherapy. Median length of psychotherapy was 12.5 1-hour sessions. The therapeutic approach was eclectic and humanistic.

Findings.—During and after psychotherapy, the frequency of visits to family physicians declined. This reduction was especially apparent in comparisons of visits before and after therapy. The psychotherapy, provided as part of an overall medical intervention, appeared to follow the pattern of the "offset effect," which has been demonstrated in other medical settings.

Conclusions.—Psychotherapy can be an effective part of total medical care. Although further research is needed, accessible, appropriate psychological care can apparently be a useful component of a healthy medical system.

► It is well known that most visits to a doctor's office are related to emotional distress. This project examines, in a sense, whether the psychotherapist's most grandiose fantasy is true—Does psychotherapy have an overall effect on health care utilization? The results clearly showed that brief psychotherapy, when provided as part of an overall medical intervention, clearly reduced the frequency of visits to family physicians. Although this offset effect has been reported for several decades, it is worth revisiting in the present environment.

A. Tasman, M.D.

A Cognitive Behavioural Approach to Preventing Anxiety During Magnetic Resonance Imaging

Lukins R, Davan IGP, Drummond PD (Murdoch Univ, Perth, Western Australia)

J Behav Ther Exp Psychiatry 28:97–104, 1997 4–27

Background.—Undergoing MRI can cause psychologic reactions ranging from nervousness to intense fear or terror. A relaxation intervention designed to prevent anxiety during MRI was assessed.

Methods and Findings.—Patients scheduled for MRI were assigned to no intervention, relaxation before imaging, or relaxation before and during imaging. The 3 groups included 52, 44, and 43 patients, respectively. Anxiety during imaging was reduced in the patients in the relaxation groups compared with those in the control group. At 7 or more months after MRI, anxiety experienced during imaging was positively associated with MRI-related fears. The intervention did not prevent the development of fears related to MRI.

Conclusions.—The relaxation intervention in this study clearly reduced patient anxiety during MRI. However, the intervention did not prevent patients from subsequently developing MRI-related fears.

► Radiologists are well aware that a significant proportion of patients scheduled for MRI cannot complete the study, contributing to both increased cost and diagnostic problems for the patient. This study clearly indicates that cognitive–behavioral therapy can be useful in alleviating anxiety during MRI.

A. Tasman, M.D.

Cognitive-Behavioral Group Therapy for Irritable Bowel Syndrome: Effects and Long-term Follow-up

van Dulmen AM, Fennis JFM, Bleijenberg G (Univ of Nijmegen, The Netherlands; Univ Hosp Nijmegen, The Netherlands)

Psychosom Med 58:508–514, 1996 4–28

Background.—The efficacy of cognitive-behavioral therapy for patients with irritable bowel syndrome on a group basis has not been well studied. Past research has included only small groups of patients, and long-term follow-up studies are lacking. The efficacy of a cognitive-behavioral group treatment compared with a wait-list control group in relieving abdominal symptoms, as well as the long-term efficacy of cognitive-behavioral group treatment, was studied.

Methods.—The 2-part investigation consisted of a controlled trial and a follow-up study. In the controlled study, 25 patients in a treatment group and 20 on a waiting list were compared. Treatment included 8 2-hour group sessions over 3 months. All patients were then followed up for a mean 2.25 years after treatment completion.

Findings.—The abdominal symptoms of the patients undergoing treatment were significantly more improved than those of patients on the waiting list. The number of successful coping strategies increased more and avoidance behaviors decreased more in the treatment group than in the control group. These positive changes persisted in the long term.

Conclusions.—Cognitive-behavioral group therapy effectively relieves the symptoms of irritable bowel syndrome, stimulates coping strategies, and reduces avoidance behavior. At long-term follow-up, improvements in the treatment group as compared with pretreatment assessment were still evident.

► Although individual cognitive-behavioral therapy has been found of use for irritable bowel syndrome in the past, there have been few studies of group cognitive behavior therapy. The positive findings in this study indicate that this may be a useful and cost-effective intervention, especially in the medical environment.

A. Tasman, M.D.

Technology and Psychotherapy

Virtual Reality Exposure Therapy

Rothbaum BO, Hodges L, Kooper R (Emory Univ, Atlanta, Ga; Georgia Inst of Technology, Altanta)

J Psychother Prac Res 6:219–226, 1997 4–29

Overview.—Because virtual reality immerses the individual in a computer-generated, real-time, position-trackable environment, the technology may be useful for treating anxiety disorders.

Using Virtual Reality to Treat Phobias.—Exposure therapy is based on the theory that fears must be activated so that the processes of habituation and extinction can be applied to modify the fear structure and improve symptoms. In a controlled study, virtual reality exposure therapy has been used successfully to treat acrophobia in a time- and cost-effective manner. A case study of an individual who had a fear of flying demonstrated a reduction in fear and avoidance behavior after virtual reality exposure therapy.

Discussion.—There are unique issues surrounding the use of virtual reality exposure therapy. Although the therapist is physically present, the patient is "alone" in the virtual environment. At present, virtual reality applications require the presence of a programmer to adjust the sequence of "realities" during therapy. Development of a turnkey system would eliminate this need. Equipment is very expensive (in excess of $150,000) and much of the software must still be developed. However, virtual reality exposure therapy can provide in vivo exposure to anxiety-producing situations in the privacy of the therapist's office rather than in a public place.

Conclusion.—Virtual reality exposure should be added to the therapist's armamentarium. Additional research is needed to examine the effectiveness of treatment in other areas.

▶ Millions of parents who fear that their children have been wasting hundreds of hours playing computer games would be reassured by this article. This is an exciting use of computer technology in treating phobia related to fear of flying. I would guess that this marks the very beginning of what will be a major increase in the use of sophisticated technologies for therapeutic purposes in the future.

A. Tasman, M.D.

Comparison of Palmtop-Computer-assisted Brief Cognitive–Behavioral Treatment to Cognitive–Behavorial Treatment for Panic Disorder

Newman MG, Kenardy J, Herman S, et al (Stanford Univ, Calif; Univ of Queensland, Australia)

J Consult Clin Psychol 65:178–183, 1997 4–30

Objective.—Cost-containment considerations have forced a re-examination of the minimum number of cognitive-behavioral sessions needed to achieve maximum benefit to the patient. The effectiveness of 12 cognitive-behavioral therapy sessions (CBT12) was compared with the effectiveness of 4 computer-assisted therapy sessions (CBT4-CA) for panic disorder.

Methods.—Eighteen patients (3 men), aged 25 to 62 years, with panic disorder of 7.5 years' average duration, were randomly allocated to receive either 12 weekly 1-hour individual therapy sessions or 4 computer-assisted therapy sessions. The 12-session treatment included homework and weekly readings directed at cognitive restructuring, breathing retraining, progressive muscle relaxation, exposure to interoceptive cues, and exposure to feared situations. Patients used the computer in the diary mode to rate anxiety levels and number of panic attacks. The computer-assisted therapy sessions consisted of 4 weekly individual sessions (a total of 6 hours). Patients used the computer in diary mode during the first session, and in the treatment-plus-diary mode in subsequent sessions, and on their own for an additional 8 weeks. Baseline measurements were compared with measurements taken at 3 assessment points during treatment.

Results.—One-way analysis of variance showed no differences between the treatments in internal validity. Patients rated both treatments as equally and highly credible and satisfactory. Multivariate analyses of variance revealed that behavior avoidance at baseline was significantly greater in the CBT12 than in the CBT4-CA patient groups. All other baseline scores were similar. Multivariate analysis showed that both treatments were equally effective for all major panic symptoms. Whereas patients in the CBT12 showed posttest improvement that was clinically significantly superior to that of patients in the CBTA-CA, no differences were observed at follow-up.

Conclusion.—Although the small size, lack of a no-computer comparison group, and lack of a control group limit the conclusions that can be drawn from this study, these results indicate that the 2 therapies were equally effective.

► This is a small and methodologically flawed study which is, nonetheless, interesting. Patients in the CBT12 had 12 sessions, but those in the CBT4-CA had only 4 sessions. These differences in patient contact in treatment make it very difficult to interpret the results of this study, which showed that CBT12 was superior in some measures. This study, however, is interesting because it describes how computers can be used for therapeutic interventions.

A. Tasman, M.D.

Telepsychotherapy: Psychotherapy by Telephone, Videotelephone, and Computer Videoconferencing

Kaplan EH (Univ of South Carolina, Columbia)

J Psychother Prac Res 6:227–237, 1997 4–31

Background.—Telepsychotherapy involves real-time counseling of patients via telephone, videotelephone, or computer videoconferencing. Two videophone cases were presented.

Types of Telecommunication Equipment.—Telephone contact has been used in the past mainly to facilitate therapy sessions for patients who travel or who are unwilling to come into the therapist's office. Videophone conferencing provides visual contact that improves communication for patients who are isolated because of health or distance problems. The better systems are expensive, costing in excess of $4,000. Costs are decreasing, and makers of various systems are striving for compatibility. Currently, prices vary from $20,000 to $30,000 per site.

Discussion.—Telepsychotherapy is best introduced after a long period of office treatment. Telepsychotherapy should not be used as a distancing mechanism by the patient but can be helpful with patients who are threatened by physical nearness. Videoconferencing is preferable to telephone counseling because with the former, the patient is visible, although physical affective manifestations are not always apparent during videoconferencing.

Conclusion.—Telepsychotherapy is indicated when a nearby psychotherapist is not available, when the patient travels and changes schedules frequently, or when the patient is physically or psychologically unable to travel to the office or has relocated. Telepsychotherapy is contraindicated when the patient is vulnerable to self-harm or harm to others or when psychiatric backup is unavailable. The use of telepsychotherapy is increasing. Some states require a license. Practitioners should seek legal advice regarding liability. Privacy is less easily assured on telephone lines, although encryption systems and unlisted lines for videotherapy sessions are available.

► Twenty years ago, a colleague of mine described to me how his psychoanalysis was continued via telephone after he had moved from the city in which his analyst lived. There are doubtless many other examples of such use of electronic communications for ongoing therapy. Given the geographic maldistribution of psychiatrists, I would expect to see this technique used more, especially when videotelephone and computer videoconferencing are less expensive and more widely available.

A. Tasman, M.D.

Education and Training

Difficulties in Integrating Spirituality Into Psychotherapy

Schultz-Ross RA, Gutheil TG (Univ of Hawaii, Honolulu; Harvard Med School, Boston)

J Psychother Prac Res 6:130–138, 1997 4–32

Objective.—Increased interest in spirituality can be defined as "deeply held beliefs that explain human nature, human relationships, and the course of events (or fate) in life and death, and that provide an underpinning for more loosely held thoughts or ideas." It has raised the issue of how to include such beliefs in psychotherapy.

Discussion.—Each therapist and each patient has an individual set of spiritual beliefs that needs to be assessed when trying to integrate spirituality into psychotherapy. The patient's basic belief system colors his or her perceptions of the value of psychotherapy and the patient's ability to reveal beliefs. The therapist's belief system may color perceptions of what is normal or abnormal and may affect the therapist's ability to help the patient. For the psychotherapist, separating the patient's psychopathologic and spiritual beliefs can become a daunting task. The therapist's view of progress as seen from his or her own belief system may differ from the patient's view, which is based on a different belief system. Other confounding factors included the fact that only 5% of psychotherapists have spiritual training, and many psychotherapists are uncomfortable with their own spirituality.

Recommendations.—Spirituality needs to be included in psychotherapy curricula, and spirituality must be separated from psychopathology. The impact on patients of the belief system of a therapist in training might benefit from exploration in a forum or symposium. Training in overcoming difficulties occurring when beliefs of patient and therapist diverge or converge can be provided. Through a framework of exploration, therapists can learn how to integrate spiritual factors into psychotherapy.

► Although this article is not solely about educational issues, it does address an issue regarding which all therapists need to become more educated. One issue involves the role of spiritual beliefs in individuals' lives. For too long, spiritual beliefs have been viewed as outside the purview of psychotherapeutic inquiry. Given the important role that spirituality plays for many people, such a view seems increasingly inappropriate. This article also highlights important concerns regarding the changing nature of psychotherapy. Increased emphasis on brief interventions, according to the authors, makes it less likely that spiritual issues will emerge and be adequately addressed. They suggest that this is unfortunate for many reasons, not the least of which is the adaptive function of spirituality for many individuals.

A. Tasman, M.D.

Countertransference: Its Continued Importance in Psychiatric Education

Rao NR, Meinzer AE, Berman SS (Brookdale Univ, Brooklyn, NY)
J Psychother Prac Res 6:1–11, 1997 4–33

Objective.—Because psychotherapy training is becoming a less important aspect of psychiatric training, countertransference training is in danger of falling by the wayside. Countertransference—all of the physician's reactions to the patient—can affect the physician's feeling about self, patient, and third parties and result in treatment failure, lawsuits, license revocation, and patient decompensation and suicide.

Discussion.—Raising awareness of countertransference and teaching management of such issues is an important part of resident training. Supervision of psychotherapy treatment by residents has been a longstanding training vehicle for dealing with boundaries in the relationship between therapist and patient. Training groups that support raising awareness of countertransference among residents are now offered in only 48% of residency programs. The benefits and efficacy of personal psychotherapy or psychoanalysis have not been objectively studied.

Conclusion.—Issues of countertransference arise in all areas of psychiatric practice—psychopharmacologic treatment, emergency situations, and managed care. Countertransference can give rise to sexual misconduct issues. Without training, residents will have difficulty recognizing countertransference when it arises. Training programs that enable residents to recognize and manage countertransference should be maintained and emphasized.

► This article exhorts training directors to not abandon thinking psychodynamically when training residents in psychotherapy. The importance of the concept of countertransference and the attendant requisite self-reflective abilities of the therapist should not be underemphasized. Clearly, countertransferential responses occur whether one is conducting psychoanalysis, brief psychodynamic therapy, cognitive behavioral therapy, or behavior therapy. The need for ongoing attention to countertransference in education is well highlighted in this article.

A. Tasman, M.D.

The Synergy of Group and Individual Psychotherapy Training
Dagg PKB, Evans JB (Univ of Ottawa, Ontario, Canada)
Am J Psychother 51:204–209, 1997 4–34

Objective.—Although traditional psychotherapy has emphasized the importance of individual sessions, some practitioners believe that training in group therapy can add another dimension to the trainee's therapy process by revealing aspects of a patient's behavior that can be manifested only in a group setting. Others believe it is important that a patient-centered focus should develop first and a relationship-centered focus second.

Cotherapy.—Cotherapy provides an opportunity for beginning therapists to practice in the presence of a supervising therapist or to compare their therapeutic decisions with those of other, more experienced practitioners.

Awareness of Dynamic Issues.—Learning to deal with group dynamics and increased anxiety levels, being able to observe a patient functioning in a variety of roles, and developing increased sensitivity to underlying issues are valuable experiences a beginning therapist can glean in group therapy training.

Conclusion.—Beginning therapists can practice under the supervision of another more experienced therapist, develop important listening skills, and compare their professional judgments with those of other practitioners. Group therapy training can heighten the skills that a beginning therapist will be called upon to use in individual therapy sessions.

► This brief article posits an interesting hypothesis, that is, whether simultaneous training in 2 separate modalities facilitates individual psychotherapy skills. Although the evidence for their position is given in only 3 brief vignettes, it is certainly an interesting hypothesis.

A. Tasman, M.D.

The Ecology of Psychotherapy Research

Anderson T, Strupp HH (Vanderbilt Univ)

J Consult Clin Psychol 64:776–782, 1996 4–35

Objective.—In psychological research, the experimental situation has an effect on the results of a study. The effects of the ecology of the experimental situation—as defined by the demand characteristics of the situation and the research instrumentation used—on the outcome of time-limited dynamic psychotherapy were examined using patient reports.

Methods.—Eighty patients with significant distress received short-term psychotherapy. Of the 80, 32 patients were seen by 16 private-practice therapists before the therapists were trained in time-limited dynamic psychotherapy (TLDP); 32 were seen after therapists were trained in TLDP; and 16 were seen during therapists' training. Interviews were conducted with the 59 patients who completed the study. Blinded raters compared outcomes with ecology ratings, patients' awareness of the goals of the experiment and the degree to which they identified with those goals (demand characteristics), and patients' experiences with tape recorders and questionnaires used in clinical settings (instrumentation variables).

Results.—Among patients who were highly aware of their roles as "subjects," patients in the posttraining group improved more than patients in the pretraining group. There was no difference between the pretraining and posttraining groups who had a low awareness of their role as subjects. Among patients who were highly aware of their roles as subjects, patients in the posttraining group had higher therapeutic exploratory process scores than did patients in the pretraining group. Many high-awareness patients in the pretraining group felt used and manipulated during the study, whereas high-awareness patients in the posttraining group wanted more involvement and found the study valuable. Therapists were less likely to adhere to TLDP-specific strategies with high-awareness patients but may have accidentally reassured them by not using recommended interventions, thereby drawing attention away from the study. Alternatively, therapists, after training, may have developed better techniques for answering patients' concerns so that patients no longer felt manipulated and used.

Conclusion.—Outcomes can be influenced by patients' fears that they are not performing correctly, feelings that they are being manipulated, curiosity about the instruments used, delight in the attention received as "subjects," or desire to be helped by the study. Studies of these ecological influences can benefit both therapist and patient.

► This important study highlights the effect on outcome of awareness of being in a research study. Clearly, this is an area in which further research must be done, especially psychotherapy outcome research, as patient expectations affect psychotherapy outcome in many ways. It should not be surprising, therefore, that awareness of being part of a research study would have an impact on outcome.

A. Tasman, M.D.

Random Versus Nonrandom Assignment in Controlled Experiments: Do You Get the Same Answer?

Shadish WR, Ragsdale K (Univ of Memphis, Tenn)

J Consult Clin Psychol 64:1290–1305, 1996 4–36

Background.—Many psychotherapy researchers use both randomized and nonrandomized (nonequivalent control group) designs to conduct their studies. But do both types of studies give the same results? These researchers analyzed both individual studies and meta-analyses to see if the results with randomized and nonrandomized designs are indeed the same.

Methods.—The authors reviewed 100 studies of marital or family psychotherapy (n = 84) or enrichment (n = 16) that met the following criteria: (1) posttest treatments were compared with control conditions rather than other treatments, (2) data were sufficient to allow calculation of an exact standardized mean difference, (3) the direction of a positive outcome was clear, and (4) the assignment of participants to groups was clear and orderly. The effect size and 12 different factors were coded, including the assignment method (random or not), self-selection vs. other means of selection for assignments, and sample size.

Findings.—The 64 randomized experiments had a significantly larger weighted effect size (d = 0.60) than that of the 36 nonrandomized designs (d = 0.08). Not only were mean posttest results higher in the randomized studies, but also they varied less. Even when other covariates were controlled for in regression analysis, randomized experiments still achieved a significantly larger weight effect size (d = 0.75) than nonrandomized studies (d = 0.48).

Conclusions.—Results of randomized studies are not the same as those of nonrandomized studies. This finding has particular ramifications for meta-analyses that include both types of studies. When they can be conducted, randomized studies remain the best method for collecting and analyzing data.

► Many individuals suggest that the double-blind, placebo-controlled design of many psychopharmacologic trials is the appropriate ideal model for psychotherapy research. Further, the use of meta-analysis has been increasing as a method for adding power to findings from numerous small studies. These authors call into question both aspects of these approaches to research and suggest that perhaps outcome is influenced in ways that have not been given adequate attention. The implications of their thinking for design of future research studies is not insignificant and should be given greater thought.

A. Tasman, M.D.

Contribution of the Therapeutic Alliance to Outcome in Active Versus Control Psychotherapies

Carroll KM, Nich C, Rounsaville BJ (Yale Univ, New Haven, Conn)
J Consult Clin Psychol 65:510–514, 1997 4–37

Background.—Although therapeutic alliance is generally considered a robust predictor of positive outcome, few data exist about its role in active vs. control psychotherapeutic interventions. These authors used a randomized trial of coping skills in cocaine treatment (CB) vs. medical management alone (CM) to determine whether the level of the therapeutic alliance had different effects on outcome in active vs. control treatments.

Methods.—Over a 12-week trial, 121 people with cocaine dependence were randomly assigned to 4 groups: CB + desipramine, CM + desipramine, CB + placebo, or CM + placebo. Participants were long-time users of cocaine (average 4.2 years, 4.4 g/week), and almost a third had received prior dependency treatment. Outcome measures were how long the participants remained in treatment, how long they abstained from cocaine while in treatment (measured by urinalysis), their Addiction Severity Index score, and how many urine toxicology screenings were free of drugs during treatment. Five trained raters provided process ratings of therapeutic alliance according to the Vanderbilt Therapeutic Alliance Scale.

Findings.—Raters found significantly higher therapeutic alliance in CB sessions than in CM sessions. This effect was not explained by differences in therapists. Regression analysis showed that the level of the therapeutic alliance had a small, but significant, effect on outcomes.

Conclusions.—Therapeutic alliance and outcome differed between the treatments, with active treatment showing better results than the control treatment. On most outcome measures, therapeutic alliance scores were significantly associated with outcome in active treatments but not in control treatments. The relation between the therapeutic alliance rating and the level of active treatment was significantly stronger than that between the therapeutic alliance rating and the level of control treatment, which suggests that processes in active and control treatments may differ.

▶ This is another study that begins to address the role of therapeutic alliance in outcome and how this might be a confounding variable even in control groups. Clearly, further research is needed to better elucidate this issue.

A. Tasman, M.D.

Psychotherapy of Depression: Implications of Reform of the Health Care System

Clarkin JF, Pilkonis PA, Magruder KM (New York Hosp-Cornell Univ, White Plains, NY; Univ of Pittsburgh, Pa; Natl Inst of Mental Health, Bethesda, Md)

Arch Gen Psychiatry 53:717–723, 1996 4–38

Objective.—Depression can be treated by medication and by psychotherapy. The role of psychotherapy and an overview of research into new areas of psychotherapy that enhance the cost effectiveness of treatment in the emerging health care system were discussed.

Evidence Supporting a Role for Psychotherapy.—Psychosocial therapy during the acute phase of depression has been shown to improve interpersonal, behavioral, and cognitive functioning more than short-term dynamic psychotherapy. Improvements after cognitive therapy plus drug therapy last longer than after drug therapy alone. During the maintenance phase, interpersonal therapy combined with drug therapy is effective in hindering recurrence. Results of continued treatment with a combination of psychosocial and drug therapies vary because the modality affects different functional areas. To elevate the status of psychosocial treatment from an experimental intervention to standard practice, treatments must be proven to be effective in large populations and in a variety of settings. Minimum standards of care must be established, guidelines must be developed, and the intervention must be embraced by managed care companies.

Implications for a National Health Care System.—Additional research needs to be conducted to provide information regarding individualizing treatment, better detection of depression and provision of treatment, effective use of psychotherapy, consideration of patient treatment preferences, and the duration and cost effectiveness of treatment.

Conclusion.—Additional large studies are needed to establish the effectiveness and cost effectiveness of psychotherapy for depression.

► We are all well aware that we have significant gaps in our knowledge regarding psychotherapy outcome. This valuable study provides an overview of what it known and what is yet to be discovered. It provides an important voice supporting the notion that valid reform of our health care delivery system cannot be adequately accomplished without this knowledge base.

A. Tasman, M.D.

Patients' View of the Alliance in Psychotherapy: Exploratory Factors Analysis of Three Alliance Measures

Hatcher RL, Barends AW (Univ of Michigan, Ann Arbor)

J Consult Clin Psychol 64:1326–1336, 1996 4–39

Introduction.—The basis of important findings in psychotherapy research has been measures of the alliance in psychotherapy. Alliance measures have been able to predict therapeutic outcome, and there is a high correlation between the components of alliance and the subscales within each measure; however, more investigation is needed on the association between the individual and the joint dimensionality of these measures. Little is known about patients' ratings of alliance measures using exploratory factor analysis. Patients' responses to 3 widely used measures of the alliance—the Working Alliance Inventory, the California Psychotherapy Alliance Scales and the Penn Helping Alliance Questionnaire—were explored.

Methods.—There were 231 outpatients and therapists who participated in the 5-year study. Most patients had neurotic problems, such as depression, anxiety, and relationship problems, and they had treatments ranging from less than 1 month to 4 years. They were measured with the 3 alliance measures as a measure of improvement to date. The factor structures that emerged from the exploratory factor analysis of patients' responses were compared to the a priori structures (the subscales) established by the measures' authors, and the importance of these factors was assessed in relation to the patients' estimates of improvement to date in therapy.

Results.—There were high correlations between the total scores of the 3 measures, indicating the presence of a strong general factor. Patients' estimate of improvement correlated with 2 of 6 factors, Confident Collaboration and Idealized Relationship, with the substantial general factor removed. The core of the alliance was viewed by patients as a purposive mutual collaboration, or working alliance. Patients did better in therapy if they acknowledged some hostility. Established subscales were resembled by 3 other factors—Goals and Tasks, Bond, and Dedicated Patient; they were unrelated to improvement beyond the general factor.

Conclusion.—In alliance theory and measurement, the collaborative working alliance should be given prominence. Limitations of this study included the fact that the therapists have varying amounts of experience and that therapies were sampled at various stage of development. Views from patients of diverse socioeconomic and cultural groups should be sampled in the future, as this sample was predominantly white and middle class.

► This is another study looking at the role of the alliance in psychotherapy outcome. The authors highlight, correctly, I believe, that research into the therapeutic alliance should include both patient's and therapist's views of the alliance, as well as views assessed longitudinally rather than just cross-sectionally. How the view of the alliance changes across therapy and its effect on outcome are not yet known.

A. Tasman, M.D.

The Role of Avoidance and Obsessiveness in Matching Patients to Cognitive Interpersonal Psychotherapy: Empirical Findings From the Treatment for Depression Collaborative Research Program

Barber JP, Muenz LR (Univ of Pennsylvania, Philadelphia)

J Consult Clin Psychol 64:951–958, 1996 4–40

Introduction.—One of the main goals of psychotherapy is matching patients to specific psychotherapies, not a simple task. There are ongoing treatment development studies on 2 different therapies of 2 specific personality disorders: obsessive-compulsive personality disorder and avoidant personality disorder. Cognitive therapy and supportive-expressive dynamic therapy are the treatments used for these independent studies. The initial results showed that cognitive therapy was somewhat more effective than supportive-expressive dynamic therapy for the avoidant personality disorder, whereas supportive-expressive therapy was somewhat more effective for the obsessive-compulsive personality disorder. The implications from the ongoing study were tested by examining data from the Treatment for Depression Collaborative Research Program. In this program, the efficacy of cognitive therapy, interpersonal psychotherapy, and pharmacotherapy for patients was examined.

Methods.—There were 250 outpatients included in the study with a minimum score of 14 on the 17–item Hamilton Rating Scale for Depression. They were randomly assigned to cognitive therapy, interpersonal therapy, imipramine plus clinical management, or placebo plus clinical management. The completer sample included patients who completed at least 12 sessions and 15 weeks of treatment. To assess treatment efficacy, the Hamilton Scale and the Beck Depression Inventory were used.

Results.—The expected interactions between cognitive therapy and interpersonal therapy and avoidance and between treatment and obsessiveness were found. Marital status and treatment was also found to be a significant interaction, showing that married patients did better after cognitive therapy, whereas noncohabitating and single patients improved more after interpersonal therapy. Similar results were found with the Hamilton Rating Scale for Depression and the Beck Depression Inventory.

Conclusion.—These results contradict previous studies, which assumed that all psychotherapies are effective. These results show that, although 2 treatments may appear to be equivalent, they may be differentially effective for different kinds of patients. Further, empirical attention is needed to match patients to treatment and to examine the dimensions of obsessiveness and avoidance.

► This is a useful contribution to our ongoing quest to find factors in patients that have predictive value regarding psychotherapy outcome with different modalities. These investigators highlight the need for more research in this area so we can more rationally prescribe psychotherapy.

A. Tasman, M.D.

Theory Building

Bridging Barriers Between Paradigms: Making Cognitive Concepts Relevant for Behavior Analysis

Hawkins RP, Forsyth JP (West Virginia Univ, Morgantown)

J Behav Ther Exp Psychiatry 28:3–6, 1997 4–41

Introduction.—The behavior therapy movement was consistent with behavioral science, emphasizing the stimulus-response relations, or Pavlovian conditioning, and this began in 1919. Another approach began in the 1950s. It was called applied behavior analysis and used the findings of basic research. Behavior analysts do not prefer mixing paradigms, but rather prefer to stick with one consistent paradigm. There have been disputes about the values of using a consistent behavior approach vs. a mixed cognitive-behavior approach.

Working Together.—The Association for Advancement of Behavior Therapy has members that include cognitive-behavior therapists and applied behavior analysts, and both groups strive to enhance constructive communication between each other to develop effective, responsible science-based clinical practices. Although the 2 approaches may not be integrated, there is much to learn from each method.

Differences.—The concept of "attachment" or "bonding" is viewed differently by the 2 camps. Behavior analysts would say that, in a child's first year of life, the environment comprises attachment, whereas cognitive therapists would use terms such as "reflecting," "indicating," or being "symptomatic." Nevertheless, behavior analysts cannot ignore the components that comprise the phenomenon.

Collaboration.—Behavior analysts can learn from looking at the cognitive literature, and their cognitive colleagues can learn by examining the behavior analytic literature. The field of psychology can be enhanced by contributions from both groups.

Cognition in Behavior Therapy: Agreements and Differences

Wilson KG, Hayes SC, Gifford EV (Univ of Nevada, Reno)

J Behav Ther Exp Psychiatry 28:53–63, 1997 4–42

Introduction.—At a theoretical and philosophical level, the differences between cognitive and behavior analytic approaches to cognition are irreconcilable. However, the therapists possess a large body of shared values in spite of the major differences between these positions, and the potential for unified effort still exists. At the level of a mutual interest in cognition and shared empirical values, a rapprochement may be possible.

Behavior therapy.—Methodological behavior and behavior analysis are 2 important streams in behavior therapy. Methodological behavior advocates object to introspection because all variables must be publicly observable. Later, this evolved into modem cognitive theory, which has more flexible association models, and more flexible cognitive mediational constructs in the form of attitudes, beliefs, and schemata were added. Behavior analytic theorists said that thinking, imagining, feeling, and other private events were open to direct scientific analysis, but this did not lead to a psychology of cognition, perhaps because the earliest behavior therapists worked primarily with children, the developmentally disabled, and institutionalized adults.

Cognition.—With the demands of working with adults, the focus turned to what clients think, and flexible cognitive mediational constructs have developed. Cognition means "to know," and with this method, human beings relate events and symbols mutually and in combination. Cognition is behavior that can readily alter the functions of other events symbolically. Cognition does not have a causal role, but plays an important role in the regulation of other forms of behavior. The analytic task is understanding the context in which the irrational cognition occurred when an irrational cognition leads to destructive forms of social behavior.

Conclusion.—A core of shared values exists in behavior therapy, and even controversial topics have an arena for reconciliation. What used to be a difference in content between these 2 theories is now a difference in approach to the same content. More thorough analyses may be possible with rapprochement around agreed-upon content areas.

► Perhaps it is merely my chauvinistic point of view, but it seems to me that in no area of medicine has progress been more impeded than in psychiatry by disputes over theoretical concepts. Of course, my position could be the result of a lack of knowledge about other areas of medical research. These 2 articles (Abstracts 4–41 and 4–42) discuss the nature of the theoretical debate between cognitive and behavior therapists. Both sets of authors argue that the need to move beyond theoretical argument is essential for clinical progress to occur. This is a position that I wholeheartedly support.

A. Tasman, M.D.

An Information Processing Model of Anxiety: Automatic and Strategic Processes

Beck AT, Clark DA (Univ of Pennsylvania, Philadelphia; Univ of New Brunswick, Fredericton, Canada)

Behav Res Ther 35:49–58, 1997 4–43

Introduction.—Information processing paradigms derived from experimental cognitive psychology and social psychology have increasingly been turned to for the treatment of anxiety disorders to understand the cognitive basis of anxiety. Specific anxiety disorders, such as panic disorder, social phobia, obsessive-compulsive disorder, and generalized anxiety disorder, have been associated with cognitive theories. Some of the research questions raised about the cognitive basis of anxiety include whether selective processing of threat is specific to anxiety vs. other emotional states; whether automatic or strategic modes of information processing dominate in anxiety, and whether threat bias in anxiety should be considered a state or trait phenomenon.

Registration and Preparation.—A very rapid, automatic recognition of a stimulus is the first stage of processing threat information. At this stage, there are low levels of cognitive processing, with very little higher level or semantic analysis occurring. The next stage in processing threat is immediate preparation, which seeks to ensure the individual's survival by maximizing safety and minimizing danger. Responses include autonomic arousal, behavioral mobilization and inhibition, primal thinking, a feeling of fear, and hypervigilance for threat cues. At this stage, processing is rigid and dichotomous, with a corresponding intolerance for ambiguity or uncertainty.

Secondary Elaboration.—Elaborative semantic processing is the next stage, which is characteristically slow, effortful, yet involuntary, because of the activation of the primal mode. There is more reflective consideration of the correct context and coping resources. The effectiveness of coping resources is re-evaluated. An important process in maintaining clinical anxiety may be failing to elaborate and process the attributes or features of the threatening stimulus at the strategic level. By a constructive reappraisal of the situation, an individual can downgrade the probability of the severity of the threat and can upgrade the ability to cope.

Conclusion.—In an effective treatment of anxiety, some degree of verbal mediation is necessary. More elaborative, strategic processing of information resulting from the activation of the constructive, reflexive modes of thinking is one of the most effective ways of deactivating the primal threat mode. Exposure is important in anxiety reduction. Anxiety is excessive or inappropriate generation of threat meaning assigned in response to a situation that is innocuous.

► The development of effective treatments best occurs when specific information about the cause of the illness is available. Unfortunately, the presence of psychiatric symptoms is a clinical phenomenon that thus far has defied the gathering of a body of indisputable data regarding etiology of nearly every psychiatric disorder. The understanding of the cause of anxiety, although attempted as far back as Sigmund Freud's early writings, still eludes us, but Beck provides yet another model for understanding anxiety. It remains to be seen whether this model will be more useful than previous ones, but it should be of interest to all those who are interested in better understanding clinical phenomena.

A. Tasman, M.D.

Factors in the Etiology and Pathogenesis of Panic Disorder: Revisiting the Attachment-Separation Paradigm

Shear MK (Univ of Pittsburgh, Pa)

Am J Psychiatry 153:125–136, 1996 4–44

Introduction.—Separation anxiety may be at the root of panic disorder, and there may be genetic factors that predispose to panic attack. One definition of the panic attack is the driving force for anticipatory anxiety and phobic avoidance. Conditioning, avoidance, and mental representations are psychological mechanisms that take on a secondary role. The current status of attachment theory as it relates to patients with agoraphobia or panic disorder and the early neurobiological theory of panic disorder were reviewed, along with recent neurobiological studies indicating that disturbances in early attachment produce long-lasting effects on neurotransmitter systems implicated in anxiety.

Attachment.—In the generation and relief of anxiety, attachment and separation have specific roles. A stimulus for acute anxiety and a predisposing factor for a variety of fear reactions is separation from an attachment figure. A foundation for development of a sense of controllability and predictability is the maternal-infant relationship. An intensely distressing affective response called separation anxiety can be regularly evoked by separation from an attachment figure during early childhood. Aberrant family interaction patterns may be the basis for agoraphobia, a clinical condition explained as a disorder of anxious attachment. Frequent absence of parental figures, threats of abandonment, or parental quarreling are related to anxious attachment.

Childhood Anxiety.—There is support for an association between adult panic disorder and childhood separation anxiety disorder. In families significantly more frequently in panic disorder, a study found an association with chronic anxiety in childhood, childhood depression, and affective disorder and alcoholism. Another review of the literature found more childhood separation anxiety among agoraphobic subjects than among normal controls. There is a strong relationship between general and childhood separation anxiety and adult anxiety disorder.

Conclusion.—More dysfunctional parenting or a higher frequency of parental loss and greater relevance of childhood anxiety was found among subjects with panic disorder than with normal controls. The nature of the relationship between early attachment and adult cognitive functioning should be refined to develop a detailed classification system that may help with predictions.

► This is a very good and readable review of what we know about the neurobiology of panic. Shear focuses her efforts on work relating to attachment and childhood anxiety. This thorough overview, however, highlights how much we still have left to learn.

A. Tasman, M.D.

Affect, Attachment, Memory: Contributions Toward Psychobiologic Integration

Amini F, Lewis T, Lannon R, et al (Langley Porter Psychiatric Inst, San Francisco)

Psychiatry 59:213–239, 1996 4–45

Introduction.—A sophisticated understanding of the physiology of the human brain has only recently surfaced to help treat emotional dysfunction. The complex relationships between the psychological and biological dimensions of human emotional dysfunction are now better understood, but need to be more integrated. The basic brain functions of affect, attachment, and memory have biological and physiologic substrates and have interrelationships. Clinically meaningful psychodynamic conceptualizations should result from illustrating findings from neurobiology.

Affect.—Powerful motivators of behavior, affects also have an important biological component noticed in the heart rate, blood pressure, and respiratory rate. Charles Darwin viewed affects as a behavioral function to advance survival and reproductive fitness. This view includes affects as an intrinsic part of the neurobehavioral repertoire. Later, it was brought out that there is a set of universal basic emotions and that the same set of facial expressions exist universally for sadness, anger, disgust, contempt, surprise, happiness, and fear. The brain is divided into 3 parts—the brain stem, the neocortex, and the lymbic system. The brain stem contains systems that have been implicated in the pathophysiology of depressive and anxiety syndromes The lymbic system is interrelated to the endocrine system and involved in learning and memory processes. Complex social behaviors have been localized to limbic regions, including the separation cry, affiliative behaviors, and maternal and rearing behaviors. The neocortex is involved in language, abstraction, strategic planning, and symbolic representation.

Attachment.—Attachment behaviors have predictable outcomes of maintaining proximity and contact with the mother and promote the security of an infant by forming a bond with its mother. The attachment figure is used by the child as a secure base from which to explore the world. The problem-solving styles of 2-year-olds, teachers' rating of the children's general affect and social competency of 3½-year-olds, and behavioral problems of 6-year-olds can be predicted by the children's previously evaluated attachment pattern. Short-term effects of separation from attachment figures manifest in the protest response and the despair response. Long-term effects result in the isolation syndrome or individuals are socially incompetent and cannot engage in normal reciprocal interactions with others. The long-term effects of partially inattentive mothering include being less able to engage in affiliative social contacts as adults, timidity, subordination, and more vulnerability to depression.

Conclusion.—An enduring neural structure that influences both emotional self-regulation and behavior concerning relatedness is implicit memory of the early attachment relationship, communicated via the language of affect. Psychotherapy will need to integrate the workings of the brain to findings of emotional life as they are manifested in clinical psychiatric settings. Further studies should explore the interplay between emotional experience and neurophysiology.

► These authors also focus on the interface of neurobiology and experience of relationships, especially early in life. We need to have more research, which I am sure will be forthcoming over the coming decades, to elucidate whether or not this approach to understanding is valid.

A. Tasman, M.D.

Reliability and Convergence of Three Concepts of Narcissistic Personality

Perry JD, Perry JC (Harvard Med School, Boston)

Psychiatry 59:4–19, 1996 4–46

Introduction.—A number of clinical descriptions of narcissistic traits, conditions, and pathologic processes have been reported, but little empirical investigation has been conducted of these constructs. Three descriptive systems for assessing narcissistic personality were examined for their reliability, convergence, and factor structure. This was an independent attempt to identify narcissistic features that are most useful for describing patients with narcissistic personality.

Methods.—There were 107 patients, ranging in age from 18 to 45 years, who participated in this study and who agreed to be videotaped during a dynamically conducted interview. The patients were selected from emergency room and outpatient settings, advertisements in the local newspaper, and the probation department of the local district court. The interviews were semistructured and diagnostic and lasted more than 2 hours in which 20 major areas were explored, such as family of origin, work, and intimate relationships. Participants were then given a narcissistic personality disorder score. The 3 descriptions compared were: DSM-III-R, Akhtar and Thomson, and Kernberg.

Results.—There were 7 patients with definite narcissistic personality disorder, 27 with significant narcissistic features, and 73 with few or no narcissistic features. There were fair to moderately good reliabilities that indicated stability of the DSM-III-R description, and there was fair reliability overall of the Akhtar and Thomson's description. There were moderately good reliabilities with Kernberg's description

Conclusion.—Even though the reliability of individual criteria varies widely, narcissistic features can be reliably assessed from videotaped interviews. Although there was great variability within individual items, the reliability of each scale was acceptable. Each scale was highly correlated with each of the other scales and was moderately, but not highly, internally consistent and homogeneous. In the clinical constructs underlying each scale, there are discrete differences, according to factor analysis. The evidence for the convergent, discriminant, and predictive validity of the factors derived from the 3 constructs still needs to be examined.

▶ The authors note that, although the criteria for a borderline personality disorder diagnosis has become well documented and validated, research in other personality disorders has lagged far behind. One reason for this is the lack of an agreed-upon underlying construct that has etiologic and treatment significance. The authors take on this task in narcissistic personality disorder. One hopes that this approach could be used for a variety of personality disorders and lead to well-designed clinical studies.

A. Tasman, M.D.

Change in Object and Self-representations in Long-term, Intensive, Inpatient Treatment of Seriously Disturbed Adolescents and Young Adults

Blatt SJ, Stayner DA, Auerbach JS, et al (Yale Univ, New Haven, Conn)
Psychiatry 59:82–107, 1996 4–47

Introduction.—In psychoanalytic theory and research and in developmental psychology, mental representation is a central theory. Early interactions with primary caregivers are transformed by children into cognitive-affective schemas of self and other that direct and regulate subsequent behavior. The imprint of significant interpersonal interactions and the developmental level and other important aspects of the individual's psychic life are borne by the cognitive-affective schema of self and other. How one thinks and feels about others and about oneself are influenced by the templates or prototypes of cognitive-affective schemas. There are some connections between specific disturbances in the structure of cognitive-affective schemas and different forms of psychopathology. In the first 18 months of life, the child establishes internal working models of attachment relationships according to the behavioral and cognitive consistency of attachment patterns. During the treatment process, the relationship of changes in the structure and content of schemas of self and significant others is studied and compared to an independent assessment of change in clinical functioning.

Methods.—There were 40 seriously disturbed inpatients with a complex array of diagnoses, such as conduct disorder, major depression with and without psychotic features, schizophrenia, and substance abuse disorders. Open-ended descriptions of self and significant others were solicited from these patients during intensive, long-term, inpatient treatment that included psychotherapy 3 times weekly. Changes in cognitive-structural and qualitative-thematic dimension of these descriptions of self and significant caregivers, such as other, father, and therapist, were examined every 6 months thereafter until termination. Changes in these representations were compared with changes in the level of psychological functioning.

Results.—There was a significant negative correlation with the initial level of clinical function and the conceptual level of the descriptions of both mother and father. At the beginning of hospitalization, increased investment in the description of significant others was characteristic of more disturbed patients. There was a highly significant positive correlation between the degree of differentiation-relatedness for the self-description and the initial level of clinical functioning. Highly significant relationships were found between the descriptions of mother, therapist, and self and the degree of clinical improvement and increased differentiation-relatedness. Increased articulation in the descriptions of father, mother, and therapist showed a relationship with the degree of clinical improvement. An increase in the benevolent factor for the description of the therapist correlated significantly with clinical improvement in the description of the father; however, improved clinical functioning correlated with a decrease in the benevolent factor, with the father described as less constructively involved, less warm, and less nurturant. With the mother, improved clinical functioning was related to a description of her as being warmer.

Conclusion.—With seriously disturbed patients, more reciprocal relationships should be established with the mother and therapist, but a greater sense of separation and individuation should be established from the father. Understanding of both the psychopathology and the therapeutic process with seriously disturbed young adults has been facilitated by the clinical research procedure of asking patients periodically throughout treatment to describe self and significant others.

▶ The notion of the capacity to form mental representations forms, as these authors accurately point out, much of the way we understand psychological development. This article demonstrates that this theoretical construct can be operationalized and used to carry out clinical research. It is just this type of study, in which psychoanalytic theoretical concepts are studied clinically, that will provide the most important advances in our understanding of mental life. One would hope that many more such studies would be forthcoming.

A. Tasman, M.D.

Additional Reading

Caligor E: Annotated psychodynamic bibliography for residents in psychiatry. *J Psychother Pract Res* 5:318–340, 1996.

▶ This paper is just what it states: an annotated bibliography. It includes both current and historically interesting papers and covers the field in a reasonable way. Any resident who managed to read all of these articles by the end of residency would be well-grounded in the literature regarding psychodynamic psychotherapy.

McCarthy MK: Fast forward: The need for videotaping in psychotherapy training today. *Harvard Rev Psychiatry* 3:166–168, 1995.

▶ It seems surprising, given the advances in electronic communications, that videotaped psychotherapy supervision is not more widely utilized. Dr. McCarthy suggests that this can be a useful approach to psychotherapy supervision, especially, in my view, with residents in training.

A. Tasman, M.D.

5 Alcohol- and Substance-Related Disorders

Introduction

Recent trends in the addiction field include an increase in the use of marijuana, tobacco, and cocaine in the teenage years, and an explosion in public interest in tobacco addiction. The problem with tobacco addiction is culminating in agreements which are being worked out as tobacco companies settle large claims made by states and the federal government resulting from years of unsavory practices by the industry. There has been an increase in penetration of managed care into treatment of addictions with greater restrictions on care at all levels, especially inpatient and outpatient detoxification. There has been increasing controversy about trying to find alternatives to prison as a principal approach to treating addiction in the United States.

This year's selections cover topics related to: etiology (Abstracts 5–1, 5–2 and 5–3), diagnosis and comorbidity (Abstracts 5–4 through 5–10), pharmacologic treatment (Abstracts 5–11 through 5–15), and treatment and outcomes (Abstracts 5–16 through 5–21). There have been no new major discoveries about the etiology of addictive disorders. However, this year's selections deal with some of the usual issues, such as the contribution of genetics vs. environmental influences (Abstract 5–1), means of subtyping alcoholics on the basis of central serotonergic functions (Abstract 5–2) and the self-medication hypothesis (Abstract 5–3). One major focus of addiction psychiatry relates to diagnosis and comorbidity issues, and Abstracts 5–4 through 5–10 cover innovations in this area.

Abstract 5–4 highlights the value of keeping severity criteria in the diagnostic system. Abstracts 5–5 and 5–6 deal with primary and secondary diagnostic issues. Abstract 5–7 looks at comorbidity and opioid abusers and Abstracts 5–8 and 5–9 deal with schizophrenia and substance abuse. It has always fascinated me that American writers tend to develop alcoholism, while Japanese writers tend to suicide, and Abstract 5–10 deals with the relationship between creativity, depression, and alcoholism.

A high priority for research in the addiction field has been the development of new pharmacologic treatments (Abstracts 5–11 through 5–15). A fine review article by Marc Schuckit summarizes results in this area while playing to a need for the development of further studies in order to develop better pharmacologic treatments for alcoholism. Naltrexone, a promising new drug to treat alcoholism, has not yet been proven to warrant widespread use, according to Schuckit. An exciting new development has been the report of positive results in relapse prevention for acamprosate, a drug that has received favorable reviews in Europe but is not yet approved by the Food and Drug Administration in the United States. Abstracts 5–13 and 5–14 point to the promise of buprenorphine as giving good results for opioid dependence and the possibility that primary care–based buprenorphine maintenance could rapidly expand the amount of treatment availability for opioid addiction. Abstract 5–15 deals with the importance of having intravenous drug users with HIV disease adhere to taking zidovudine and some of the problems that occur with psychiatric comorbidity leading to treatment resistance.

The last section deals with perhaps the most important issue facing the addiction field, which is studying treatments and outcomes (Abstracts 5–16 through 5–21). Ambulatory detoxification is rapidly becoming a first choice treatment for alcoholism, as well as other drug abuse, based on the kind of research reviewed in Abstract 5–16. Wrap around support treatments can be vital in achieving retention in prenatal substance abuse treatment programs (Abstract 5–17). Relapse prevention in alcohol programs can be aided by using the laboratory test described in Abstract 5–18. Abstract 5–19 emphasizes the importance of needle exchange programs in preventing HIV transmission and makes suggestions for changes in laws that can lead to greater community safety. The high success rates of impaired physicians' programs is well illustrated in Abstract 5–20. Wouldn't it be wonderful if we could get such high success rates for all categories of addicted patients? Unfortunately, patient characteristics seem to have bigger effects than advances in effecting treatment outcome. Abstract 5–21 provides a survey of cost of employee assistance programs which gives a sense of how cost effective and worthwhile these kinds of programs have been for the 54,000 work sites that use them. We need to continue the search for better psychopharmacologic agents that help both in the treatment of addictions and comorbidity, as well as in further studying which combinations of treatment work best for which individuals. The fact that efforts at treatment matching to date have not panned out as well as some of us would hope should not stop us from doing research which can serve as a sound basis for developing better treatment guidelines. Only as we improve our empirical base will the guidelines we develop achieve a level of validity that leads to productive results

Richard J. Frances, M.D.

Etiology

Indicators of Genetic and Enviromental Influences in Drug Abusing Individuals

Johnson EO, van den Bree MBM, Uhl GR, et al (Natl Inst on Drug Abuse, Baltimore, Md)

Drug Alcohol Depend 41:17–23, 1996 5–1

Background.—Estimates of liability variance caused by genes and shared and nonshared environment do not show the relative contribution of genetic and environmental factors to drug dependence. Methods have been proposed for determining the contributions of genetic and environmental influences using simulation and blood pressure data. A recent report proposed that separate scales be used to estimate genetic and environmental influences in alcohol-dependent individuals. The scales were based on alcohol symptom items from the National Institute of Mental Health Diagnostic Interview Schedule (DIS). The development of separate scales for estimating genetic and environmental influences in individuals with drug dependence was reported.

Methods.—Data were obtained from 73 male twin pairs who met Diagnostic and Statistical Manual of Mental Disorders, ed III criteria for drug abuse or dependence. There were 38 monozygotic (MZ) pairs and 35 dizygotic (DZ) pairs. Items were included in the genetic scale if they had significant MZ/DZ differences in probandwise concordance. Items were included in the environmental scale if they did not have significant MZ/DZ differences.

Results.—As predicted, there were significant differences between MZ and DZ twins in intraclass correlations for the genetic scale, but not for the environmental scale. A correlation was seen between genetic scores on drug and alcohol scales, but no such correlation was seen between environmental scores. A comparison of scores on genetic scales showed that the correlation between drug and alcohol scores within individuals was

TABLE 4.—Cross-Twin Partial Correlation Analysis of Genetic and Environmental Drug Abuse/Dependence Scales and Alcohol Dependence Scales

	Within twin*,†	Cross-MZ	Cross-DZ
Gentic drug with genetic alcohol	0.47‡	0.41§	−0.17
Environmental drug with environmental alcohol	0.19	0.09	0.39

*One-tailed test.

†All correlation coefficients are partial Spearman rank correlations controlling first for environmental and then genetic scales, respectively.

‡$P = 0.001$.

§$P < 0.05$.

(Reprinted from Johnson EO, van den Bree MBM, Uhl GR, et al: Indicators of genetic and environmental influences in drug abusing individuals. *Drug Alcohol Depend* 41:17–23, copyright 1996 with kind permission from Elsevier Science Ireland Ltd., Bay 15K, Shannon Industrial State, Co. Clare, Ireland.)

similar to the correlation across MZ twins. Both of these correlations were higher than the correlation across DZ twins (Table 4).

Discussion.—These findings indicate that the relative contribution of genetic and environmental factors to drug dependence can be evaluated in affected individuals and that common genetic factors may be at work in both alcohol and drug dependence.

▶ A number of twin studies and other studies have demonstrated familial and genetic contributions to alcoholism and addictive disorders. This study finds a common genetic mechanism for both alcoholism and other drug dependence. Parceling out the amount of environmental and genetic influence can be helpful in subtyping individuals based on the relative contributions of genetic and environmental influences.

R.J. Frances, M.D.

Behavioral and Neuroendocrine Responses to *m*-Chlorophenylpiperazine in Subtypes of Alcoholics and in Healthy Comparison Subjects

George DT, Benkelfat C, Rawlings RR, et al (Natl Inst on Alcohol Abuse and Alcoholism, Bethesda, Md; Natl Inst of Mental Health, Bethesda, Md; Natl Inst of Mental Health, Rockville, Md, et al)

Am J Psychiatry 154:81–87, 1997 5–2

Background.—In a recent study, the serotonin (5-HT) uptake inhibitor clomipramine was administered to abstinent alcohol-dependent patients and healthy control subjects. There were no significant differences in behavioral or neuroendocrine response between these groups. It was hypothesized that alterations in 5-HT function may only occur in certain types of 5-HT receptors or certain subgroups of alcohol-dependent individuals.

Methods.—The subjects were 40 male alcohol-dependent patients, 16 type I (late onset) and 24 type II (early onset with antisocial traits), and 22 healthy control subjects. Before and after infusion of *m*-chlorophenylpiperazine (*m*-CPP), psychological, physiologic, and neuroendocrine responses were measured.

Results.—The subtypes of alcoholics displayed different behavioral responses after infusion of *m*-CPP. Type I alcoholics reported more anger and anxiety and type II alcoholics reported more euphoria and drinking (Fig 1). The control subjects had a greater increase in plasma corticotropin response to *m*-CPP than either subtype of alcoholics.

Discussion.—Subgroups of alcoholics displayed differential behavioral effects in response to *m*-CPP. These findings show that differences in central serotonergic functions may be key co-factors with age of onset and impulsive antisocial traits in alcohol-dependent individuals. The study of such serotonergic differences may result in the development of different

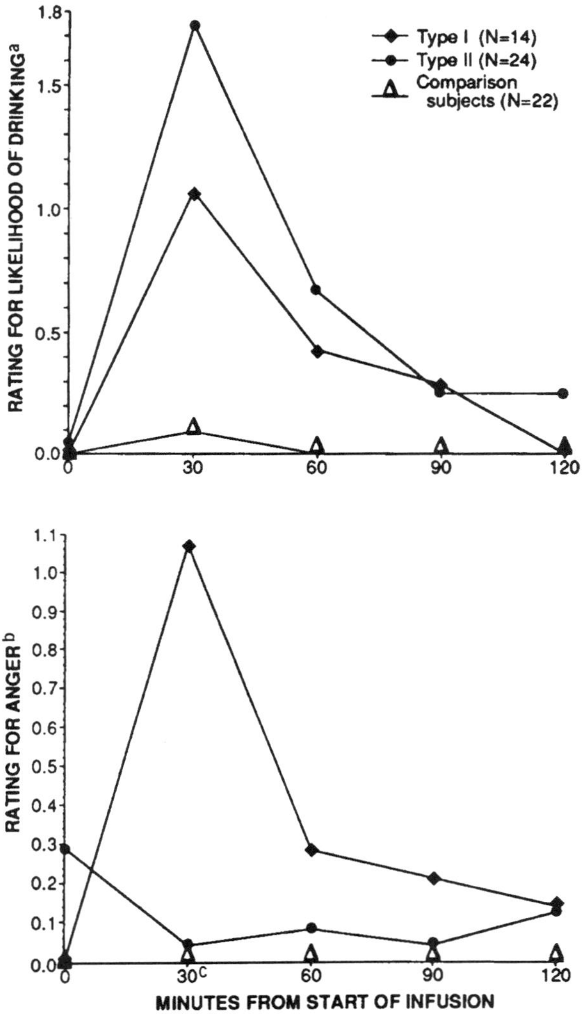

FIGURE 1.—Effects of *m*-chlorophenylpiperazine on the likelihood of drinking and on anger in type I and type II alcoholics and healthy comparison subjects.[a] indicates significant group differences ($F = 6.2$, $df = 2, 57$, $P = 0.004$); effect for type II alcoholics significantly greater than for comparison subjects ($t = 3.5$, $df = 57$, $P < 0.001$).[b] indicates significant time-by-group interaction ($F = 6.3$, $df = 6, 171$, $P < 0.001$).[c] indicates significant group differences ($F = 8.1$, $df = 2, 58$, $P < 0.001$); effect for type I alcoholics significantly greater than for type II alcoholics ($t = 3.6$, $df = 58$, $p < 0.001$) and for comparison subjects ($t = 3.7$, $df = 58$, $P < 0.001$). (Courtesy of George DT, Benkelfat C, Rawlings RR, et al: Behavioral and neuroendocrine responses to *m*-chlorophenylpiperazine in subtypes of alcoholics and in healthy comparison subjects. *Am J Psychiatry* 154:81–87, copyright 1997, the American Psychiatric Association. Reprinted by permission.)

pharmacologic and psychotherapeutic interventions for different subtypes of alcohol-dependent individuals.

► This study attempts to discover whether subtypes of alcoholics can be differentiated on the basis of central serotonergic functions. Looking for biological markers for subtyping can be a way to distinguish early onset alcoholics, indicating a possible central serotonergic etiologic factor in early onset alcoholism.

R.J. Frances, M.D.

The Self-medication Hypothesis of Substance Use Disorders: A Reconsideration and Recent Applications

Khantzian EJ (Harvard Med School, Boston; Cambridge Hosp, Mass; Tewsbury Hosp, Mass)

Harvard Rev Psychiatry 4:231–244, 1997 5–3

Introduction.—Dependence on addictive drugs or alcohol can be persistent and unrelenting for some individuals. Those caught in the process of addiction are not deterred by loss of control, health, self-respect, friends and relatives, or even the threat of loss of life. Much debate occurs over the root causes and etiology of these addictions. One hypothesis is the notion of "self-medication," in which the individual takes the drugs or drinks the alcohol as a partially successful attempt to assuage painful feelings. This hypothesis addresses important emotional and psychological dimensions.

Hypothesis.—Psychological suffering is relieved by this self-medication hypothesis. Some degree of psychopharmacologic specificity is involved with the person's preference for a particular drug. There is a close reciprocal relationship between the personality and inner state of suffering and the type of drug chosen. After experimenting with several drugs, patients may choose one particular drug because it relieves, heightens, or ameliorates the state they find painful. For example, opiates are chosen to counter the effects of rage; central nervous system depressants, such as alcohol, are chosen to mask fears of closeness, to soften rigid defenses, and ameliorate states of isolation; stimulants are chosen to relieve boredom and to act as augments for hypomanic, high-energy individuals as well as those with atypical bipolar disorder. Difficulties in regulating affects, self-esteem, relationships, and self-care are factors that lead individuals toward self-medication. Individuals who are overwhelmed with painful affects or who seem not to feel their emotions at all are persons who have substance use disorders.

Recent applications.—This theory also applies to nicotine dependence, shizophrenia, and posttraumatic stress disorder with a substance abuse disorder. To alleviate or remedy subjects' state of distress involving dysthymia, depressive symptoms, or dysphoria, nicotine is used. To relieve the negative symptoms associated with schizophrenia, alcohol, stimulants, and other drugs are used. To self-medicate the affective flooding or numbing involved with posttraumatic stress disorder, alcohol and other drugs are used.

Conclusion.—The neurobiological aspects and the psychological correlates of addiction must be addressed and integrated into a unified theory of substance use disorder. To improve understanding and treatment of the target symptoms and subjects' distress, the self-medication hypothesis can be used. Studies are still not consistent in their results about the cause–consequence controversy involving psychopathology and substance use/abuse.

► The self-medication hypothesis has been with us since the days of Hippocrates and has been expanded by Kraepilin, Weider, and Caplan and Frosch. In modern times, the leading exponent of this hypothesis is Edward Khantzian, M.D., who does the most up-to-date and clear review of the field in this article, as well as adding further insight. In my opinion, it is more often the "wrath of grapes than the grapes of wrath" that causes problems for people who use alcohol and other substances. The observations contained in this article certainly are applicable to an important subsegment of patients with addictive disorders, and a good knowledge of how to apply this wisdom clinically is useful to have for any clinician in the addiction field.

R.J. Frances, M.D.

Diagnosis—Comorbidity

An Adoption Study of DSM-IIIR Alcohol and Drug Dependence Severity

Yates WR, Cadoret RJ, Troughton E, et al (Univ of Iowa, Iowa City)
Drug Alcohol Depend 41:9–15, 1996 5–4

Background.—Adoption studies published more than 20 years ago reported a link between risk for alcoholism and genetic factors. Since then, evidence supporting this link has been reported by family, twin, and molecular genetic studies. Results of these studies have been inconsistent, possibly because of the heterogeneous nature of alcoholism and discrepancies in the methods used to diagnosis alcoholism.

Methods.—There were 95 adopted individuals who had biological parents with alcoholism, drug dependence, or antisocial personality disorder. Another group of 102 adopted individuals served as control subjects. All subjects were interviewed for presence of alcohol abuse/dependence, drug abuse/dependence, or dependence using the Diagnostic Interview Schedule (DIS-III-R).

Results.—Using DSM-III-R criteria for alcohol dependence, a genetic effect was seen in adoptees with 5 or more DSM-III-R criteria for alcohol dependence. A genetic effect was also seen in adoptees with 1 or more DSM-III-R criteria for drug dependance compared with individuals who met no criteria. There were no significant gender differences.

Discussion.—These findings indicate that genetic factors affect the risk for alcoholism and drug dependence at various levels of severity. These findings are consistent with previous studies of alcohol abuse reporting a genetic effect for more severe alcohol dependence. These findings extend to drug dependence. A confounding factor may be the effect of exposure in utero to alcohol or drugs.

► This paper is supportive of an earlier work by Goodwin which found that severity correlated with alcohol dependence. However, with drug dependence, the correlation of genetic contribution can hit at a lower threshold of number of DSM-III-R dependence criteria. Indirectly, the paper supports the value of keeping severity criteria continued in the diagnostic system.

R.J. Frances, M.D.

Reference

1. Goodwin DW: *Is Alcoholism Hereditary?* New York, Ballantine, 1988.

The Relationship Between DSM-IV Alcohol Use Disorders and DSM-IV Major Depression: Examination of the Primary-Secondary Distinction in a General Population Sample

Grant BF, Hasin DS, Dawson DA (Natl Inst on Alcohol Abuse and Alcoholism, Bethesda, Md; Columbia Univ, New York)

J Affect Disord 38:113–128, 1996 5–5

Background.—The clinical value of the primary-secondary distinction in predicting familial aggregation of alcoholism and major depression has been investigated. In current studies, the definitions of primary and secondary disorders vary, as do the subgroups of patients with and without alcoholism and major depression. In current studies, the rates of secondary depression among alcoholics also vary, but rates of primary depression are less varied. The variations have resulted from differences in patient samples, diagnostic criteria, psychiatric assessments, and study methods. The major limitation of previous studies is that they were conducted in clinical or treated populations.

Methods.—Data were obtained from the 1992 National Longitudinal Alcohol Epidemiologic Survey. Personal interviews were conducted with 42,862 adult, noninstitutionalized individuals in the United States. The household response rate was 91.9% and the sample person response rate was 97.4%. Details of sociodemographic, diagnostic assessment, alcohol-related, depression-related, and drug-related variables are included.

Results.—Respondents with primary, secondary, or concurrent depression made up the 3 co-morbid groups. Data from these groups were compared with data from respondents with major depression only and respondents with alcohol use disorders only. There were significantly more women in the group with major depression only than in the other 4 groups. There were significantly more men in the group with alcohol use disorders only than in the other 4 groups. Patients in the 3 co-morbid groups were younger and less likely to be black than patients with major depression only. Patients in the 3 co-morbid groups did not have any less severe alcohol use disorders than patients with alcohol use disorders only. The co-morbid groups did not experience any less severe major depression than patients with major depression only. The length of the longest episode of major depression and the number of depressive symptoms during the worst episode were similar among patients in the 3 co-morbid groups and

and in patients with major depression only. A history of a drug use disorder was seen in about 40% of patients in each co-morbid group. This percentage was significantly higher than in patients with major depression only and in patients with alcohol use disorders only. Patients with alcohol use disorders only also had a higher incidence of lifetime drug use disorders than patients with major depression only.

Discussion.—Among patients from the general population in these 3 co-morbid groups, the rate of primary depression was 41.0%, the rate of concurrent depression was 16.5%, and the rate of secondary depression 42.5%. These findings are inconsistent with most findings from the treatment literature regarding familial aggregation of alcohol use disorders and sociodemographic, alcohol, and depression profiles. This inconsistency occurs because most previous studies were conducted among alcoholics receiving treatment. The findings of this study are discussed in detail in this extensive article.

▶ Recent writers have believed that alcoholism and depression are discretely inherited disorders whereas researchers, such as Winokur, have hypothesized that alcohol use disorders and major depression can be ultimate manifestations of the same underlying disorder and that both are familial. This study finds that those who have alcoholism after depression have often had a positive family history of alcoholism. The controversy continues.

R.J. Frances, M.D.

Reference

1. Winokur G: Alcoholism and depression in the family, in Goodwin DW, Erickson CK (eds): *Alcoholism and Affective Disorders: Clinical, Genetic and Biochemical Studies*. Jamaica, NY, Spectrum Publications, 1979, pp 49–56.

Aetiology of Secondary Depression in Male Alcoholics

Roy A (Veteran's Affairs Med Ctr, East Orange, NJ)

Br J Psychiatry 169:753–757, 1996 5–6

Introduction.—Negative life events have been shown to be more prevalent in patients who are depressed than those who are not depressed. Depression in alcoholic patients is important because of the additional psychiatric morbidity and poorer outcome of alcoholism. Risk factors for depression and recent life events were compared in 40 males with primary alcoholism and secondary major depression and 40 matched never-depressed primary male alcoholic controls.

Methods.—All research subjects had been abstinent for at least 2 weeks before undergoing a structured interview regarding medical and psychosocial history, family and marital history, life events in the previous 6 months, and early parental loss. The Beck Depression Inventory was completed by all participants.

Results.—Compared to nondepressed controls, depressed alcoholic patients had significantly more first or second degree relatives who had been treated for depression or had exhibited suicidal behavior; suicide attempts themselves; life events in the previous 1, 3, and 6 months; life events with severe, marked, or mild negative impact; and dependent events caused by drinking. Twenty-two of 40 depressed alcoholic participants were unemployed before depression onset, compared to 18 of 40 nondepressed controls. Twenty depressed alcoholic patients had separation from a parent before age 17 years and 4 had a death of a parent, compared to 18 and 4, respectively, among controls. Twelve of 13 married depressed alcoholic patients had a poor marital rating for the year before depression onset, compared to 14 of 18 married controls.

Conclusion.—Males with primary alcoholism with major depression were significantly more likely to have recent adverse life events and family history of depression than nondepressed alcoholic controls.

▶ Depressed alcoholic patients can have a positive family history of suicidal behavior and recent negative life events that may predispose them to a secondary depression. It is not surprising that alcoholic patients, who may be more vulnerable to depression because of life events or biological vulnerability, would succumb to alcohol-induced secondary depression.

R.J. Frances, M.D.

Psychiatric and Substance Use Comorbidity Among Treatment-seeking Opioid Abusers

Brooner RK, King VL, Kidorf M, et al (Johns Hopkins Univ, Baltimore, Md)
Arch Gen Psychiatry 54:71–80, 1997 5–7

Introduction.—Earlier reports of psychiatric comorbidity in opioid abusers underrepresent women, report opioid and alcohol dependence while excluding other substances commonly used by opioid abusers, and have given diagnoses at times when patients have not been stabilized in treatment. Rates of psychiatric and substance use disorder were compared using a wider range of substance use and other psychiatric diagnoses, a standardized time frame after treatment entry for conducting diagnostic evaluation, and a larger proportion of women.

Methods.—Seven hundred sixteen opioid-dependent men and women admitted to an outpatient methadone maintenance clinic underwent interview and evaluation at 4–5 weeks after admission and stabilization on methadone. Diagnoses were based on the Structured Clinical Interview for the Diagnostic and Statistical Manual of Mental Disorders, ed 3, revised. Rates of substance use and other psychiatric diagnoses in men and women and in patients with and without psychiatric comorbidity were compared.

Results.—Forty-seven percent of the cohort (48% men and 47% women) had a lifetime psychiatric diagnosis other than substance use disorder. Of the 340 patients with psychiatric comorbidty: 61.5% had 1 diagnosis, 21.8% had 2 diagnoses, 10.6% had 3 diagnoses, and 6.1% had 4 or more diagnoses. The most common diagnoses were antisocial personality disorder (25.1%) and major depression (15.8%). Lifetime rates of nonsubstance use disorders in the general population (Epidemiological Catchment Area Study; Baltimore) were compared with those of opioid abusers. The rates of major depression and antisocial personality, respectively, were 3 and 8 times greater in drug abusers than in the general population. There was a strong association between psychiatric comorbidity and a more severe substance use disorder.

Conclusion.—Major depression and antisocial personality were common psychiatric comorbidity diagnoses observed in both male and female opioid abusers. Psychiatric comorbidity and severity of substance use and other psychosocial problems were more commonly observed in patients with antisocial personality.

► Rates of psychiatric comorbidity among opioid abusers tend to be high, and among those with opioid dependency, probably higher. This 1997 study gives an update of rates of comorbidity and finds that they are particularly high for antisocial personality disorder and major depression. A pathology professor of mine once said, "Them that has, gets."

R.J. Frances, M.D.

Relationships Between Symptoms of Schizophrenia and Substance Abuse

Brunette MF, Mueser KT, Xie H, et al (Dartmouth Med School, Concord, NH)

J Nerv Ment Dis 185:13–20, 1997 5–8

Introduction.—The association between severity of substance abuse and schizophrenia is not well understood. Some reports suggest a tendency for patients with schizophrenic symptoms to use alcohol or drugs to self-regulate symptoms. The correlation between severity of schizophrenic symptoms and severity of substance abuse among outpatients who abused primarily alcohol and cannabis was evaluated in 172 patients with *Diagnostic and Statistical Manual of Mental Disorders*, ed 3, revised diagnoses of schizophrenia or schizoaffective disorder.

Methods.—Separate measures were used to rate the severity of schizophrenia psychopathology and severity of substance use disorder. Patients' lifetime and current substance use diagnosis were determined.

Results.—The relationships between symptoms of schizophrenia and substance abuse were weak or nonexistent and had no consistent pattern. Patients did not seem to use other substances to self-regulate symptoms.

Conclusion.—There was no significant relationship between schizophrenic symptoms and substance abuse. Patients did not seem to self-regulate symptoms with alcohol or drugs. Findings suggest that substance abuse may trigger higher rates of institutionalization by means other than exacerbating symptoms.

► This study did not show support for the self-medication hypothesis in an outpatient sample. The authors' data were more consistent with the hypothesis that higher rates of institutionalization had more to do with comorbid substance problems than with exacerbations of schizophrenic symptoms.

R.J. Frances, M.D.

Gender Differences in Patients With Schizophrenia and Substance Abuse

Brunette MF, Drake RE (Dartmouth Med School, Lebanon, NH)

Compr Psychiatry 38:109–116, 1997 5–9

Background.—The co-occurrence of substance abuse with chronic mental illness, such as schizophrenia, is common. Although gender differences have been documented among substance abusers in the general population and among schizophrenic patients, little is known about such differences among individuals with both schizophrenia and substance abuse problems.

Methods.—A total of 118 patients with *DSM-III-R* diagnoses of schizophrenia and 54 with schizoaffective disorder were studied. Thirty-four also had antisocial personality disorder. All 172 patients had comorbid substance use disorders. Thirty-seven patients were women, and 135 were men.

Findings.—Women with chronic mental illness and substance use disorder had more social contact and fewer legal problems than their male counterparts. However, the women had more problems with victimization and medical illnesses, compared with the men. Men and women were found to have similar courses and severities of substance abuse, which was unexpected.

Conclusions.—Overall patterns of substance abuse in schizophrenic women and men may be influenced more by factors associated with their schizophrenia than by factors influencing gender differences in substance abusers in the general population. The current data should be considered when planning services explicitly addressing women's family and social needs, issues related to victimization, and higher rates of medical problems.

► One interesting finding in this study is that schizophrenia shaped substance abuse in both men and women and that women had higher than expected rates of substance use when they were schizophrenic. In other ways, some of the same characteristics that distinguish men from women in the general population also distinguish men and women with dual diagnosis. In this study, women had more social contact, fewer legal problems, greater victimization, and more medical illness than men. My impression is that women with dual diagnosis have not suffered from less stigmatization than men. Rather, women with substance problems and psychiatric illness are less likely to be seen as eccentric and more likely to be stigmatized, perhaps in part leading to a greater vulnerability toward victimization.

R.J. Frances, M.D.

Verbal Creativity, Depression and Alcoholism: An Investigation of One Hundred American and British Writers

Post F (Bethlem Royal Hosp, London)

Br J Psychiatry 168:545–555, 1996 5–10

Background.—A previous study of world-famous men demonstrated that only visual artists and creative writers had a higher prevalence of pathologic personality traits and alcoholism than the general population. Depressive disorders were found in writers almost twice as often as in men with other high creative achievements. Depression and alcoholism were further explored among male creative writers.

Methods.—The postmortem biographies of 100 American and British writers were reviewed. When possible, DSM diagnoses were made. The frequencies of various abnormalities and deviations among poets, prose fiction writers, and playwrights were compared.

Findings.—Overall, the writers studied had a high prevalence of affective disorders and alcoholism. The prevalence of bipolar affective psychoses among poets exceeded population norms. Despite this, poets had a lower prevalence of all types of affective disorders, alcoholism, personality deviations, and psychosexual and marital problems than prose fiction and play writers.

Discussion.—It was hypothesized that the high levels of emotional imagination and the associated excessive activity in neural networks needed for writing, as well as the frequency of depressive personality traits, distinguishes male writers from other men with high creative achievements. Cognitive therapy may be more suitable than Prozac for creative writers and other artists.

► The mythologic flying horse Pegasus tripped over a mountain and unleashed the springs of creativity of the muse as well as the source of wine often said to be the inspiration of poets. It has always struck me that many American writers seem to develop alcoholism, whereas Japanese writers suffer depression and often suicide. This speculative article combines data with hypotheses about the greater frequency of alcoholism in playwrights and prose writers in comparison with poets.

R.J. Frances, M.D.

Pharmacologic Treatment

Recent Developments in the Pharmacotherapy of Alcohol Dependence

Schuckit MA (Univ of California, San Diego; Veterans Affairs Med Ctr, San Diego)

J Consult Clin Psychol 64:669–676, 1996 5–11

Background.—Assessing the efficacy of treatments for alcohol abuse or dependence is difficult for many reasons. This article discusses recent developments in the pharmacotherapy of alcohol dependence after careful consideration of these difficulties.

Discussion.—The efficacy of alcohol dependence treatment can only be determined after controlling for the usual clinical course of the disease, subgroups of alcohol-dependent individuals, and placebo effects. Side effects and costs must be considered when interpreting the results of treatment trials. There must be assurances that the overall improvement in functioning associated with the treatment outweighs its liabilities. Also, medication use is almost always combined with education, counseling, and behavioral therapies, the effects of which must be taken into account. With these considerations in mind, the following 3 medications appear promising in the treatment of alcoholism: naltrexone, buspirone, and acamprosate.

Naltrexone has been studied extensively in the United States. Intriguing data also have been published on the effects of medications affecting serotonin and dopamine brain activity and on alcohol-sensitizing agents such as disulfiram. However, none of these agents has been proven clinically effective in the routine treatment of the average alcoholic. Future research needs to help identify the subgroups of alcohol-dependent men and women most likely to respond to specific pharmacologic treatments.

▶ The enthusiasm over new treatments for alcohol dependence is tempered by cautions about their routine use at this point in the field's development. This is a careful review of the recent developments, and it has a conservative slant in terms of recommendations. Although reliable studies have indicated the value of using naltrexone, its use has not been widespread. Perhaps this review reflects a consensus of the field that tends to be conservative, although this might change when large-scale, double-blind trials have been done, and many have had wide experience with this drug. Perhaps other elements, such as high cost and lack of patient acceptance, have contributed to its limited use. The final plea is for more research that can answer the question of whether routine use of psychopharmacologic agents for alcoholism is warranted.

R.J. Frances, M.D.

Relapse Prevention by Acamprosate: Results From a Placebo-controlled Study on Alcohol Dependence

Sass H, Soyka M, Mann K, et al (Psychiatric Clinic, Rheinisch Westfälische, Technische Hochschule, Aachen, Germany; Univ of Munich, Germany; Univ of Tübingen, Germany; et al)

Arch Gen Psychiatry 53:673–680, 1996 5–12

Background.—Studies of the interaction between ethanol with dopaminergic, serotonergic, and γ-aminobutyric acid–ergic (GABAergic) systems and glutamate-*N*-methyl-D-aspartate and opiate receptors have prompted the creation of new approaches to the pharmacotherapy for alcoholism. Acetyl-3-aminopropanesulfonic acid as calcium bisacetylhomotaurinate (acamprosate) recently has been shown to suppress alcohol intake in animals, without changing alcohol toxicity. The efficacy of acamprosate in maintaining abstinence in alcohol-dependent patients was evaluated.

Methods.—A total of 272 patients were included in the randomized, double-blind, placebo-controlled trial. After short-term detoxification, the patients received routine counseling and acamprosate or placebo for 48 weeks. The patients were monitored for another 48 weeks without medication.

Findings.—Acamprosate recipients had a significantly higher continuous abstinence rate within the first 60 days of treatment, compared with placebo recipients (67% and 50%, respectively), and until completion of the treatment period (43% and 21%, respectively). The acamprosate group also had a significantly longer mean abstinence duration—224 days, compared with 163 days. However, psychiatric symptoms did not differ between the groups. Of the patients receiving acamprosate, 41% dropped out of the study, compared with 60% of those receiving placebo. There were few adverse effects. Diarrhea and headache were the primary ones. At the end of the 48-week follow-up period without medication, 39% of the acamprosate recipients and 17% of the placebo recipients had remained abstinent.

Conclusions.—Acamprosate appears to be safe and effective in preventing relapse in a comprehensive alcoholism treatment setting. The optimal time for treatment initiation and treatment duration, as well as possible combination with other psychotropic medications, have yet to be established.

► Acamprosate is a promising medication that is not yet FDA approved in the United States. However, it has shown good results in helping improve outcomes for patients with alcoholism. Acamprosate, which works through a different mechanism than naltrexone, might be useful for patients who are refractory to other treatments. This article also underlines the value of American psychiatrists becoming familiar with advances that take place in Europe. Whether acamprosate will be deserving of more widespread use will depend on further study of larger population samples.

R.J. Frances, M.D.

A Placebo Controlled Clinical Trial of Buprenorphine as a Treatment for Opioid Dependence

Johnson RE, Eissenberg T, Stitzer ML, et al (Johns Hopkins Univ, Baltimore, Md)

Drug Alcohol Depend 40:17–25, 1995 5–13

Background.—Large-scale placebo-controlled clinical studies of the efficacy of pharmacotherapy for drug dependence generally have been limited to alcohol, cocaine, and nicotine dependence. The current study evaluated the early clinical efficacy of buprenorphine, compared with placebo, in the treatment of opioid dependence.

Methods and Findings.—A total of 150 male and female opioid-dependent volunteers participated in the 14-day study. The study design was parallel-group with a behavioral choice component. By random assignment, 60 subjects received placebo; 60 received 2 mg daily of sublingual buprenorphine; and 30 received 8 mg of daily sublingual buprenorphine. Dose administration was double-blind. Between days 6 and 13, the subjects could ask for a change in treatment, knowing that their new treatment would be selected randomly from the remaining 2 alternatives. Subjects receiving either dose of buprenorphine spent more time on the initial dose, requested fewer treatment changes, used fewer illicit opioids as assessed by urinalysis, and rated dose adequacy as higher than those given placebo.

Conclusions.—Buprenorphine was found to be more effective than placebo in the treatment of opioid dependence. Furthermore, this study showed that the current methodological design is an effective way to assess the potential efficacy and acceptability of new drug treatments for opioid dependence.

► Studies such as this one are generating interest in the use of buprenorphine as a treatment for opioid dependence that leads to less illicit opioid use as well as less use of other drugs such as cocaine. Buprenorphine poses the possibility of having an opioid agonist and antagonist, which might be a viable alternative to methadone and conceivably could be packaged in ways that might lead to lower chances of diversion and more widespread means of distribution, possibly in primary care settings. Given buprenorphine's opioid antagonist actions, I wonder whether it also reduces alcohol abuse in opioid addicts.

R.J. Frances, M.D.

A Pilot Study of Primary-Care-based Buprenorphine Maintenance for Heroin Dependence
O'Conner PG, Oliveto AH, Shi JM, et al (Yale Univ, New Haven, Conn)
Am J Drug Alcohol Abuse 22:523–531, 1996 5–14

Background.—In traditional drug treatment settings, the management of heroin dependence with opioid maintenance has typically included methadone and, more recently, buprenorphine. In this pilot study, buprenorphine maintenance in the treatment of heroin dependence was assessed in a program administered by primary-care providers in a primary-care setting.

Methods.—Seven patients were enrolled in the nonblinded, open-label study for 6 months of primary-care–based buprenorphine maintenance therapy. The drug was given in 16 mg doses on Monday and Wednesday and in a 32 mg dose on Friday. Primary-care providers examined the patients each week. In addition, the patients attended self-help meetings.

Outcomes.—Five (71%) patients completed the 6-month study. The remaining 2 were removed from the study. Urine toxicologic assessment indicated that 4 of the 5 patients completing treatment were clear of opioids.

Conclusions.—Primary-care–based opioid maintenance with buprenorphine appears to be feasible in the management of opioid dependence. Large, randomized studies comparing primary care with traditional drug treatment settings are now needed to verify these results.

► This study suggests a method that might increase availability of drug treatment through developing a technique that can be used by primary-care clinics, that would not lead to diversion, and that may be effective in managing opioid dependence. A thrice weekly buprenorphine regimen, with 6 months of retention rates that are comparable to traditional methadone maintenance settings, is a promising result, which warrants further study with larger patient samples.

R.J. Frances, M.D.

Psychiatric Morbidity, Illicit Drug Use and Adherence to Zidovudine (AZT) Among Injection Drug Users With HIV Disease
Ferrando SJ, Wall TL, Batki SL, et al (Cornell Univ, New York; Univ of California, San Diego)
Am J Drug Alcohol Abuse 22:475–487, 1996 5–15

Background.—Adherence to prescribed medical therapies may be problematic among HIV-infected injection drug users in methadone maintenance treatment (MMT) programs. The relationship between need for psychiatric consultation, illicit drug use, and zidovudine (AZT) compliance in this population was investigated.

Methods.—The records of 57 injection drug users receiving MMT, who were prescribed AZT between May and August of 1991, were reviewed. The 46 patients needing psychiatric consultation (group 1) were compared with the 11 not requiring such consultation (group 2).

Findings.—Group 1 patients were less likely than group 2 patients to adhere to AZT therapy. Fewer patients in group 1 had a mean corpuscular volume out of the normal range. Also, group 1 patients had a lower mean monthly increase in MCV since AZT initiation. The 2 groups did not differ in recent illicit drug use and CD4 lymphocyte count changes from the beginning to the end of AZT treatment.

Conclusions.—Psychiatric morbidity is common among HIV-infected injection drug users receiving MMT. Psychiatric disorders may contribute to poor AZT adherence in this population. Psychiatric screening and compliance-enhancing interventions should be targeted to injection drug users entering drug treatment programs.

► Now that treatments are available that can markedly alter treatment outcome for HIV infection, the treatment of psychiatric disorders, which can affect patients' compliance with their medical treatment, including taking AZT, is essential. Psychiatric comorbidity is common in HIV-infected injection drug users, and these problems can affect his or her motivation to adhere to other medical treatments. This is complicated by the fact that both HIV infection and AZT can cause psychiatric symptoms and can contribute to poor adherence to treatment.

R.J. Frances, M.D.

Treatment and Outcomes

Outcomes of Patients in a VA Ambulatory Detoxification Program

Wiseman EJ, Henderson KL, Briggs MJ (Little Rock Veterans Affairs Med Ctr, Ark)

Psychiatric Serv 48:200–203, 1997 5–16

Background.—Although outpatient medical detoxification is known to be safe and cost-effective for patients with mild to moderate alcohol withdrawal symptoms, little is known about the outcomes of ambulatory detoxification programs. The results of one Veterans Affairs ambulatory detoxification program were reported.

Methods.—Outcomes were assessed for 517 of the 577 patients referred consecutively to the program during 9 months in 1995. All met the criteria for mild to moderate alcohol withdrawal syndrome.

Findings.—A total of 453 patients successfully completed outpatient detoxification. Thirty-seven patients were re-enrolled; 25 were admitted for inpatient detoxification; 20 dropped out; and 19 were discharged. Of those completing outpatient detoxification, 434 were referred for further treatment. A total of 415 entered, and 322 completed the next phase of treatment.

Conclusions.—The rates for program completion and for continuing in and completing further treatment in this study were higher than rates in previous studies. The unique factors that contributed to these favorable outcomes were systematic screening, medical protocols for detoxification, psychosocial treatment, program-supported housing, and attention to patient satisfaction.

► Cost-savings and studies such as these are fueling efforts to promote outpatient detoxification and have led to increased limitations in the use of inpatient detox. We should remember that all the patients in this study met the criteria for mild to moderate alcohol withdrawal syndrome, which implies that there is still a significant number of patients with severe withdrawal syndromes who require inpatient treatment. There are patients who drop out or lack a connection to outpatient detox, which necessitates admission to inpatient detoxification. This program also provided program-supported housing, which is not available to all patients, and this may be another factor that led to the positive success rates.

R.J. Frances, M.D.

Effects of Case Management on Retention in Prenatal Substance Abuse Treatment

Laken MP, Ager JW (Wayne State Univ, Detroit)

Am J Drug Alcohol Abuse 22:439–448, 1996 5–17

Background.—Pregnancy outcomes are improved in substance abusers who participate in treatment programs during pregnancy. Case management has been suggested as a way to decrease barriers to treatment. One community-based case-management program designed to retain pregnant women in treatment was reviewed.

Methods and Findings.—A total of 225 pregnant women was included in the study. All received case-management services, which consisted of home visits, telephone counseling, transportation, and referral. During their pregnancy, all the women contacted a substance abuse treatment center, and 56% received treatment. Path analysis identified the following 5 factors associated with prenatal attendance at the substance abuse treatment center: (1) history of protective services involvement, (2) number of drugs ever used, (3) current methadone treatment, (4) intensity of case management, and (5) the provision of transportation to drug treatment appointments.

Conclusions.—Case management contributes significantly to the retention of pregnant drug abusers in treatment programs. Additional research is needed to further explore which elements of case management assist substance-abusing women during and after pregnancy.

► We should carefully study anything that helps pregnant women stay in substance abuse treatment, and we should make efforts to make it available.

This study finds that wraparound supports, such as providing transportation, methadone, intense case management, and involving protective services, are all helpful.

R.J. Frances, M.D.

Superiority of Carbohydrate-deficient Transferrin to γ-Glutamyltransferase in Detecting Relapse in Alcoholism

Schmidt LG, Schmidt K, Dufeu P, et al (Benjamin Franklin Univ, Berlin; Free Univ of Berlin; Inst of Clinical Chemistry and Biochemistry, Berlin; et al)

Am J Psychiatry 154:75–80, 1997 5–18

Background.—The value of carbohydrate-deficient transferrin is generally accepted in screening male population samples for heavy alcohol intake. However, its role in detecting relapses has not been definitively established.

Methods.—A total of 101 male alcoholics entering a 6-month rehabilitation program after hospital detoxification was studied. Drinking status was assessed by self-report and collateral reports during regular contacts with the rehabilitation team. Blood samples also were obtained at the periodic visits for measurement of carbohydrate-deficient transferrin and γ-glutamyltransferase (GGT).

Findings.—A mean 25.6% of the men reported relapse per scheduled contact. Positive predictive values showed that carbohydrate-deficient transferrin values exceeding the upper normal limit identified relapse with a 76.2% probability, compared with 32.9% with GGT. Carbohydrate-deficient transferrin was especially useful for detecting early relapses in the initial rehabilitation phase, before GGT values normalized. Because of its longer half-life, however, GGT was of some value with a four-week monitoring schedule for detecting new drinking episodes in patients with previously normal results.

Conclusions.—Carbohydrate-deficient transferrin was better than GGT in detecting relapses in this group of alcoholics receiving outpatient treatment. γ-Glutamyltransferase gained some diagnostic efficiency for alcoholics with normal values in previous tests when monitoring was performed at 4-week intervals.

► Clearly, carbohydrate-deficient transferrin can be useful in relapse prevention programs and as a screen for heavy alcohol consumption. In spite of a positive experience with this test for close to a decade in Europe and the United States, I still have not seen widespread availability for its use in inpatient or outpatient settings. I am not sure whether the problem relates to too little marketing or too high a price for the test.

R.J. Frances, M.D.

Prevention of HIV/AIDS and Other Blood-borne Diseases Among Injection Drug Users: A National Survey on the Regulation of Syringes and Needles

Gostin LO, Lazzarini Z, Jones S, et al (Havard School of Public Health, Boston; Ctrs For Disease Control and Prevention, Atlanta, Ga)

JAMA 277:53–62, 1997 5–19

Background.—Injection drug use is the second most common risk factor for AIDS. A national survey on the regulation of syringes and needles was reported.

Survey Findings.—State or local laws or regulations restricting the sale, distribution, or possession of syringes exist in every state, the District of Columbia (DC), and the Virgin Islands (VI). Forty-seven states, DC, and VI have drug paraphernalia laws prohibiting the sale, distribution, and possession of syringes known to be used to introduce illicit drugs into the body. Eight states and VI have syringe prescription laws that prohibit the sale, distribution, and possession of syringes without a valid medical prescription. In 23 states, pharmacy regulations or practice guidelines limit access to syringes.

Suggestions for Increasing Access.—To improve the availability of sterile syringes to prevent bloodborne disease among injection drug users, the legitimate medical purpose of sterile syringes to prevent HIV and other bloodborne infections should be clarified; drug paraphernalia laws should be modified to exclude syringes; and syringe prescription laws should be repealed. In addition, pharmacy regulations and practice guidelines limiting the sale of sterile syringes should be repealed; professional training of pharmacists, other health care professionals, and law enforcement officers about the prevention of bloodborne viruses should be promoted; local discretion in establishing syringe exchange programs should be permitted; and community programs for safe syringe disposal should be designed.

Conclusions.—Evidence suggests that deregulating the sale and possession of syringes would decrease the morbidity and mortality associated with bloodborne diseases among injection drug users, their sexual partners, and their children. Such deregulation can be done without harmful social repercussions.

► Over the years, the data supporting needle exchange programs as an effective means of reducing HIV transmission among IV drug users has grown. However, progress has been too slow in modifying state laws in ways that can make needle exchange programs more available and widely used. This article provides useful information regarding varying patterns of regulating syringes and needles across the country and makes suggestions for changing laws and designing safe community programs.

R.J. Frances, M.D.

Substance Abuse and Dependence in Physicians: The Missouri Physicians' Health Program

Bohigian GM, Croughan JL, Sanders K, et al (Missouri State Med Association's Physicians' Health Program, St Louis)

South Med J 89:1078–1080, 1996 5–20

Background.—The medical community is increasingly concerned about substance abuse and dependence among physicians. The Missouri Physicians' Health Program was established to help such physicians resume healthy personal and professional lives. This program and its outcomes were described.

The Missouri Physicians' Health Program.—The main purpose of the program is to facilitate impaired physicians' return to healthy functioning. It is an independent, voluntary, and confidential service for Missouri physicians with alcoholism, drug abuse, or psychiatric illness. The program is sponsored by the Missouri State Medical Association, working in conjunction with the Licensing Board of the State of Missouri. Between 1990 and 1994, 194 of the 11,930 licensed physicians practicing or residing in Missouri were referred to the program. At present, 146 physicians are enrolled. The remaining 48 either completed the program, moved from Missouri, or did not enroll after referral. As of December 1994, 94% of the enrollees were stable and recovering (Table 4).

Conclusions.—The Missouri Physicians' Health Program has been successful in aiding physicians with substance abuse and dependence, with 94% of the enrollees compliant with the monitoring requirement and stable in recovery. Early intervention followed by appropriate treatment and follow-up often enable such physicians to resume healthy lives.

► This article was picked from among a number of articles describing very high success rates in physicians' health programs across the country. In this program, the recovery rate for 146 participants was a remarkable 94%, which almost sounds too good to be true except for the fact that other states report high rates as well, ranging from greater than 80% to this rate of 94%. The importance of getting treatment to impaired professionals and people of achievement cannot be emphasized enough, especially given the high suc-

TABLE 4.—Current Status of Participants (n = 146)

	No.
Stable and working well within the program	137 (94%)
License currently suspended but in stable recovery	2 (1%)
Currently being retreated or having recent relapse	7 (5%)

(Courtesy of Bohigian GM, Croughan JL, Sanders K, et al: Substance abuse and dependence in physicians: The Missouri Physicians' Health Program. *South Med J* 89:1078–1080, 1996. Reprinted by permission from the *Southern Medical Journal*.)

cess rates when participants are high functioning and likely to comply with monitoring requirements to achieve a stable recovery.

R.J. Frances, M.D.

Costs of Employee Assistance Programs: Findings From a National Survey

French MT, Zarkin GA, Bray JW, et al (Univ of Miami, Fla; Research Triangle Inst, NC)

Am J Health Promot 11:219–222, 1997 5–21

Background.—Many employers have created employee assistance programs (EAPs) to address the problems associated with substance abuse among workers. The annual cost per eligible employee of EAP services by type of EAP, worksite characteristics, and other factors were documented.

Methods.—A stratified random sample of all private nonagricultural worksites in the United States with 50 or more full-time employees was surveyed. Interviewers contacted 3,204 worksites, obtaining an overall response rate of 90%. Internal and external models were compared, the former being staffed by company employees and located at the worksite or a short distance away, and the latter providing services to worksite employees on a contract basis.

Findings.—The estimated mean cost per eligible employee for internal EAPs was $26.59. These cost estimates were U-shaped from smaller to larger worksites. Variation was moderate to high, based on industry and region. For external EAPs, the mean cost per employee was $21.47. These cost estimates were fairly stable across most factors, except for primary industry. The median costs of internal and external EAPs differed significantly across a wide range of worksite characteristics, with internal EAPs being generally more expensive.

Conclusions.—Although EAP coverage at worksites is increasing rapidly, many firms have yet to implement such programs. The current cost estimates will be useful in companies' exploration of EAP options.

► This article provides a nice review of the availability and cost of EAPs, which now serve approximately 54,000 worksites nationally. A good understanding of what EAP services do provide and how much it costs can be very useful to both industry and human resource departments in deciding whether to have an EAP. The costs seem reasonable and worth an effort that can save companies significantly with regards to not only health costs but the corporate damage done by employees who have psychiatric and substance abuse problems.

R.J. Frances, M.D.

6 Law and Psychiatry

Introduction

Forensic psychiatry is coming of age as a field with the development of added qualifications in forensic psychiatry administered through the American Board of Psychiatry and Neurology, and with fellowships in forensic psychiatry requiring residence review committee and Accreditation Council for Graduate Medical Education approval. While forensic psychiatrists will be heading up forensic programs, doing consulting, and spending a high percentage of their time testifying on cases, there will still be a need for psychiatrists without this qualification to do some forensic work. In fact, all general psychiatrists need to keep up an interest in forensic psychiatry. I have found in my everyday work as a psychiatrist, and as an administrator and CEO of Silver Hill Hospital, that I am constantly keeping forensic issues in mind.

Abstracts 6–1 through 6–4 deal with the right to refuse treatment and end-of-life issues. Abstracts 6–1 and 6–2 deal with patients' refusal of medications and attitudes about being forcibly medicated. Abstract 6–3 highlights issues related to advance directives, an area that requires further study. This year the Supreme Court decided not to uphold a patient's right to physician-assisted suicide, and Abstract 6–4 was part of the material the court reviewed in making that decision.

This year's section on criminality, Abstracts 6–5 through 6–14, includes studies of laboratory measures of violence (Abstract 6–6), importance of screening for androgenic steroid use in evaluating criminal behavior (Abstract 6–5); Abstracts 6–7 to 6–9 relate to the issue of violence in psychiatric settings and the kinds of threat and physical harm that happen to mental health care workers. These issues are of major concern to all who work in psychiatric settings. They emphasize the importance of substance abuse and point to the alarmingly high rate of assaults in psychiatric hospitals against employees. These articles provide useful hints that reduce danger to staff. As a hospital administrator, I have come to appreciate the courage of staff working in psychiatric hospitals and that, while the threat of violence is an occupational hazard, there are strategies that can help reduce risks.

Abstracts 6–10 through 6–14 cover a variety of issues related to criminality, including child molestation (Abstract 6–10), criminal behavior in males with affective disorder (Abstract 6–11), sexual harassment (Abstract

6–12), collaboration of mental health workers with police officers (Abstract 6–13), and the insanity defense (Abstract 6–14).

Abstracts 6–15 to 6–18 relate to a variety of issues that involve risk and claim. Abstract 6–15 points out some of the stress that develops from being a plaintiff in litigation. Abstract 6–17 discusses malpractice issues and some of the stresses that relate to funerals and funeral homes. The issue of restricting sexual behavior of hospitalized psychiatric patients is surveyed in Abstract 6–16. Abstract 6–18 deals with the conflicts which forensic psychiatrists have in their own personal lives between meeting career and personal obligations.

A current climate of high litigation, high numbers of risk and claim issues, increased numbers of psychiatric patients finding their way into the prison system, and increased controversy around issues related to assisted suicide and end-of-life decisions, are all leading to a heightened interest among psychiatrists in pursuing careers in this fascinating field.

Richard J. Frances, M.D.

Right to Refuse Treatment and End of Life Issues

Prospective Study of Patients' Refusal of Antipsychotic Medication Under a Physician Discretion Review Procedure

Kasper JA, Hoge SK, Feucht-Haviar T, et al (Univ of Virginia, Charlottesville)
Am J Psychiatry 154:483–489, 1997 6–1

Background.—Although the right of committed psychiatric patients to refuse antpsychotic medications is acknowledged, debate continues over the proper scope of the right to refuse treatment and the procedures to determine when refusal can be overriden. The rate and outcomes of treatment refusal were examined in a state facility in which psychiatrists can treat objecting patients when deterioration seems likely.

Methods.—Three hundred forty-eight patients admitted to three acute psychiatric inpatient units in Virginia were studied. Newly admitted patients were given a questionnaire to elicit their attitudes toward admission and were administered the Brief Psychiatric Rating Scale (BPRS). Data was collected on patients refusing antipsychotic medication and on patients compliant with such treatment.

Findings.—Patients refusing treatment had significantly greater BPRS scores than patients complying with antipsychotic treatment. The former group also had more negative attitudes toward hospitalization and toward past, present, and future treatment. Refusal episodes were brief, lasting a mean of 2.8 days. All patients refusing treatment were eventually treated. Treatment refusers were more likely to be assaultive, to require seclusion and restraint, and to have longer hospitalization.

Conclusions.—The psychiatrists used their discretion to promptly treat patients refusing antipsychotic medications. However, such patients had more morbidity than compliant patients.

▶ This article is a balanced discussion of the policy implications of dealing with refusal of antipsychotic medication. Rapid treatment may reduce, but will not eliminate, the negative sequelae of in-hospital treatment refusal. The rights of patients to refuse treatment should be weighed against the possible danger to self and others, which leaving patients untreated can cause. Patients who refuse treatment generally have more severe problems, and their refusal of treatment will lead to longer and more costly hospitalizations.

R.J. Frances, M.D.

Patients' Attitudes Toward Having Been Forcibly Medicated
Greenberg WM, Moore-Duncan L, Herron R (Hahnemann Univ, Philadelphia; Greystone Park Psychiatric Hosp, Paramus, NJ)
Bull Am Acad Psychiatry Law 24:513–524, 1996 6–2

Background.—Forced antipsychotic medication procedures are generally considered necessary in certain circumstances. Although past research has investigated patients' attitudes toward being forcibly medicated, such patients were interviewed while still in the hospital, which may have influenced their responses. Interviews with consecutively forcibly medicated acute-care inpatients were conducted after discharge to the community.

Methods.—Sixty-five patients were eligible for the study. Telephone interviews were attempted by a clinician not involved in the patient's treatment. Thirty patients were interviewed successfully.

Findings.—Forty-seven percent of the patients interviewed had received forced injections. The rest had taken oral medication under duress. In

TABLE 2.—Patient Interview Responses (n = 30)*

	Agree	Disagree	Unsure
	(%)	*(%)*	*(%)*
Rationales for refusal			
Feared side effects	17 (57)	9 (30)	4 (13)
Believed nothing was wrong with me	9 (30)	16 (53)	5 (17)
Feared being weakened by medication	6 (20)	19 (63)	5 (17)
Felt medication was "poison"	6 (20)	22 (73)	2 (6)
Did not want anyone telling me what to do	5 (17)	18 (60)	7 (23)
Feared getting "addicted" to medication	5 (17)	20 (67)	5 (17)
Was confused at time	3 (10)	22 (73)	5 (17)
Another patient urged me to refuse	1 (3)	25 (83)	4 (13)
Family member urged me to refuse	0 (0)	24 (80)	6 (20)
Recalled emotions at time of forced medication			
Angry	12 (40)	13 (43)	5 (17)
Helpless	10 (33)	15 (50)	5 (17)
Fearful	7 (23)	17 (57)	6 (20)
Relieved	7 (23)	15 (50)	8 (27)
Embarrassed	4 (13)	21 (70)	5 (17)

*In addition to sometimes providing ambivalent answers to a given question, patients also occasionally failed to answer at all or gave only an irrelevant response. For this table, all such responses are included under the "unsure" column.

(Courtesy of Greenberg WM, Moore-Duncan L, Herron R: Patients' attitudes toward having been forcibly medicated. *Bull Am Acad Psychiatry Law* 24:513–524, 1996.)

recalling their experiences, 57% had feared side effects, 17% had feared "addiction," and 17% objected to being controlled by others. Forty percent reported feeling angry; 33%, helpless; 23%, fearful; and 13%, embarrassed. Twenty-three percent recalled feeling relieved (Table 2). In retrospect, 60% agreed with having been coerced. Fifty-three percent said they were more likely to take medication voluntarily in the future.

Conclusions.—Weeks after hospital discharge, two thirds of interviewable patients who expressed a clear opinion supported having been forced to take medications. Patients with poorer outcomes, such as rapid readmission or discharge to a state hospital, may have more negative feelings toward forcible medication.

► Often patients would rather be forcibly medicated than restrained when asked after the event, but this is clearly not universally the case. There are patients who are traumatized as a result of forced medication, and whenever possible efforts should be made to help patients to willingly accept the need for medication. However, there is a value in forcibly medicating patients when this is necessary, and the need seems to be appreciated by patients and their families.

R.J. Frances, M.D.

The Illusion of End-of-Life Resource Savings With Advance Directives

Teno J, for the SUPPORT Investigators (George Washington Univ, Washington, DC; Univ Hosps of Cleveland, Ohio; Univ of California, Los Angeles; et al)

J Am Geriatr Soc 45:513–518, 1997 6–3

Background.—It is not known whether increasing documentation of advance directives (ADs) would result in decreased resource utilization. This possibility was examined.

Methods.—Five U.S. teaching hospitals enrolled 9,105 seriously ill patients in the Study to Understand Prognoses and Preferences for Outcomes and Risks of Treatments (SUPPORT). Between 1989 and 1991, before the Patient Self-Determination Act (PSDA), 4,301 patients were enrolled. In the two years after PSDA implementation, 4,804 were enrolled. This Act required that health care facilities ask about and document existing ADs at the time of admission. The SUPPORT intervention, in which a nurse facilitated communication among patients, surrogates, and physicians about preferences for and outcomes of treatments, was provided to 2,652 patients in the later period, the remaining 2,152 serving as control subjects.

Findings.—Both the PSDA and SUPPORT interventions increased chart documentation of existing ADs. Patients in the intervention group were more likely to have pre-existing ADs documented. However, there was no corresponding change in hospital resource use for patients who died during hospitalization. Patients in the intervention group with early documentation of ADs had a trend toward greater cost.

Conclusions.—These findings cast doubt on whether policy interventions aimed at increasing AD documentation will decrease hospital resource use among dying patients. Increasing the documentation of preexisting ADs did not result in decreased hospital resource use.

► This article is part of a series which demonstrates that not enough study has been done on advance life directives before they have been widely implemented. In this study, AD documentation did not reduce hospital resource use for dying patients. Other findings from this group demonstrated that ADs did not facilitate communication or clarification of patient preferences. Very often physicians were not aware of the AD. What is really needed are ways to improve communication between patients' families and physicians rather than focusing solely on documentation.

R.J. Frances, M.D.

American Geriatrics Society on Physician-assisted Suicide: Brief to the United States Supreme Court

Lynn J, Cohn F, Pickering JH, et al (George Washington Univ, Washington, DC; Wilmer, Cutler, & Pickering, Washington, DC)

J Am Geriatr Soc 45:489–499, 1997 6–4

Background.—In 1996, the American Geriatrics Society (AGS) filed a brief with the United States Supreme Court opposing the legalization of physician-assisted suicide (PAS). The AGS stated that legalizing PAS would pose a moral dilemma for geriatricians. They reasoned that most elderly persons, before dying, have serious and progressive illness for extended periods which require significant social, financial, and medical support, resources that are too often unavailable or inadequate. By collaborating in PAS, geriatricians would be complicit in a social policy that conserves community resources by eliminating the persons who need them. By refusing to assist with their patients' suicide because their relative poverty and disadvantaged social situation are believed to be coercive, geriatricians would condemn their patients to live through undesired difficulties at the end of their lives. Because of this conundrum, the AGS opposes the legalization of PAS.

Summary of Argument.—The AGS brief argued that the Second and Ninth Circuits overturned state laws prohibiting PAS on the basis of three serious misperceptions. First, the courts were misinformed as to how most people in the United States live while dying. In fact, severe pain and symptoms in persons nearing death can be managed. Also, end-of-life health care is currently undergoing major changes. Second, the courts mistakenly concluded that PAS and foregoing life-sustaining treatments are not significantly different. Third, the courts mistakenly assumed that certain criteria or safeguards could be easily identified and implemented: that a patient be terminally ill, competent, suffering, acting voluntarily, seeking assistance in obtaining a means of suicide, and seeking assistance that would be available only from a physician. The medical profession does not have adequate definitions for some of these criteria and lacks experience with all six of them. Thus, it is not reasonable to believe that legislatures or courts could easily design procedures to ensure that each criterion is met. For all these reasons, the AGS argued that a decision to constitutionalize PAS would be, at best, seriously premature.

► A geriatric physician perspective is an important part of any public discourse on PAS. Geriatricians have firsthand views that give them special expertise in understanding aging and dying, and they are especially concerned that limits on PAS will be difficult to establish and sustain. The geriatricians in this article suggested that the Supreme Court should not, at this time, make a decision regarding the constitutional right to PAS. In fact, since this article was written the Supreme Court did just that: they did not uphold a patient's right to PAS.

R.J. Frances, M.D.

Criminality and Comorbidity

Studies of Violent and Nonviolent Male Parolees: I. Laboratory and Psychometric Measurements of Aggression

Cherek DR, Moeller FG, Schnapp W, et al (Univ of Texas-Houston)

Biol Psychiatry 41:514–522, 1997 6–5

Background.—Recent definitions of aggression focus on the causing of harm or injury to another individual who is motivated to avoid such treatment. This harm need not be physical, as long as the other individual experiences some type of aversive consequence. There must also be intent to do harm. Using the Point Subtraction Aggression Paradigm (PSAP), a laboratory procedure, the relationship among previous aggression, psychometric measures of aggression, and behavioral measures of aggressive responding was investigated in male parolees.

Methods.—Thirty male parolees were divided into violent and nonviolent groups based on their criminal history. In the PSAP procedure, subjects are paired with a fictitious other person in experimental sessions and provided with two or three response options: earning money; taking money from another individual earning money (the aggressive response); and protecting their earnings from the other individual (an escape response). The subjects are provoked by having money taken away from them and attributing these substractions to the fictitious other person.

Findings.—The violent group of parolees had significantly more aggressive responses than the nonviolent group. The number of aggressive responses was significantly associated with most psychometric measures of aggression.

Conclusions.—These findings support the external validity of the PSAP. There was a direct relationship between the history of violence among male parolees and the frequency of aggressive responses on the PSAP in a laboratory setting.

► Development of laboratory tests that could be used to measure aggressive response may help us to develop tests that could predict response outside the laboratory. In this study, the concordance between aggressive behavior in and outside of the laboratory supports the value of laboratory study of aggression. These tests could be helpful in determining whether pharmacologic agents could help reduce aggressive behavior outside the laboratory and whether laboratory tests would predict violence outside of the laboratory. Considering the amount spent on the prison system, society does not spend enough money studying human aggression.

R.J. Frances, M.D.

Laboratory

Anabolic-Androgenic Steroid Use Among 133 Prisoners
Pope HG Jr, Kouri EM, Powell KF, et al (McLean Hosp/Havard Med School, Belmont, Mass; Correctional Psychiatric Services, Acton, Mass)
Compr Psychiatry 37:322–327, 1996 6–6

Objective.—Anabolic-androgenic steroids are widely abused, especially among athletes. There is evidence that steroids may cause behavioral symptoms, especially aggressive or violent behavior. Previous reports have described men who committed violent or murderous acts while taking steroids, in the absence of any history of violence or psychiatric disorder. Prompted by experience with such a case, the frequency of steroid use among male prisoners was assessed.

Methods and Findings.—One hundred thirty-three male prisoners at a state correctional institution were interviewed about steroid use. The men had a mean age of 31 years; 50% were white, 23% were black, and 20% were Hispanic. Nine of the men either admitted using steroids or, in two cases, were strongly suspected of doing so. Just two of these men had committed criminal acts that they attributed to steroid use. Another prisoner reported acts of violence while taking steroids, although he had not been arrested for them. The remaining prisoners reported no psychiatric changes with steroid use (Fig 1).

Conclusions.—The findings suggest that 2% of crimes leading to incarceration may be caused by steroid use. Thus, steroid use appears to be an uncommon but sometimes significant factor in criminal behavior. It may be useful to assess history of steroid use in men being evaluated for criminal activities.

► This study points to the importance of screening for steroid use in cases of violence. It points to the fact that steroid use is now attributed to some crimes and that approximately 2%, or as many at 20,000, convicts in the United States may have committed crimes related to steroid use.

R.J. Frances, M.D.

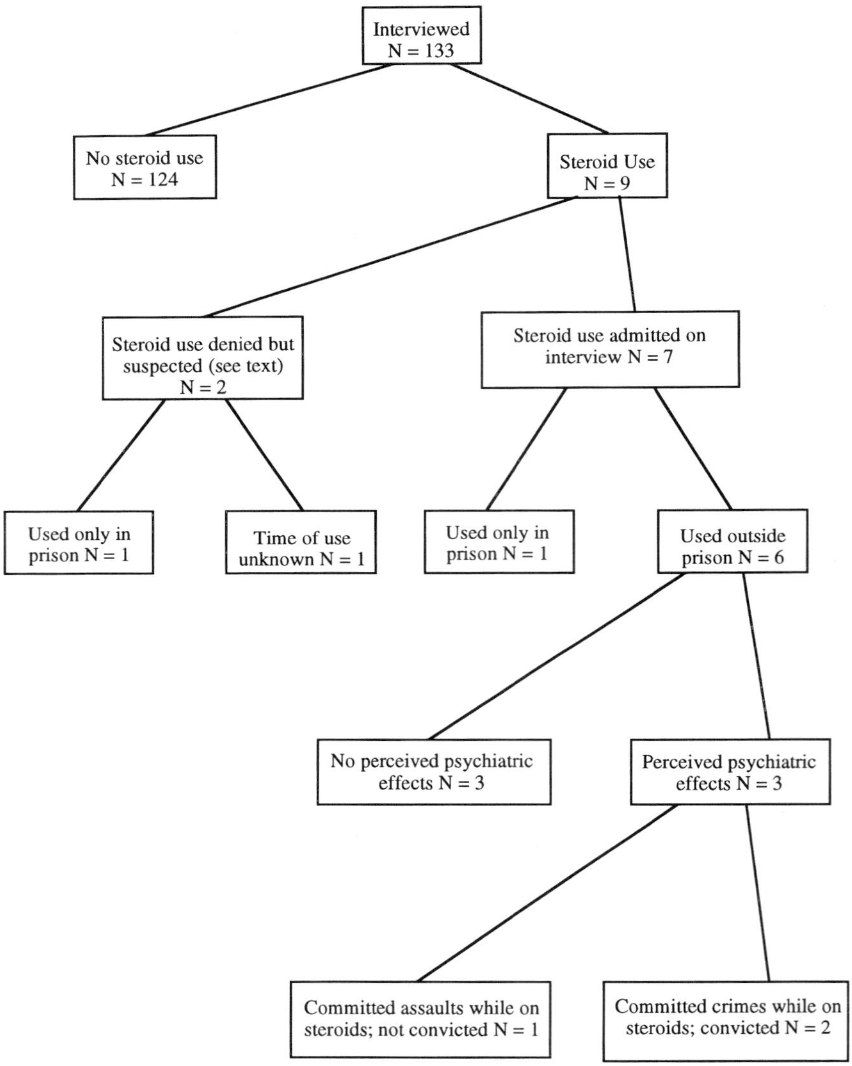

FIGURE 1.—Outcome of prisoner interviews. (Courtesy of Pope HG Jr, Kouri EM, Powell KF, et al: Anabolic-androgenic steroid use among 133 prisoners. *Compr Psychiatry* 37:322–327, 1996.)

Criminality and Violence

Threats Against Clinicians: A Preliminary Descriptive Classification
Brown GP, Dubin WR, Lion JR, et al (Univ of Rochester, NY; Univ of Nevada, Las Vegas; Temple Univ, Philadelphia)
Bull Am Acad Psychiatry Law 24:367–376, 1996 6–7

Purpose.—Clinicians have always been subject to various types of threats, yet few clinical studies have examined this problem. There are few data on how and in what context threats occur, or on how the threats are managed and resolved. A series of threats against clinicians is described, and a preliminary classification of threats is proposed.

Methods.—The analysis included 19 cases of threats against clinicians: 16 psychiatrists, two surgeons, and one clinical psychologist. Any hostile statement or action short of physical contact was considered a threat (Table 1).

Findings.—The threats fell into two basic categories, depending on whether there was a therapeutic relationship between the patient and clinician. *Situational threats* were those occurring when the clinician was functioning as an administrator or temporary care provider, such as in the general psychiatric ward or emergency department. These incidents often involved the denial of a wish by the clinician, to which the patient responded immediately with a threat. *Transferential threats* usually occurred in the course of a psychotherapeutic relationship, most often on an outpatient basis. The threat seemed to grow out of the intimacy inherent in

TABLE 1.—Threat Overview Data

	Total Threats n = 19	Situational n = 10	Transferential n = 9
Average clinician age	40	40	39
Clinician male:female	11:8	7:3	4:5
Incident when resident	6	3	3
Prior training in aggression management	4	3	1
Threatened or assaulted on other occasion	9	4	5
Inpatient:outpatient	8:11	6:4	2:7
Average patient age	32	34	31
Patient male:female	15:4	9:1	6:3
Psychotic disorder	8	5	3
Personality disorder	7	3	4
Known substance abuse	5	5	0
Legal action taken or attempted	8	3	5
Precipitating event	16	10	6
Weapon used	2	0	2
Change in professional life	13	6	7
Change in personal life	5	0	5

(Courtesy of Brown GP, Dubin WR, Lion JR, et al: Threats against clinicians: A preliminary descriptive classification. *Bull Am Acad Psychiatry Law* 24:367–376, 1996.)

such a relationship. Though there was often a precipitating event for the threat itself, these incidents seemed to evolve in an insidious manner.

Both types of threats included threats of death and assault. Threats of revenge, harm to family members, and defamation occurred only with transferential threats. Weapons (guns) were involved in two of the nine transferential threats. Though the threatened clinician often took legal action, follow-through proved difficult. Legal action did not provide the expected relief in situations involving ongoing threat. Most threatened clinicians reported changes in their personal or professional lives after the threat, including taking a more thorough history of violent behavior and increased measures related to personal safety. Though most of the threats eventually ceased, three transferential threats were still ongoing.

Conclusions.—Threats against clinicians can be divided into situational and transferential types. Further analysis will tell whether this classification system is accurate and adequate. The American Psychiatric Association and others have reported steps that clinicians can take to make the workplace safer.

► This is an accurate description of the kinds of threats made against clinicians. Healthcare work safety is an important issue, and a better understanding of threats against clinicians may lead to steps that can help therapists make their jobs safer. This article contributes a system to classify threats as either situational or transferential. The strategies for managing the kinds of threats are given, with specific case examples. Recognition for the occupational hazard of staff working in psychiatric hospitals can best be achieved by the kind of data provided in this study. Means of reducing risks from violence through efforts at quality improvement and training can be vital to the safety of employees, as well as to the reputation of the hospital. Isolated work conditions are a factor that increases danger. Good security alarm systems and a staff well trained in defusing dangerous situations are also crucial.

R.J. Frances, M.D.

Injuries Due to Assaults on Psychiatric Hospital Employees in Washington State

Bensley L, Nelson N, Kaufman J, et al (Washington State Dept of Health, Olympia; Washington State Dept of Labor and Industries, Olympia)

Am J Ind Med 31:92–99, 1997 6–8

Background.—Workers at health care facilities—especially staff at psychiatric hospitals—are at high risk for assault by patients. There is little information on the extent of violence in psychiatric hospitals, or on the potential risk and protective factors. Toward filling this gap, rates of assaults on staff were studied at a state psychiatric hospital.

Methods.—Data for the analysis were drawn from workers' compensation claims, hospital incident reports, and an employee survey. The ques-

TABLE 2.—Results of Multiple Regression Analysis Predicting Injuries Due to Assaults on Psychiatric Hospital Ward Staff (Standardized Betas)

Measure	Working in isolation from other employees	Occupation as mental health technician	Occupation as registered nurse	Work on geriatric medical unit	Work on adult psychiatric unit	Training in past year	Duration of employment
Most severe assault in the past year	.33*	.40†	.18	.41†	.16	.19§	.03
Number of assaults in the past year	.27‡	.42‡	.30*	.40†	.29‡	.17	.07
Most severe assault during total employment	.30*	.41†	.33‡	.22§	.09‡	n/a	.36*
Number of assaults during total employment	.30‡	.34§	.32§	.33‡	.31§	n/a	.40*

*$P < 0.0001$.
†$P < 0.001$.
‡$P < 0.01$.
§$P < 0.05$.
Abbreviation: na, not available.
(Courtesy of Bensley L, Nelson N, Kaufman J, et al: Injuries due to assaults on psychiatric hospital employees in Washington State, *Am J Ind Med* 31:92–99, 1997.

tionnaire examined assault experiences, isolation from other employees, training in the management of assaultive patients, availability of help during assaults, and various employment characteristics. The potential risk and protective factors addressed in the survey were studied for their relationships with the numbers and seriousness of assaults committed.

Results.—According to the workers' compensation data, the frequency of assaults was 13.8 claims per 100 employee-years. Sixty percent of all workers' compensation claims resulted from assaults. The hospital incident reports suggested a rate of injuries caused by assault of 35 per 100 employee-years.

According to the survey, 415 injuries were caused by assault per employee-year. Nearly three fourths of employees reported at least one minor injury caused by assault during the previous year. Injuries were less severe for employees who had received assault management training during the previous year. Factors associated with more severe injuries included working in isolation, working as a mental health technician, and working on the geriatric-medical unit (Table 2). Fifty-six percent of employees who called for help during an assault reported that help arrived quickly.

Conclusions.—Injuries from assaults are a common hazard for workers at psychiatric hospitals. The study identifies risk and protective factors for injuries caused by assaults; more work is needed to develop effective strategies to reduce the frequency and impact of such assaults. The frequency of assaults varies according to the data used, suggesting that assault-related injuries are underreported.

► This article surveys the high rate of assaults experienced by staff in psychiatric hospitals. The costs in terms of compensation, missed work days, morale, and disability make this a bigger problem than most people in hospitals want to know. Such issues as isolated working conditions, lack of adequate training in managing violent patients, and adequate strategies for dealing with certain patient populations are highlighted. We clearly need to develop more effective interventions and better strategies to aid staff in reducing violent patient behavior.

R.J. Frances, M.D.

Violence by Patients Admitted to a Private Psychiatric Hospital

Tardiff K, Marzuk PM, Leon AC, et al (Cornell Univ, NY; Payne Whitney Clinic, NY)

Am J Psychiatry 154:88–93, 1997 6–9

Introduction.—Studies conducted during the 1980s suggested that as many as 10% of patients had behaved violently in the month before admission to a psychiatric hospital. The risk of violence was greater for patients with schizophrenia than for those with other disorders and greater for young men than for women. Violence has been an increasing problem in American society. Rates and patterns of violence committed by patients before admission to a private psychiatric hospital were examined.

Methods.—Seven hundred sixty-three inpatients were interviewed for the study. The interview assessed demographic and socioeconomic information, history of violence, and alcohol and drug use. Psychiatric diagnoses were assessed according to DSM-III-R criteria. Episodes of violence in the month before admission were assessed in detail, including the target, place, use of a weapon, and severity of injury. The data was analyzed to determine the rates and patterns of such violence, and to identify factors associated with a greater risk of violence.

Results.—About 14% of male patients and 15% of female patients had physically attacked another person in the month before hospital admission. Compared with similar studies performed at the same hospital during the 1980s, this reflected a 50% increase in violence by male patients and a 150% increase in violence by female patients. The sexes were similar in terms of the targets of the attack, the severity of injuries, the use of a weapon, and the place of the attack. The attacks were often directed against family members at home. Weapons were used infrequently, but more than one third of the attacks resulted in injuries. For male patients, youth was the only factor significantly related to violence on univariate analysis. For females, violence was associated not only with youth but also with low socioeconomic status, substance abuse, and axis II diagnoses. After controlling for age, socioeconomic status, and axis II pathology in logistic regression analyses, violence by female patients was significantly associated with cocaine use. Recent heroin use was associated with an increased risk of violence by male patients.

Conclusions.—This study suggests a rising frequency of violence committed by patients in the month before admission to a psychiatric hospital, particularly among female patients. Substance abuse is strongly correlated with violence by patients in the community. The findings underscore the need to recognize and address the link between violence and psychiatric disorders.

► It is useful to chart the likelihood and risk of violence in hospitals, and this Cornell group has been a leader in studying this area. The increases noted in violence were especially high among women, which may relate to an increase in drug abuse, an increase in acuity of illness of those admitted, and perhaps a shift in the population that tend to be seen at the Payne Whitney clinic. The specific association between cocaine use and violence, especially in women, is the most striking finding in this study.

R.J. Frances, M.D.

Criminality—Other

Risks Factors Associated With Recidivism Among Extrafamilial Child Molesters

Prentky RA, Knight RA, Lee AFS (Joseph J Peters Inst, Philadelphia; Brandeis Univ, Philadelphia; Boston Univ)

J Consult Clin Psychol 65:141–149, 1997 6–10

Objective.—Surprisingly few studies have attempted to assess the risk of recidivism among child molesters. Factors analyzed as predictors of recidivism have included the sex of the victims, the number of previous offenses, and the intensity of the offender's fixation on children as sex objects. Factors affecting the risk of recidivism were evaluated in a follow-up study of 111 male child molesters.

Methods.—The offenders were released from 1 treatment center during a 25-year period. Data from the offenders' prison records was analyzed to assess potential risk factors, such as amount of contact with children, degree of sexual preoccupation with children, impulsivity, juvenile and adult antisocial behavior, frequency of previous sexual offenses, paraphilias, social competence, and sex of the victims. Data on criminal offenses during follow-up were obtained from law enforcement sources. These were divided into serious sexual charges, nonsexual victim-involved offenses, and victimless offenses. Discriminant analysis was performed to determine the ability of risk-assessment variables to distinguish between recidivists and nonrecidivists.

TABLE 1.—Discriminant Function Analysis Using Sexual Reoffense as the Criterion

	M/σ* for:			
Scale variable	Group 1 (n = 73)	Group 2 (n = 40)	r†	F(1, 111)
Amount of contact	0.411/0.49	0.475/0.51	.13	0.42
Fixation	0.767/0.43	0.925/0.27	.41	4.52†
Impulsivity	−0.076/0.67	0.100/0.72	.25	1.68
Paraphilias	−0.129/0.33	0.440/1.69	.53	7.70§
Juvenile antisocial behavior	0.020/0.91	0.097/0.99	.08	0.17
Adult antisocial behavior	0.027/0.50	0.005/0.65	−.04	0.34
Alcohol use history	−0.106/1.02	−0.211/0.92	−.10	0.29
No. of prior sexual offenses	3.475/3.56	5.425/3.51	.65	11.19‖
Sex of victim	0.757/0.70	0.825/0.81	.07	0.14
Social competence	−0.101/0.87	0.100/0.76	.24	1.51

**Group 1*, No evidence of sexual recidivism; *group 2*, charged with one or more new sexual offenses.
†Correlation between component and criterion.
‡$P < 0.05$.
§$P < 0.01$.
‖$P < 0.001$.

(Courtesy of Prentky RA, Knight RA, Lee AFS: Risk factors associated with recidivism among extrafamilial child molesters. *J Consult Clin Psychol* 65:141–149, 1997. Copyright 1997 by the American Psychological Association. Reprinted with permission.)

Results.—Forty subjects were charged with one or more new sexual offenses during follow-up. Variables significantly associated with recidivism were fixation, paraphilias, and number of previous sexual offenses (Table 1). These three variables correctly identified 73% of subjects as recidivists or nonrecidivists. Factors associated with nonsexual victim-involved and violent recidivism were juvenile and adult antisocial behavior, paraphilias, and low amount of contact with children. In all of these analyses, discriminatory ability was significantly better than chance—0.73 to 0.79 on analysis of area under the receiver-operating characteristic curve. Sexual recidivism rate did not differ significantly according to the sex of the victims.

Conclusions.—Factors predicting recidivism among child molesters depend on the type of recidivism being considered. Variables associated with sexual recidivism are degree of sexual preoccupation with children, paraphilias, and number of previous sexual offenses. For nonsexual and violent recidivism, the predictive variables are those reflecting impulsive, antisocial behavior. In contrast to past studies, this study found no predictive efficacy for victim sex.

► Among types of criminal behavior, none has been singled out for more attention than have sex offenses committed against children. However, not until recently has there been systematic study of factors that might predispose sex offenders toward recidivism of sexual and violent crimes. Perhaps the best predictor of future offenses for both sexual and aggressive crimes is number of previous offenses. Sexual preoccupation with children and sexual deviancy are two other important factors.

R.J. Frances, M.D.

Criminal Behavior in Males With Affective Disorders

Modestin J, Hug A, Ammann R (Psychiatric Univ Hosp Zürich, Switzerland; Psychiatric Univ Hosp, Berne, Switzerland)

J Affect Disord 42:29–38, 1997 6–11

Purpose.—Though there is an increased emphasis on the link between mental illness and criminal behavior, relatively little is known about criminality in patients with affective disorders. The available data suggests that people with mental disorders are much more likely to be involved in violent or illegal conduct; however, there have been no comprehensive studies of affective disorders. Criminality was assessed among a sample of male inpatients with affective disorders.

Methods.—The study included 261 male inpatients with affective disorders. All met the Research Diagnostic Criteria for bipolar affective disorder or for major, minor, or intermittent depressive disorder. Criminality was assessed through conviction records. The findings were compared with those of a group of matched subjects from the general population. Mean age was about 42 in both groups.

Results.—Forty-two percent of the patients and 31% of the control subjects had criminal records. Except for sexual offenses and traffic violations, the inpatients were more likely to have violations of all different types, including various types of violent crime. Compared with noncriminal patients, criminal patients with affective disorders tended to be younger, single, and of lower social class. Thirty percent of the patients and 15% of the control subjects had been sentenced to prison. A criminal record was found for 48% of patients with bipolar disorder and 60% of those with unipolar minor or intermittent depression, significantly more than in the general population. The patients with major depression were no more likely than population control subjects to have a criminal record. Personality disorder was common among criminal patients with minor or intermittent depression and among noncriminal patients with the same disorders. Forty-four percent of criminal patients with bipolar disorder were drug abusers, compared with 12% of noncriminal patients with bipolar disorder.

Conclusions.—Inpatients with affective disorders are more likely than are matched population control subjects to have criminal records. The increase in criminality is significant only for patients with bipolar disorder and minor or intermittent depression, not those with major depression. Drug abuse is common among patients with bipolar disorders and criminal behavior. Though the social significance of the findings is unclear, they warrant further attention.

▶ The finding that criminal behavior is more common in bipolar disorder than unipolar disorder is not surprising. In the midst of a manic episode, disinhibition is frequently associated with criminal behavior. Often bipolar disorder is associated with drug use, and the combination contributes to criminality and also to high rates of hospitalization.

R.J. Frances, M.D.

Factitious Sexual Harassment

Feldman-Schorrig S (UCLA, Los Angeles, Calif)
Bull Am Acad Psychiatry Law 24:387–392, 1996 6–12

Background.—In factitious disorders, the person intentionally produces or fakes signs or symptoms of a disorder to assume the sick role. The symptoms may be predominantly psychologic, predominantly physical, or a combination. Reports suggest that the desire to acquire victim status can also lead to factitious disorders. Recent years have seen increasing numbers of complaints of sexual harassment. Some cases of sexual harassment maybe factitious, prompted by a person's need for portrayal as a victim. The problem of factitious sexual harassment is reviewed.

Factitious Sexual Harassment.—Factitious sexual harassment may sometimes explain apparently discrepant findings in sexual harassment claims, such as an apparently sincere accusation that is proved false, trivial allegations leading to an intense reaction, and strong evidence that the alleged harassment was encouraged. In examining such cases, it is important to understand motives underlying the wish to be perceived as a victim. These may include the need for validation of the plaintiff's self-perception of victimhood, often related to childhood sexual abuse. Complaints of sexual harassment may also elicit sympathy or emotional support, particularly in the therapy setting. Some plaintiffs may characteristically harbor a great deal of anger or feel trapped in a situation such as an abusive relationship. Such women may project their anger onto a male target they view as abusive. In another mechanism, repetition compulsion may lead women with a history of childhood sexual abuse to reenact the victim role in their relationships with men. It is important to note, however, that a history of repetition compulsion does not necessarily mean that harassment has not taken place.

Factitious disorders have previously been linked with borderline personality disorder. One characteristic shared by these disorders is *pseudologia fantastica,* or pathologic lying. It can be difficult to distinguish between factitious disorder and malingering, especially because the possibility of financial reward is inherent in litigation.

Discussion.—The problem of factitious sexual harassment stems from the desire for victim status. The plaintiff in factitious sexual harassment cases is usually very convincing in her allegations, and the correct diagnosis can be difficult to make in the absence of contradictory evidence. The possibility of factitious disorder should be considered in sexual harassment cases in which there is a discrepancy between the plaintiff's apparently sincere accusations and the objective facts.

▶ Having seen cases similar to those described in this article, I am convinced that this is a growing problem. It can be difficult to investigate the veracity of a claim of sexual harassment. It takes a combination of "bloodhound" and good psychiatric skills to discover when the accusation of sexual harassment is factitious and arises from intentional production or feigning of signs to assume a sick role. Discriminating factitious disorder from malingering may be especially hard, because economic gain is usually involved in these lawsuits and it can be hard to tell when secondary gain is the principal feature, as would be the case in a factitious disorder. Assuming the injured role with an opportunity to release anger and repeat or reenact some earlier experience of abuse is common in these cases. Careful gathering of the facts is a valuable tool in making the correct diagnosis in this situation.

R.J. Frances, M.D.

Collaboration With Police Officers Within a Partial Hospital Program
Steiner JL, Berg DN, Sledge WH (Yale Univ, New Haven, Conn)
J Nerv Ment Dis 185:269–273, 1997 6–13

Introduction.—Safety is a major concern in the psychiatric treatment setting. Police officers commonly interact with mentally ill patients in the community, where they have the authority to arrest patients or bring them to the emergency department. Once patients are in the health care setting, the psychiatrist's evaluation takes precedence. Prompted by a violent incident—the stabbing of a staff member by a recently discharged patient—an urban community mental health center hired city police officers to provide extraduty coverage to its day hospital. This arrangement was undertaken without discussing the role expectations beforehand. The one-year experience with this arrangement is reported.

Phases of the Relationship.—The police and day hospital personnel both entered into the relationship with unspoken assumptions about what constituted appropriate interventions for disruptive behavior and who would be carrying out those interventions. At the start of the arrangement, there was a "honeymoon period," with quick camaraderie between the staff and police. During this period of mutual appreciation, however, the balance of power and psychologic authority rested with the police. Before long, the roles were brought into conflict by an incident of verbal, racially based abuse by a patient. The police officers wanted to arrest the patient for breach of the peace, whereas the clinical personnel insisted on a clinical intervention. Contact between the officers and staff was civil but strained for a few months after that event. Rather than being dependent, the clinical staff had asserted their power to make decisions regarding interventions for disruptive behavior. With time, and without formal discussion, the roles of the police and staff gradually became reconciled. The police came to accept advice from the clinical staff about interventions and to recognize the staff's right to make decisions about their roles in a given situation. In this way, the staff regained their sense of control and competence, which had deteriorated since the stabbing. The officers reported that their own ability to deal with mentally ill persons was improved by watching the staff in action. The relationship moved from one of power imbalance to one of mutual interdependence and collaboration. The officers' assistance in specific incidents with out-of-control patients was invaluable. Their mere presence aided in deescalating situations, without any need for force.

Discussion.—The unfolding relationship between police officers and clinical staff in a day hospital program for the mentally ill is described. Though roles and responsibilities were unclear at first, this relationship evolved into one of mutual support and benefit. An effective and respectful approach to security can be achieved, despite the different structures and missions of the police and clinical staff.

▶ Any means of increasing communication and collaboration between police and psychiatric hospitals warrants attention, because both sets of professionals frequently deal with the same kinds of problems. Cross-training and cross-functional teamwork was fostered by the collaboration set forth here. This kind of cooperation can lead to better security for all.

R.J. Frances, M.D.

Insanity Defense Pleas in Baltimore City: An Analysis of Outcome

Janofsky JS, Dunn MH, Roskes EJ, et al (Univ of Maryland, Baltimore; Johns Hopkins Univ, Baltimore, Md)

Am J Psychiatry 153:1464–1468, 1996 6–14

Background.—There is a long history of debate over the use of the insanity defense. The rate of insanity pleas, and the success rate of such pleas, varies considerably. However, the insanity plea is generally used much more rarely than perceived by legislators or the general public. In Maryland, every defendant who pleads insanity is referred for a pretrial screening, and data on insanity pleas is systematically compiled. A one-year analysis of the outcomes of insanity pleas in Baltimore was performed.

Methods.—The analysis included all defendants who pleaded not criminally responsible in Baltimore City during 1991. The law at that time, a modification of the American Law Institute Test, stated that defendants were not criminally responsible if they lacked the capacity to appreciate the criminality of their conduct, or to conform to the requirements of the law, because of a mental disorder or mental retardation. Each defendant received a psychiatric evaluation at the medical service of the court. Information on the defendants' demographic characteristics, crimes committed, diagnoses, and psychiatric opinions regarding criminal responsibility was analyzed. The outcomes of their trials were determined as well.

Results.—A total of 60,432 indictments were filed during the year studied. Of those defendants, 190 pleaded not criminally responsible, for a rate of 0.31 per 100 indictments. On psychiatric evaluation, 55% of the defendants were believed to be criminally responsible, 2% were believed to be definitely not responsible, and 33% were believed to be possibly not responsible; an opinion was deferred in the remaining 8% of cases. By the time their case went to trial, all but eight defendants dropped this plea. All eight defendants were found criminally not responsible at trial, and the plea was uncontested. In all other cases, the charge was dropped before trial, the defendant remained not competent to stand trial, or the defendant withdrew the plea of not criminally responsible. The final rate was therefore 0.013 per 100 indictments, or 4.2% of the cohort originally pleading not criminally responsible.

Conclusions.—In this large series of "criminally not responsible" pleas, there were no contested insanity trials. This means that, for all defendants who still made this plea by the time their case went to trial, the state and defense agreed that the person was not criminally responsible. The findings are evidence against the perception that insanity pleas are overused and misused. The pretrial screening program used in Maryland is not only clinically valuable but provides for easy collection of research data.

▶ Although the insanity defense frequently comes under attack, articles like this one regularly appear in the forensic literature, pointing to the very low rate at which the insanity defense is used and the very low rate, in this case "0," in which trials contested the plea of not criminally responsible. These conclusions are not novel. It is useful for those who argue against the McNaughton rule to be familiar with these data.

R.J. Frances, M.D.

Risk and Claims

Perils of Being a Plaintiff: Impressions of a Forensic Psychiatrist
Halleck SL (Univ of North Carolina, Chapel Hill)
Clin Orthop 336:72–78, 1997 6–15

Introduction.—Although litigation has obvious negative emotional effects on the defendants, there has been relatively little attention to the impact on the plaintiffs. These are people who have been victimized by the alleged negligence of others, and who are seeking compensation through litigation. A forensic psychiatrist has drawn on his impressions to discuss the psychological risk to plaintiffs in litigation.

The Stresses of Litigation for Plaintiffs.—The psychological risks of litigation for the plaintiff are illustrated in a series of case reports. It is often assumed that if a patient in litigation gets worse, it must be because of monetary incentives for not improving. When the patient does not improve after the end of the case, other reasons must be sought. One possible reason is the high level of stress experienced by the plaintiff, sometimes lasting a period of years as the case wears on through the courts. A great part of this stress arises from questioning the authenticity and severity of the patients' symptoms during the process of litigation.

Unlike physical symptoms, psychological symptoms can be evaluated only by listening to the patient's version of the suffering or by making observations of the patient's behavior. If the patient's level of function drops, that disability must be explained to the patient and to all those around him or her. There is considerable pressure to convince oneself and others that the new behavior pattern is involuntary, whereas the opposite is generally assumed. Confirmation that the behavior is involuntary generally requires a medical diagnosis. The pressure to justify the dysfunctional behavior rises even higher in the presence of litigation for damages. This pressure is intensified when the patient's disability is evaluated by medical experts on either side of the case. Plaintiffs will probably be afraid of being examined by the expert employed by the defense, especially afraid that they will be accused of malingering. This situation invokes the concept of negative reinforcement, in which the best way to refute allegations that the patient could be doing better is for the patient to become even more symptomatic. This can be a conscious or subconscious process. Thus, even the most benign evaluation by a defense expert can lead to acceleration of symptoms.

Discussion.—Being the plaintiff in litigation can take a serious emotional toll, sometimes serving to make the patient's condition worse. Everyone involved in the litigation process must understand the possible harm involved with entering into litigation. Attorneys for the plaintiff must make sure that the plaintiff is aware of these risks, and should be aware that settling for a lesser amount may be better for their client's well-being than going before a jury. Defense attorneys might consider being more generous with settlement offers if they see that the patient is becoming more disabled. Plaintiff's experts should be careful not to exaggerate the patient's disability, and should encourage the patient to function at the highest possible level. Defense experts should be sure that patients understand their role.

► This is a sensitively written article, which points out that plaintiffs can also, to some degree, be victimized by the process of litigation and experience significant amounts of stress. It points out that being a plaintiff is not without risk of complicating one's problems, including developing secondary pain that can cause additional psychiatric distress. Just raising awareness of these problems among physicians, attorneys, and the plaintiff can lead all to try to make greater efforts to do no harm to the patient. Perhaps it is not surprising that a physician has written this article, not a lawyer.

R.J. Frances, M.D.

State Hospitals' Responses to the Sexual Behavior of Psychiatric Inpatients

Buckley PF, Hyde JL (Northcoast Behavioral Healthcare System, Northfield, Ohio; Case Western Reserve Univ, Cleveland, Ohio)

Psychiatric Serv 48:398–399, 1997 6–16

Purpose.—Sexual behavior by the severely mentally ill—whether normal or deviant—can pose difficult emotional and social problems. Policies must protect patients and promote a therapeutic milieu while meeting official mores and public expectations. There is evidence that sexual activity among psychiatric patients has been greatly underestimated. State psychiatric hospitals were surveyed regarding their policies toward sexual activity among patients.

Methods.—A questionnaire was sent to the directors of 86 state psychiatric facilities across the United States. Most of the hospitals were acute, long-stay facilities. The directors were asked whether their hospital had a formal policy on patient sexual behavior, whether they saw such behavior as a problem, whether they had a psychoeducational program to deal with patient sexual behavior, and whether the hospital had mixed- or single-sex units.

Results.—There were 57 responses. Eighty-three percent of respondents said that they had a formal policy regarding patient sexual behavior. Eighty-eight percent reported that such behavior was a problem, and 26% that it was a significant and persistent problem. Seventy-five percent of the hospitals had relevant psychoeducational activities, covering such areas as HIV prevention, prenatal care, and personal relationships. Others had such policies under development. Sixty percent of the hospitals had mixed-sex units.

Conclusions.—State psychiatric hospitals report problems related to patient sexual behavior. A surprisingly large percentage of hospitals have a policy regarding patient sexual behavior; it remains to be seen whether they are able to implement guidelines that are sensible and sensitive. The development of regional or national guidelines, encouraged by greater acknowledgment of and sharing information about the problems associated with patient sexual behavior, is needed.

► This paper gathers data on how hospitals around the country deal with sexual behavior of psychiatric patients and could form a basis for beginning to develop guidelines regarding methods of dealing with this problem. Benchmarking revealed that most hospitals have developed policies on sexual behavior; however, they have not widely applied guidelines that are sensible and sensitive.

R.J. Frances, M.D.

Tales of the Crypt for Psychiatrists: Mourning, Melancholia, and Mortuary Malpractice

Eth S, Leong GB, Garrick TR (New York Med College; Univ of California, Los Angeles; Univ of Missouri, Columbia)

Bull Am Acad Psychiatry Law 24:483–492, 1996 6–17

Objectives.—In the United States, every death eventually involves bringing the body to a mortuary or funeral home. With its emotional implications, the funeral process has great potential for difficulties. These sometimes come out in the form of litigation against the mortuary or cemetery involving mishandling of the dead body. A number of cases involving civil litigation for negligence between grieving families and the mortuaries handling the bodies of their loved ones were reviewed.

Methods.—The authors acted as defense psychiatric experts by evaluating 25 individual plaintiffs in nine lawsuits involving mortuaries and/or cemeteries. The defendants were accused of negligence resulting in psychological harm to a grieving family member. In each case, the defense sought an academically based forensic psychiatrist to help defuse the emotional issues related to death.

Results.—Each of the 25 plaintiffs reported psychiatric and somatic complaints. Nine had undergone evaluation by plaintiff's experts, leading to various diagnoses to account for the symptoms reported. The cases involved such incidents as wrong caskets, improper closed-casket services, burial in the wrong plot, and lost cremated remains. The defense evaluation suggested that the plaintiffs were sincerely grief stricken over the loss of their loved one, and angry about the defendants' perceived insensitivity. However, in no case was there a supportable Axis I or II diagnosis. The emotional reactions were explained by the plaintiffs' angry bereavement, as influenced by the circumstances of the funeral process and cultural and religious factors. The most appropriate DSM diagnosis for these cases was the V-Code "bereavement," although this term was imprecise.

Conclusions.—The emotions involved in grieving, along with cultural and religious factors, play an important role in the psychology of civil litigation involving mortuaries and malpractice. The emotional state of the grieving family members makes them highly vulnerable to lapses of expected routine and perceptions of disrespect toward the deceased. The risk of problems may be heightened if the death was a traumatic one or the relationship with the diseased was ambivalent. Multiple DSM diagnoses should not be assigned simply to account for every symptom in the grieving relative. A diagnosis of "bereavement NOS," signifying an unusual occurrence in the grieving process but not necessarily a psychiatric disorder, may be the best approach in this situation.

▶ Having treated funeral home directors, I am not surprised that mistakes are made that can lead to mortuary malpractice, and that psychiatrists are likely to be drawn into litigation related to these situations. Psychiatrists' knowledge of mourning and grief may give them special insight into aspects of funeral home activities that can lead up to litigation. Cultural and religious factors can play a role in how bereavement is handled and can play a role in civil litigation.

R.J. Frances, M.D.

Forensic Career

Trading Forensic and Family Commitments

Kearney AJ, Gutheil TG, Commons ML (Harvard Med School, Boston)

Bull Am Acad Psychiatry Law 24:533–546, 1996 6–18

Background.—Like other professionals, expert witnesses must find a balance between their commitments to family and profession. For forensic experts, case schedules frequently come into conflict with family activities. There have been no systematic studies of these difficult choices. The decisions made by forensic experts when they have to make a choice between family and profession were examined in a pilot study.

Methods.—The study used consumer preference theory, which measures the importance of a particular commitment in terms of the value attached to it by the individual, or the utility derived from the activity. Fifteen forensic experts completed an instrument designed to assess the trade-offs made in choosing between family and professional commitments. The decision-making process behind the balance between the conflicting sets of commitments was evaluated as well.

Results.—Five of the 15 participants traded commitments to maximize their satisfaction with the outcome. The trading function was particularly significant considering the multidimensional nature of the commitments under consideration. Another four participants chose one alternative or the other—family in one case and profession in three—and stuck with it. Rather than basing their decisions on the utility level of any given situation, these professionals felt obligated to maintain a particular level of devotion to family or profession. Of the remaining six participants, four showed ill-defined trading patterns, whereas only two followed an apparently random pattern of choices. On analysis of some personal characteristics, politically liberal individuals and those who attended church regularly seemed to sacrifice less for their professions than political conservatives and nonchurchgoers.

Conclusions.—Forensic experts may make decisions between professional and family commitments based on the relative importance they attach to those commitments. Few such professionals appear to follow a random pattern of choices. These preliminary findings are only the initial examination of an emotionally and ethically complex topic. With better understanding, the decision-making process may be refined sufficiently to provide practitioners with guidance in making difficult choices.

► This is a wonderful paper because it has implications not only for forensic psychiatrists but for all professionals who struggle with conflicts between their professional responsibilities and their responsibilities to family commitments. Forensic psychiatrists suffer the special problem of often not being able to control the schedule of dates of trials and have to weigh their responsibilities to clients heavily in decisions about time allocation that often also affect their families. Comparing these results of forensic psychiatrists to decisions on priorities of professionals in other areas, such as CEOs in business, athletes, etc., would be interesting.

R.J. Frances, M.D.

7 Community Psychiatry

Managed Care

APA Resource Document: I. The Professional Responsibilities of Psychiatrists in Evolving Health Care Systems
Hoge SK (Univ of Virginia, Charlottesville)
Bull Am Acad Psychiatry Law 24:393–418, 1996 7–1

Introduction.—The practice of psychiatry is changing under pressure to control health care costs. Historically, the profession has been free to establish patterns of practice and ethical traditions that encourage individuals to seek treatment and to trust their physician. Some psychiatrists believe that cost containment measures require them to withhold certain treatment information and to discourage individuals from seeking needed treatment. Suggestions for resolving some of the problems created by managed care and other health care systems are given.

Principles of Psychiatric Practice.—There are 4 principles of psychiatric practice that must be preserved under any system of health care. The first is the fiduciary obligation to patients. Patients expect psychiatrists to act in their best interest even without being asked to do so. When patients seek help, they are sick, in distress, and may have cognitive impairments that prevent them from making good decisions. Without the expectation that the psychiatrist will put the patient's interest first, the integrity of the health care system cannot be maintained. The second principle is the autonomy of patients to make treatment decisions, especially to select their psychiatrist and to make decisions about specific services. The selection of a psychiatrist can be key to the success of treatment. This autonomy is based on the assumption that psychiatrists will provide all relevant information about the patient's mental health care. The third principle is access to psychiatric care and continuity of care, which can be another key element to the success of treatment. The fourth principle is quality of care. The psychiatric profession must set standards of care and ensure that practitioners are competent. The practice of psychiatry is constantly changing, and only those with expertise who are trained to evaluate research can make judgments about the quality of care. Patients cannot be expected to have this expertise and should not have to bargain with health care systems about appropriate care.

Responsibilities of Psychiatrists Under Managed Care.—Psychiatrists have several responsibilities under managed care. The first responsibility is to disclose all treatment options, regardless of insurance coverage. The patient should have the option of choosing an uncovered treatment method and paying for it out-of-pocket. The second responsibility is to openly discuss any incentive arrangements to limit care and any managed care practices that may affect the course of treatment. These arrangements create a potential conflict and threaten the doctor-patient relationship. It is vital that these and other issues be openly discussed to maintain the trust of the patient. The third responsibility is to appeal on the patient's behalf any cases of denied payment by a third-party payer when medical judgment dictates otherwise. Some specific responsibilities of the appeal process are given. Finally, there are responsibilities after coverage for recommended treatment that has been denied. These responsibilities are identical to those that existed before health insurance coverage was common: the psychiatrist must negotiate with the patient about care and payment. If the recommended care is not possible, alternative care must be provided or a referral to another psychiatrist who can provide these services must be made. These and other responsibilities are important because many patients are unaware of managed care practices.

General Regulation of Managed Care.—It is clear that managed health care systems must be regulated. General regulation must address the issues of certification of managed care and liability. Managed care companies currently make decisions about resource allocation, limits on coverage, credentialing, and health care delivery without the involvement of patients or psychiatrists. These current procedures must be improved by mandatory certification or accreditation of managed care companies with real penalties to enforce the regulations. The threat of legal liability may compel managed care companies to maintain adequate standards of care. Currently, patients may be put at risk by managed care decisions, for example, if coverage for certain services is denied to suicidal patients or if inpatient coverage is terminated before an outpatient plan is secured. Psychiatrists now fear that they may be held legally responsible for the decisions of managed care companies. Insurance companies have maintained that they are exempt from liability under existing federal law. It is imperative to combine actual responsibility and legal liability. One provision of the Employee Retirement Income Security Act (ERISA) preempts all state laws on the liability of large insurance plans and limits recovery to payment of the withheld benefits. Claims cannot be brought for damages suffered or punitive damage. This preemption portion of the ERISA should be repealed or modified.

The Role of Psychiatrists in Managed Care.—Managed care companies are corporate entities and have no obligation to observe the principles of psychiatric practice. These companies must be required to establish a medical staff structure consisting of a governing board and a medical board. The medical board would be responsible for reviewing restrictions on services, credentials, and any issues relating to quality of care. "Gag" provisions interfere with the patient's right to be informed and the right of the patient to participate in health care decisions. Psychiatrists should not sign contracts that include these gag clauses. In the future, courts may rule that gag clauses are unenforceable because they are contrary to the public interest. Legislation that protects a psychiatrists's communication is essential, and managed care companies should not be allowed to undermine the psychiatrist's allegiance to the patient.

Discussion.—This article also discusses in detail incentive provisions, the role of the psychiatrist in the review process, criteria for denial of coverage, and appeals. The article has worthwhile suggestions for the practice of psychiatry, not only for interaction with the patient but also for legislation that can bring about much needed changes in managed health care systems.

► Although the ethical issues raised by managed care have been discussed at professional meetings for at least a decade, very little has appeared in the lay or professional literature until relatively recently. Issues discussed here, such as the "responsibility to disclose . . . to appeal . . . and . . . [that] after the denial," are beautifully elucidated and should facilitate physicians' interactions with their patients and with managed care organizations.

J.A. Talbott, M.D.

The Economic Impact of Psychotherapy: A Review

Gabbard GO, Lazar SG, Hornberger J, et al (Menninger Clinic, Washington, DC; George Washington Univ, Washington, DC; Stanford Univ, Calif)

Am J Psychiatry 154:147–155, 1997 7–2

Introduction.—Several studies have shown a decrease in the use of medical care after psychotherapy, with medical inpatient stays reduced by about 1.5 days with psychotherapeutic interventions. An updated review of the literature was conducted to determine whether psychotherapy has an effect on a variety of costs, including the cost of psychotherapy itself, the cost of mortality, the cost of psychiatric hospitalization, the cost of disability and impaired work performance, and other medical and laboratory costs.

Methods.—There were 686 articles identified in a MEDLINE search, and of these, 41 articles included measures of outcome with implications for cost. Eighteen studies were selected for analysis. The others were excluded because they lacked a comparison group, there was a focus on a medical disorder instead of a psychiatric illness, and outcomes did not include cost data. Outcomes included data on medical care use or work function or actual cost accounting.

Results.—Psychotherapy reduces costs according to these studies. In 1 trial with a random assignment of participants, treatment groups showed marked improvement in depressive symptoms during 16 weeks, and the groups included amitriptyline prescribed by a psychiatrist, cognitive-behavior therapy performed by a clinical psychologist, counseling by a social worker, and routine care provided by a general practitioner that included antidepressant medication, counseling, or referral to another agency. When a social worker provided individual counseling, this was found to be statistically significant in superiority to care provided by a general practitioner.

Conclusion.—Schizophrenia, bipolar affective disorder, and borderline personality disorder showed the most evidence of a positive effect on costs with psychotherapeutic intervention. A limitation of this review is that most of these studies involved small groups of subjects. Future studies measuring the outcome of psychotherapy should incorporate cost analyses.

▶ We all know that psychotherapy is perceived as less effective and costlier than pharmacotherapy by many, including some in managed care. It is important that we demonstrate not only what this article did, that psychotherapy holds down costs, but also compare the economic impact of psychotherapy vs. other types of treatment as well as the effectiveness of combined (psychotherapeutic-psychopharmacologic) treatment.

J.A. Talbott, M.D.

Designing a Comprehensive Care Program for High-cost Clients in a Managed Care Environment

Quinlivan R, McWhirter DP (Telecare Corp, San Diego, Calif; Univ of California, San Diego)

Psychiatric Serv 47:813–815, 1996 7–3

Introduction.—Clients who use a high volume of inpatient mental health services present a challenge to managed care's goal of reducing costly hospitalizations. When the California Department of Mental Health began its reform of mental health services in 1994, San Diego Mental Health Services became the managed health care plan for San Diego County and entered into contractual agreements with 14 private psychiatric inpatient facilities to care for approximately 350,000 clients eligible for Medi-Cal, the state Medicaid agency. The Telecare Corporation, a private contractor, was engaged to develop a comprehensive care program for these clients.

The High-Cost Client.—A pre–managed care study of frequent users of inpatient services identified a small group of high-cost clients who had 3 or more admissions in 6 months. High-cost clients identified after the first 6 months of consolidated inpatient services under managed care were compared with clients included in the pre–managed care study. The 113 highest users of managed care after 6 months accounted for 22% of all admissions of clients in the system; the average annualized cost per client was $27,189. High-cost clients in the pre–managed care and post–managed care groups were generally comparable in age, sex distribution, and ethnicity. Nearly all clients in both groups had multiple axis I diagnoses, but a greater percentage in the pre–managed care group had schizophrenia (57% vs. 36%).

Targeting High-Cost Clients.—High-cost users were defined as all clients with an annualized cost for inpatient care in excess of $24,000. As a group, high-cost users account for at least 20% of budgeted resources for inpatient care. Seven problems were found to be related to frequent admissions: acute drug and alcohol use precipitating a suicidal or psychotic crisis soon after the last discharge, refusal to take medications, violent outbursts or threats of violence, suicide threats or attempts, self-mutilation, a diagnosis of borderline personality disorder, and an inability to manage financial resources.

Best-Practice Guidelines.—To develop a comprehensive care program for high-cost users of inpatient services, recommendations were made for service delivery: continuity of care, alcohol and drug abuse treatment, specialized services for targeted clients with a diagnosis of personality disorder, alternatives to acute hospitalization, residential treatment settings for those prone to violence, medication management and education, and assistance in managing financial resources. The high-cost group will be followed up to determine whether such programming will reduce inpatient stays.

► Managed behavioral health care has had it relatively "easy" so far in our field, "managing" the care of employed, relatively well-functioning individuals. However, now, providers will be dealing with the traditional "publicly-supported" populations; those covered by Medicaid, those covered by Medicare who have not already been "creamed off," and those with no coverage. Anyone going "at risk" for these populations had better have a strategy for the high-cost clients that incorporates all that we have learned since 1955, when deinstitutionalization began. Otherwise, they will be in trouble.

J.A. Talbott, M.D.

Shortening Length of Stay Without Increasing Recidivism on a University-affiliated Inpatient Unit

Thomas MR, Rosenberg SA, Giese AA, et al (Univ of Colorado, Denver)
Psychiatric Serv 47:996–998, 1996 7–4

Background.—Clinicians have become concerned that shortening the inpatient stay of individuals in psychiatric units could harm the patients and result in so-called revolving door treatment. Epidemiologic studies have reported higher rates of readmission after shorter inpatient stays, but controlled studies have reported higher rates of readmission after longer inpatient stays. More information is clearly needed. The effect of shorter inpatient stays on the readmission rates of psychiatric inpatients was investigated in an observational, retrospective study.

Methods.—All patients between 18 and 64 years old who were admitted for acute care at a psychiatric hospital between 1985 and 1992 were analyzed. Before 1990, the facility provided traditional inpatient care. In 1990, the facility was reorganized and offered an alternatives program consisting of a locked inpatient unit, an unlocked 24-hour open unit, and a partial hospitalization program. Data were divided into the 2 time periods for the traditional unit and the alternatives program.

Results.—Data from 1,008 individuals, 523 patients from the traditional program and 485 patients from the alternatives program, were analyzed. The diagnostic differences between the 2 groups were discussed. After the alternatives program was instituted, the mean length of stay was reduced from 20.2 days to 6.2 full-day equivalents, but the overall readmission rates at 1, 3, 6, 12, and 36 months after the initial admission did not increase. Readmission rates did increase from 13.7% to 35.2% for a subgroup of patients with psychotic disorders. After adjusting for differences in diagnoses, analysis showed that readmission rates remained similar for both study groups.

Discussion.—In these privately insured patients, shortening the inpatient stay did not increase recidivism. The only outcome measures in this study were length of stay and relapse; comorbidity was not analyzed. More research is needed to evaluate other outcome measures and to determine whether certain subgroups of patients are at risk of relapse after short-term inpatient treatment.

► It seems to me that there are 2 lessons to be learned here. First, shortened stays are as (if not more) effective as longer ones for patients without psychosis. Second is the converse, that patients with disorders like schizophrenia have more readmissions, although fewer than those in the "traditional" control treatment group. It is hoped that we'll be able to target, predict, and prevent, that is, target such individuals, predict who can and cannot do better with what length of stay, and prevent excess recidivism.

J.A. Talbott, M.D.

A Pharmacoeconomic Model of Outpatient Antipsychotic Therapy in "Revolving Door" Schizophrenic Patients

Glazer WM, Ereshefsky L (Yale Univ, New Haven, Conn; Univ of Texas, San Antonio)

J Clin Psychiatry 57:337–345, 1996 7–5

Background.—It is unlikely that there will be enough resources to meet the demand for health care in the United States. This is especially true in cases of chronic schizophrenia and other severe mental illnesses. It is estimated that the total cost associated with schizophrenia in the United States was $65 billion in 1991. Given that resources will always be limited, available resources must be well distributed. Psychiatrists may have to expand their role from patient advocate to allocator of care and consider the impact on society of a given treatment method in terms of quality of life and cost-effectiveness. Pharmacoeconomic models help identify, mea-

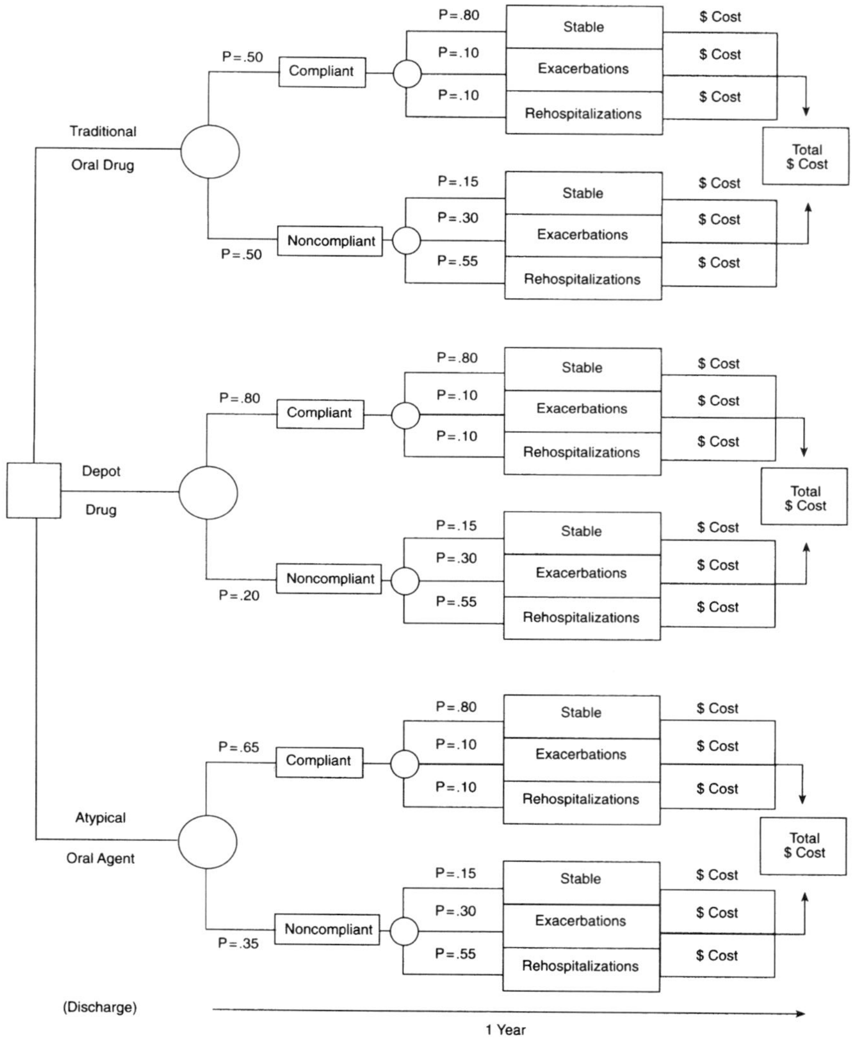

FIGURE 1.—Decision tree used in the pharmacoeconomic model (P = Probability). (Courtesy of Glazer WM, Ereshefsky L: A pharmacoeconomic model of outpatient antipsychotic therapy in "revolving door" schizophrenic patients. *J Clin Psychiatry* 57:337–345, 1996. Copyright 1996, Physicians Postgraduate Press. Reprinted by permission.)

sure, and compare the cost and outcome of pharmaceuticals. These models are not intended to replace the insight or judgment of clinicians, but rather summarize a subset of the information needed to make informed decisions. Cost-effective management strategies using pharmacoeconomic methodology were investigated in individuals with schizophrenia who require repeated hospitalization.

Methods.—Various pharmacoeconomic analysis methodologies have been used to assess the cost and quality-of-life benefits of alternative treatments. A clinical decision analysis model (Fig 1) was constructed that uses compliance rates and rehospitalization to compare the costs of direct treatment with alternate outpatient neuroleptic drugs in individuals with schizophrenia who require repeat hospitalization, known as "revolving door" schizophrenic patients. Treatment with traditional oral neuroleptics, depot neuroleptics, and atypical oral agents, such as risperidone was analyzed.

Results.—Under 5 sets of cost and outcome assumptions, switching to a depot neuroleptic in a patient with a history of relapse and rehospitalization may lower the cost of direct treatment by $650–$2,600 per year when compared with treatment with an atypical drug, and by $460–$1,150 per year when compared with treatment with a traditional neuroleptic. Under a sixth set of assumptions, the cost of treatment with an atypical drug would be $700 less than treatment with a depot drug and $1,860 less than with a traditional neuroleptic.

Discussion.—This decision analysis model takes into account the compliance rate and associated rehospitalization in calculating the outcome and direct costs of treatment. Switching to a depot drug in patients with a history of repeated hospitalization may lower the cost of treatment in the first year. This finding was consistent under different sets of probability and cost assumptions. Findings from other clinical situations may vary.

▶ This is a wonderful example of what we need to know to practice effective and efficient modern psychiatry. This sort of study and decision tree are exactly what we need across treatment modalities with varying diagnoses. The downside is, of course, that managed care will seize such data and prescribe something such as depot medications for all "revolving door" patients, regardless of whether they're suitable candidates.

J.A. Talbott, M.D.

Enrollment Duration, Service Use, and Costs of Care for Severely Mentally Ill Members of a Health Maintenance Organization

McFarland BH, Johnson RE, Hornbrook MC (Oregon Health Sciences Univ, Portland)

Arch Gen Psychiatry 53:938–944, 1996 7–6

Introduction.—There is concern that individuals with severe mental illness do not receive adequate treatment in prepaid systems. Some authors report that enrollment of HMO members with mental illness may be prematurely terminated, but few empirical data have been gathered on this question.

Methods.—The study setting was the Northwest Region of Kaiser Permanente, a group-practice HMO in Portland, Oregon. Patients with severe mental illness were selected from the 2,334 individuals who received an antipsychotic drug or lithium from an HMO pharmacy during 1986 or 1987. A review of charts identified 250 adults in this group who received a diagnosis of schizophrenia, bipolar disorder, or multiple diagnoses. These patients with severe mental illness were age- and sex-matched with control HMO members with and without diabetes mellitus. Utilization data of the state mental health agency and HMO records were reviewed to determine duration of HMO enrollment, private and public service utilization, and HMO costs of care during 4 years of follow-up.

Results.—Patients with mental illness had an average age of 32 years; 80% were white and 30% were never married. All had lengthy histories of mental illness, and 40% reported 3 or more psychiatric admissions. Seventy-nine had a chart diagnosis of schizophrenia, 93 had bipolar disorder, and 78 had multiple disorders. Control groups were 250 "pharmacy" controls who had used the HMO's outpatient pharmacy during 1986 or 1987 (and had not received an antipsychotic drug or lithium), 250 member controls selected from the HMO's membership during 1986 and 1987, and 234 HMO members with a diagnosis of diabetes mellitus.

As expected, the patients with severe mental illness used more services and had substantially higher HMO costs of care per month. Yet once previous years of HMO enrollment were taken into account, there were no statistically significant enrollment differences among those with diabetes, those with severe mental illness, and pharmacy controls. During the follow-up period, the patients with severe mental illness had 42 months of HMO enrollment; enrollment duration was 37 months for controls without diabetes and 47 months for controls with diabetes.

Conclusions.—No evidence was found in this controlled study for early termination of HMO members with severe and costly mental illness. Patients with mental illness also received care from community mental health services, thus optimizing both private and public services.

► It has long been rumored that if possible, managed care organizations "turf" enrollees who are severely mentally ill out to public systems as quickly as possible because of the expense of their care over a lifetime. This is of special concern now that managed care is moving from managing the care of the employed, relatively well population to those receiving Medicaid and Medicare. Although this study is encouraging, *total costs*, for example, those of both HMOs and community care, must be accounted for in planning and providing care in the future.

J.A. Talbott, M.D.

Medical Costs Attributed to Depression Among Patients With a History of High Medical Expenses in a Health Maintenance Organization

Henk HJ, Katzelnick DJ, Kobak KA, et al (Dean Found for Health, Research and Education, Madison, Wis)

Arch Gen Psychiatry 53:899–904, 1996 7–7

Introduction.—One study found an association between worse mental health status at the time of health insurance enrollment and increased use of general medical services. Because depression appears to be associated with increased use of non-psychiatric health services, identifying and treating patients who have depression may relieve their distress and reduce the costs of non-psychiatric medical care. To determine whether a positive screen for depression would predict continued high medical expenditures, patients enrolled in an HMO were followed up.

Methods.—Data were obtained for approximately 50,000 patients enrolled in a group-model HMO in Madison, Wisconsin. To be included, patients had to be older than 18 years, with drug coverage benefits, and have been continuously enrolled for 2 years. Medical and drug charges were collected for 3 years (1992, 1993, and 1994), with the first 2 years for identification of high users of services and the third year for follow-up. A depression screen based on the Medical Outcomes Survey was mailed to 786 enrollees identified as high users (incurring medical and drug costs of $450 or more for 1992 and $504 or more for 1993 plus estimated depression treatment costs of $1,217 for 1992 and $1,400 for 1993). Adjustment was made for medical co-morbidity, age, sex, and benefits package.

Results.—The survey was completed by 63% of those in the high-user group. Twenty of 150 in the high-user group who screened positive for depression were treated for depression. Patients who were high users and had depression were more likely than high users who were not depressed to have higher medical costs in 1994. Although expenditures for high users with and without depression were similar for 1992 and 1993, 1994 costs were significantly higher for the depressed group ($5,764 vs. $4,227). Yet a relatively small proportion (less than 9%) of third-year medical costs was associated with the direct treatment of depression. With adjustment for age, sex, benefits package, and co-morbidity, there remained a 26% higher expenditure for a positive depression screen. Treatment of depression would yield an average difference of $1,498 in third-year costs.

Discussion.—Managed care organizations may be concerned that aggressive screening and treatment of patients with depression will increase their total costs. In the long-term, however, depression treatment may reduce costs as well as relieve disability and distress.

► Despite 25 years of cost-offset data showing that psychiatric interventions reduce medical morbidity and cost, the only area of the industry that seems to have understood these studies is employee assistance programs.

You would think that insurance companies, managed care organizations and HMOs would find it in their selfish interests to provide more—not less—resources for treating conditions like depression that so clearly boost medical costs.

J.A. Talbott, M.D.

Characteristics of Managed Care Patients in a Psychiatric Emergency Service

Breslow RE, Klinger BI, Erickson BJ (Albany Med College, NY)

Psychiatric Serv 47:1259–1261, 1996 7–8

Introduction.—Treatment rationing has occurred through managed care programs in psychiatric emergency services. Problems with psychiatric managed care in emergencies include managed care entities dumping medically ill patients by redefining them as psychiatric emergencies; overuse of psychiatric hospitalization in emergencies; and discordances between resources of the managed care network and where emergency care is sought. Characteristics of patients in the psychiatric services who were enrolled in a managed care program were compared with those of patients who were not in a managed care program.

Methods.—Patient records were reviewed for 293 patients who visited a psychiatric emergency service, 69 of whom were enrolled in a managed care plan. Whether managed care patients who visit the emergency service do so primarily for hospitalization, and whether they have brief contacts with the service because of pre-approval for hospitalization, was studied.

Results.—About 44.9 % of patients who visited the psychiatric emergency service were referred to outpatient mental health and substance abuse services. There was a longer average contact time among managed care patients than non–managed care patients, but it was not statistically significant. Police and mobile teams were involved with 29.5% of the non–managed care patients and 17.4 % of the managed care patients. There were 67.9% repeat visitors in the non–managed care group, compared with 27.5 % in the managed care group.

Conclusions.—-Two different populations are found in the managed care and non–managed care groups. More emergency community intervention, more previous psychiatric hospitalizations, and more psychotic and substance use disorders were found in the non–managed care group when compared with the managed care group. This study should be repeated after most patients receiving Medicaid have been enrolled in managed care programs.

► The authors state that their study did not confirm their expectations, but the results do prove interesting. The contacts were longer, and the authors speculate that this was because of increased time spent on authorization and negotiation. This is counter to managed care's stated goal of increased efficiency. I agree that the authors should revisit the issue once Medicaid and Medicare populations come under managed care in New York.

J.A. Talbott, M.D.

The Massachusetts Medicaid Carve-Out: Managing Care in the Public Sector

Patullo E, Malpiede M (Ctr for Family Development, Boston; MENTOR, Boston)

New Dir Ment Health Serv 72:45–57, 1996 7–9

Background.—In contrast to appearances, managed behavioral health care is an industry in its infancy, particularly in the public sector. Massachusetts was the first state to place nearly all of its Medicaid behavioral health care beneficiaries into a managed care program run by a private organization. The experience with the Massachusetts Medicaid carve-out is reviewed.

The Massachusetts Medicaid Carve-Out.—The program began in 1992, when the Massachusetts Division of Medical Assistance (the Massachusetts Medicaid agency) contracted with Mental Health Management of America (MHMA), a for-profit company, to provide treatment for mental illness and substance abuse. The $165 million program was initiated in response to rising costs and inefficient care. A capitated rate per member was paid out every month. If costs rose higher than the cap, MHMA was to pay 8¢ on the dollar amount above the cap, to a maximum of $2 million. Any savings realized below the cap returned to MHMA along the same formula. The public-private partnership sought not only to cut costs but also to create a shift in thinking such that the distribution of resources was driven by the individual client's needs. A Medicaid waiver was obtained to remove the policies that traditionally favored hospitalization, in favor of promoting clinically based care. Certain providers were restricted, and new levels of care were introduced. Resources were redistributed to less expensive, clinically preferable options such as community mental health resources and free-standing clinics. Clinical protocols were revised to include mandatory assessment before admission, immediate discharge planning, and a new approach to utilization review. Activities were coordinated with those of the public human services agencies, and a new quality improvement effort was initiated.

The carve-out program realized tangible benefits, at the expense of considerable trial and error. The real measure of success was the improvement in services provided. By 1996, when the contract came up for rebid, there was an increasingly competitive market ready to respond. The contract was transferred from MHMA to another organization. However, the initial experience provided a basis for continued improvement in public delivery of behavioral health care services. It has resulted in interconnections between the public and private spheres, directing all efforts toward the goal of improving the quality of mental health care for Medicaid enrollees.

Discussion.—The Massachusetts Medicaid carve-out experiment has important implications for future efforts of this type. Important lessons were learned, including the need to be realistic regarding the potential cost savings, the need for long-term evaluation of success, and an appreciation of the need for new approaches.

▶ The Massachusetts Medicaid experiment is lauded by its architects and looked at skeptically by outsiders, but there is no doubt that its progress will be closely watched. As a harbinger of all Medicaid managed care developments, it has much to teach; the rest of us just hope the lessons learned are applicable elsewhere and lead to better patient care.

J.A. Talbott, M.D.

Managing the Whole System of Care
Hogan MF (Ohio Dept of Mental Health)
New Dir Ment Health Serv 72:13–24, 1996 7–10

Purpose.—Managed care is rapidly becoming a major factor in mental health care delivery in the public sector, and private companies seem likely to play a significant role in managing publicly funded care. The changes brought about by this trend are likely to be as significant as those produced by the deinstitutionalization movement of past decades. The growing role of managed care in public mental health services was reviewed.

Managed Care in the Public Sector.—After reviewing the scope, structure, and functions of public mental health systems, the author looks at the introduction of managed care into the public sector. Managed care is not new to the public sector, particularly in terms of the public mental health system's need to use its limited funds in the best way and to target its services carefully. A familiar example is the development of lower-cost alternatives to hospitalizations, including residential care and rehabilitation-oriented models. However, the applicability of managed care to other areas involved in public sector managed health care—such as housing, rehabilitation, or self-help—has not been tested. It has been suggested that managed care is inappropriate or irrelevant to public systems. The goal must be to combine the efficiency of private managed care with the values and services offered by the public sector. Although it is easier said than done, the "high touch, low tech" methods of the public sector must be combined with the "high tech, low touch" methods of the private sector. This fusion must be achieved in a deliberate fashion, with attention given to the complex, interrelated, episodic needs of the seriously mentally ill. Failure to carefully evaluate the fit between these 2 approaches will lead to the same kinds of problems encountered during deinstitutionalization. The best approach is to build on the Community Support Program model, to make sure that housing and other supports are provided together with treatment services. A commitment to long-term support and case management is essential as well. On the other side, managed care has a lot to offer, especially for beneficiaries who do not have long-term, disabling conditions. The challenge will be to integrate the best aspects of each approach in a system that is publicly funded but privately provided.

Discussion.—The goal of combining public and private approaches in the public mental health care system raises the possibility of eliminating broader divisions between insurance-financed and public care. The integration of managed care into the public health system must be done carefully, without the problems encountered with deinstitutionalization. If this can be done successfully, it will be a major step toward a fully integrated, 1-tiered system for mental health care in the United States.

► Mike Hogan discusses 2 essential features regarding public managed care: first, that putting all populations under managed care has the perceived advantage of arriving at a single system of care but, second, that public systems and patients traditionally covered by public systems are not amenable to the same treatments, programs, and systems as those traditionally covered by indemnity insurance. Single-episode treatment of married, employed individuals is less demanding than treatment and rehabilitation of chronically and/or episodically ill, unemployed, single individuals.

J.A. Talbott, M.D.

Creating Incentives for the Delivery of Services

Hyde PS (ComCare, Arizona)

New Dir Ment Health Serv 72:25–34, 1996 7–11

Background.—Managed care is a new and growing phenomenon in public sector mental health care. A major part of managed care is controlling access to care for patients needing expensive services. This raises important questions about the incentive to provide care for patients with complex mental health care needs, such as the seriously and persistently mentally ill. Some type of incentive is needed to protect people with complex behavioral health care needs. The author reviewed the various types of incentives posed to ensure that the persistently mentally ill are provided with services under managed mental health care.

Types of Incentives.—The proposed incentives fall into 4 categories: eligibility standards, structures, financial incentives, and advocacy. Eligibility standards can ensure that difficult-to-manage groups receive the attention they need. The population to be served can be clearly defined, with objective assessments to identify high-need patients and make sure they are not being denied services. Another approach of this type is consistent review of services provided and outcomes experienced. Eligibility approaches of this type must be combined with attention to how the care system is structured. An example of a structural approach is "carve-outs," in which payers contract with organizations to provide or manage behavioral health care services. Such organizations may be community mental health agencies, or private entities that specialize in managing behavioral health care. In another structural arrangement, eligibility determination can be separated out from treatment planning and approach and service vision. Having different units perform these tasks, under the supervision of a care manager, helps to ensure that the patient receives adequate services.

Without appropriate financial incentives, no other type of incentive is likely to have the desired effect. Financial incentives are an inherent part of the organization and delivery of managed care. The author describes 8 different types of financial incentives: paying the managed care provider per user; paying at a differential rate for patients likely to use different levels of service; paying an additional amount for persons with serious or persistent illness; attaching differential payments to certain services, rather than certain individuals; paying a differential case rate; using risk corridors to ensure that an established percentage of funds is available for services; having individualized service plans and guidelines for persons with serious mental illness; and using support services not funded by Medicaid as incentives for the patient to stay in treatment. Regardless of what approaches are used, advocacy is necessary to ensure quality outcomes. Payers and providers alike must nurture consumer groups, which should be represented on governing boards and advisory panels. Attention to grievances and appeals and customer service is needed as well.

Discussion.—Managed care has great promise for improving the costs and organization of behavioral health services. However, various types of incentives are needed to ensure that people with serious and persistent mental illness receive the services they need. Everyone involved in the managed care program must make the best of the limited resources available to patients served by the public mental health system.

► Hyde's point that efforts to reduce costs must be coupled with "incentives to care for persons with the most complex and expensive disorders" could not have hit the nail on the head better. A concern of many is that the first, and even second, "winners" of bids for care of "public populations" will undertreat or not treat them and that it will take years for this to result in adverse outcomes, disability, etc. Clearly, this greatest social experiment since deinstitutionalization must be carefully studied or we will be as late in realizing its problems as we were with the 1955 unplanned move to community care without resource provision.

J.A. Talbott, M.D.

Economic Issues/Cost Comparisons

Mental Health Expenditures for Services for People With Severe Mental Illnesses

Hollingsworth EJ, Sweeney JK (Univ of Wisconsin, Madison)
Psychiatric Serv 48:485–490, 1997 7–12

Introduction.—The components of and total expenditures for mental health services for people with severe illnesses are a concern in discussions of health care reform, rising expenditures for mental health care, and attempts at managed care. Little attention has been given to providing adequate estimates of mental health expenditures for severely mentally ill persons, particularly those served in the public sector. Previous studies have shown that expenditures for mental health treatment range from $10,826 to $29,965 in 1994 dollars. Expenditures for a 1-year period for 1,890 clients of a public mental health system were reported.

TABLE 2.—Types of Mental Health Services Used and Mean Expenditures for Services

Service type	% using service	Units of service used	Mean expenditure per client per year	% of total expenditure	Mean expenditure per year for clients using the service
Case management	75.7	44,291 hours	$ 697	6.3	$ 920
Community support	47.6	45,968 hours	833	7.6	1,535
Counseling	49.4	12,730 hours	361	3.3	791
Medication checks	37.5	1,765 hours	49	.5	130
Medication counseling	36.2	1,338 hours	158	1.4	406
Vocational services	23.3	125,047 hours	622	5.7	2,261
Day treatment	23.0	77,449 hours	804	7.3	2,251
Inpatient hospital care	17.9	10,300 days	1,386	12.6	7,741
Supervised housing	11.6	40,628 days	1,011	9.2	7,993
Evaluation	11.1	534 hours	24	.2	199
Tardive dyskinesia screen	10.7	73 hours	9	.1	16
Transportation	7.2	1,461 hours	169	1.5	1,911
Nursing home care	5.6	7,196 days	335	3.0	5,571
Care in an institute for mental disease	5.2	25,230 days	3,366	30.6	29,712
Medical day treatment	3.4	13,330 hours	403	3.7	1,582
Adult family home care	3.0	12,014 days	354	3.2	4,184
Alcohol and other drug abuse	2.6	865 hours	93	.9	1,717
Supportive home care	2.1	2,093 hours	89	.8	1,666
Detoxification	1.8	156 hours	29	.3	216
Community options program services	1.0	3,213 hours	166	1.5	3,471
Crisis care	.8	30 hours	4	.0	461
Other supportive services	.8	49 hours	20	.2	372
Daily living skills	.6	662 hours	13	.1	795
Total			$10,995	100.0	

(Courtesy of Hollingsworth EJ, Sweeney JK: Mental health expenditures for services for people with severe mental illnesses. *Psychiatric Serv* 48:485–490, 1997.)

Methods.—Ten public, nonmetropolitan mental health systems were included in the study, and 1,890 clients were reviewed. All of these clients had received 12 months of service during the study year. The evaluation included data regarding services and expenditures and unduplicated Medicaid claims for 12 months in 1989 and 1990. The direct care cost was defined as the actual dollar expenditures related to an illness or disorder, including amounts spent for hospital and nursing home care, physician and other medical professional services, drugs and appliances, and rehabilitation. Public funding from local, state and federal sources were the focus of this study and did not include any of the sometimes considerable private expenditures by individuals.

Results.—For 1 year, expenditures per client averaged $10,995, with a maximum of $95,093. A total of 53.5% of all expenditures represented community-based outpatient services, including residential care and vocational services; 12.4% represented residential care; and 5.7% represented vocational services (Table 2). Overall, 46.5% was spent for institutional care with inpatient hospital care accounting for 12.6%. Services typically not covered under managed care plans accounted for about 40.6% of total expenditures.

Conclusion.—More than half of total expenditures went to community-based care. Social and rehabilitation services have an important role and must be included in managed care plans if they are to provide adequate services for people with severe mental illness. Managed care plans often do not include community support and nonmedical counseling 2 services that are used by about half of the clients.

► This is a valuable contribution for several reasons. It shows, once again, how expensive care is for the chronic mentally ill, even in a state (Wisconsin) with a well-developed community-based care system. It also shows how only one quarter of "institutional" expenses are for hospital care. And it cautions us to beware, in the move to "manage" the care of the chronically mentally ill, not to disallow such services as rehabilitative, community support, and nonmedical counselling.

J.A. Talbott, M.D.

The Cost of Treatment of Psychiatric Emergencies: A Comparison of Hospital and Community Services

Merson S, Tyrer P, Carlen D, et al (St Mary's Hosp, London; St Charles' Hosp, London)

Psychol Med 26:727–734, 1996 7–13

Background.—The shift from hospital-based to community-based acute psychiatric services and the clinical effect of this change on patients have been examined in various randomized, controlled studies. These studies have reported no advantage in symptom outcome or social function outcome of hospital-based services for patients with severe mental illness who are seeking acute care. Some of these studies have also investigated the cost of these services, but few have used adequate methodology in comparing costs, and many have examined the cost of specific services for specialized groups of patients. Accurate information on the cost of treatment for common clinical conditions is needed. The outcome of hospital-based and community-based psychiatric services was compared in patients seeking emergency psychiatric treatment in a randomized, controlled trial.

Methods.—Patients seeking emergency psychiatric treatment during a 12-month period were randomly referred to hospital-based or community-based psychiatric services. Psychopathology and social function were assessed. Follow-up was 3 months. The cost of each item of service was calculated.

Results.—One hundred patients were included in the study; 52 received hospital-based services and 48 received community-based services. The use of nonpsychiatric services was similar for both groups. Patients who received hospital-based care used more inpatient beds, and patients who received community-based care used more home-based interventions. The total cost of hospital-based treatment was £130,000 and the total cost of community-based treatment was £56,000.). However, the median cost per patient was almost 50% higher for those receiving community-based services. About 10% of the cost of community-based treatment was from failed contacts as compared with 2% of the cost of hospital-based treatment.

Discussion.—For this group of patients there appears to be no clinical advantage to hospital-based psychiatric services. Community-based psychiatric services are a cost-effective alternative to hospital-based care. This is one of the first studies in the United Kingdom to use adequate costing methodology to compare the cost of these psychiatric services. Patients who were very severely ill and required mandatory admission were excluded, but the diagnoses and severity of illness of all other patients were typical of those at an emergency psychiatric clinic and an inner-city hospital psychiatric service. Therefore these results may be reasonably applied to other urban areas.

▶ Although not exactly a replication of Stein, Test, and Weisbrod's pioneering study[1] of the Program for Assertive Community Treatment, this study from the United Kingdom parallels their findings. I'm not sure I totally agree with their reasoning about the reasons for the difference in median patient cost; there may be other factors. Also, I am troubled by the finding that the cost-effectiveness of community care is helped by patients themselves not following up or using services—shades of managed care!

J.A. Talbott, M.D.

Reference

1. Weisbrod BA, Stein LI, Test MA: Alternative to mental hospital treatment, II. Economic benefit-cost analysis. *Arch Gen Psychiatry* 37:400–405, 1980.

Day Hospital/Crisis Respite Care Versus Inpatient Care, Part I: Clinical Outcomes
Sledge WH, Tebes J, Rakfeldt J, et al (Yale Univ, New Haven, Conn)
Am J Psychiatry 153:1065–1073, 1996 7–14

Day Hospital/Crisis Respite Care Versus Inpatient Care, Part II: Service Utilization and Costs
Sledge WH, Tebes J, Wolff N, et al (Yale Univ, New Haven, Conn)
Am J Psychiatry 153:1074–1083, 1996 7–14

Objective.—The feasibility, effectiveness, patient satisfaction, service utilization, and cost of an experimental day hospital/crisis respite psychiatric treatment program and a hospital inpatient program were compared.

Background.—The current pressure to reduce health care costs has also affected the provision of mental health care. Psychiatric treatment must now be cost-effective as well as clinically effective. There is a shift in psychiatry to provide services on an ambulatory basis and to move as much care as possible out of institutional settings. One alternative to hospitalization for many individuals with acute mental illness is day hospital programs. These treatment programs have been examined by various controlled trials and shown to be safe and effective; no significant differences in outcome measures such as postdischarge mental health service contacts, rehospitalizations, and ratings of psychiatric status by patients and families have been found between day hospital and inpatient treatment. Acute crisis residential care, or crisis respite care, is a newer alternative to hospitalization that has emerged in the United States and United Kingdom and has been used by a range of individuals seeking emergency psychiatric treatment. These alternative programs have not been widely implemented because it is assumed that hospitalization is the most effective method of treatment and because of a lack of evidence of cost-effectiveness. Few studies have compared the clinical efficacy and cost-effectiveness of crisis respite care with conventional psychiatric hospitalization.

Methods.—To compare the clinical outcome of the 2 treatment programs, 197 adult patients were evaluated by staff and judged as needing hospitalization. The enrollment period was 2 years. Patients were enrolled from an urban, poor population, had prolonged mental illness, and were at risk for hospitalization. Eligibility requirements included voluntary status and a lack of response to other treatments. Patients were randomly assigned to the experimental day hospital/crisis respite program or to inpatient psychiatric treatment. Symptoms, functioning, social adjustment, quality of life, and patient satisfaction with treatment were evaluated at baseline, at discharge, and at 2, 5, and 10 months after discharge. To compare service utilization and costs of the 2 treatment programs, data were obtained from patient records, including the number of inpatient days, day hospital days, days at the crisis respite residence, and ambulatory services from the time of admission through the 10-month follow-up.

Units of ambulatory services were measured in client hours in session. The average costs for inpatient and outpatient services were based on a full cost accounting of the resources used to provide these psychiatric services. Treatment costs were also compared by patient disorder.

Results.—Clinical outcome, symptoms, functioning, social adjustment, quality of life, and patient satisfaction with treatment were similar for both the day hospital/crisis respite program and the inpatient hospitalization program. The experimental program had a slightly higher positive effect on psychiatric symptoms, overall functioning, and social functioning. The rate of readmissions for both groups was comparable. Program effectiveness was analyzed by patient disorder, but no significant differences were found. Regarding service utilization and cost, the average cost of the day hospital/crisis respite program was less than that of inpatient hospitalization. The savings was $7,100 per patient, or 20% of the total direct cost per patient. During follow-up, service utilization and cost of the 2 programs were comparable. Costs were lower for baseline admissions because the per-unit cost for day hospital/crisis respite care was lower and the average stay was shorter than hospitalization. There were significant differences in cost among patients with psychosis, affective disorders, and dual diagnoses. Patients with psychosis had the highest costs in both programs. The direct service staff and capital costs of the 2 programs were nearly equal, but the operating costs of the day hospital/crisis respite program were 51% of the cost of inpatient treatment.

Discussion.—This study included only voluntary patients and excluded patients who required constraints, 1-to-1 surveillance, or 24-hour active medical attention, or patients who were intoxicated. There appeared to be no clinical advantage to acute psychiatric hospitalization over crisis respite care in these voluntary patients in symptoms, functioning, social adjustment, or quality of life. For some patients, day hospital/crisis respite care was less expensive, and savings may be higher for patients without psychosis. The higher overhead costs of hospitals accounted for most of the cost differences between the 2 programs. Alternative programs such as day hospital/crisis respite care are not designed to provide the highest security or medical care that hospitals provide. These alternative programs can only be effective if there are effective triage and crisis services to make accurate placements and if the program is backed up by access to hospitalization.

► As with the article by Merson et al. (Abstract 7–13), costs for patients in this study are less in the community program, and as with Thomas et al. (Abstract 7–4), patients with psychotic illness constitute a higher cost group. It is ironic that it has been about 20 years since Stein, Test, and Weisbrod[1] published their results of the Program for Assertive Community Treatment and that now the driving force in our field is economic (e.g., managed care and cost control) rather than philosophic (e.g., quality of care and return to the community).

J.A. Talbott, M.D.

Reference

1. Weisbrod BA, Stein LI, Test MA: Alternative to mental hospital treatment, II. Economic benefit-cost analysis. *Arch Gen Psychiatry* 37:400–405, 1980.

Cost-effectiveness Evaluation of Three Approaches to Case Management for Homeless Mentally Ill Clients

Wolff N, Helminiak TW, Morse GA, et al (Community Support Systems, St. Louis)

Am J Psychiatry 154:341–348, 1997 7–15

Introduction.—Case management is recommended for homeless individuals with severe mental illness, who account for approximately one third of the homeless population. Three different approaches to case management in this population were compared for client outcome and cost-effectiveness, a concern in the current environment of scarce resources.

Methods.—The 3 case management approaches used were assertive community treatment alone, assertive community treatment with community workers, and brokered care management (purchase of services). Eligible subjects were homeless or at risk for homelessness; had a serious *DSM-III-R* axis I diagnosis; had no recent convictions for rape, homicide, or serious assault; and were willing to receive services as participants in a longitudinal study. Although 165 individuals were randomized, only 85 were eligible for the cost-effectiveness study. Follow-up continued for 18 months. Case managers in the brokered care management group arranged for purchase of mental health and psychosocial rehabilitation services but saw their clients infrequently. Assertive community treatment teams had smaller caseloads; served as advocates for their clients, often meeting with then outside the office; and provided a wide range of support services.

Results.—The rate of attrition was significantly higher in the brokered condition (63%) than it was in the assertive community treatment only (44%) or the assertive community treatment with community workers (33%) conditions. Compared with the brokered condition, the other 2 conditions provided more direct client contact, led to a greater reduction in psychiatric symptoms, and produced a higher level of client satisfaction. The total cost of treating participants did not differ significantly among the 3 conditions, although the lowest reported costs for the 18-month period were for assertive community treatment with community workers ($39,913 for the average client). There were significant differences, however, in the division of costs within each program. Assertive community treatment programs spent less on inpatient services and more on case management services and maintenance.

Conclusion.—Because assertive community treatment of the homeless mentally ill has better client outcomes and no greater costs, it is more cost-effective than brokered case management.

► If assertive case management costs no more than the brokered variety, payors should be willing to support it, given the better clinical outcome.

J.A. Talbott, M.D.

Mental Health Systems and Reform

A Cross-sectional Study of Private Psychiatric Practices Under a Single-payer Health Care System

Anderson K, Catterson A, Gaudet M, et al (Univ of Ottawa, Ontario, Canada; Committee of Private Psychiatrists, Ottawa, Ontario, Canada; Massachusetts Gen Hosp, Boston)

Can J Psychiatry 42:395–401, 1997 7–16

Introduction.—In Canada, universal access to mental health services is provided, and the cost is substantially less than comparable services provided in the United States. Concerns have been raised, however, that this single-payer system may be abused by the "rich worried well," those wealthy individuals who are worried yet mentally well, while the low-income and uninsured mentally ill do not receive treatment. Ontario sets virtually no limit on outpatient psychiatric care, including the number of psychotherapy sessions provided to each patient per year, and this province was the focus of the study.

Methods.—There were 107 psychiatrists working full-time in private practice who were surveyed. They worked in Ottawa-Carleton which has a population of about 900,000. The survey probed the sociodemographic characteristics and background of the psychiatrists, their practice patterns, work hours, and sources of referral. Also surveyed were the patients' sociodemographic status, their risk of suicide, history of physical or sexual abuse, and history of substance abuse. Data were gathered on treatment modalities, frequency of visits, and length of time since the patient's first appointment. The patients were categorized according to *Diagnostic and Statistical Manual of Mental Disorders*, edition IV, criteria. Axis I includes schizophrenia, mood disorders, anxiety disorders, sexual dysfunction, eating disorders, and adjustment disorders.

Results.—One or more Axis I disorders were found in 93% of the patients, with mood and anxiety disorders being the most common. Among the patients treated by the private psychiatrists, wealthier patients were relatively underrepresented. Between patients earning below $30,000 per year and patients earning above $60,000 per year, there were no significant differences in the distribution of Axis I, Axis II, and Axis III disorders. The most widely used primary modes of treatment were psychotherapy (53%) and pharmacotherapy (35%). It was found that low-income patients were more likely to have a history of physical or sexual abuse than high-income patients.

Conclusion.—Primarily individuals with major psychiatric disorders are treated in the Canadian single-payer system. The "worried well" are not favored. To confirm these findings, larger epidemiologic studies with independent assessments of psychiatric populations are needed.

► With the collapse of the Clinton Health Plan, many of us assumed that it would be a long time before the arguments for a single-payer system emerged again. Not so! This article refutes 1 of the commonly held myths about treatment by private practitioners: that they only treat the "worried well". Granted, only 3% of these practices involved persons with schizophrenia, but the percentage of patients receiving medication (35%) or brief cognitive or supportive psychotherapy (25%) gives weight to the conclusion that these are patients deserving of treatment.

J.A. Talbott, M.D.

Mental Disorders in Public, Private Nonprofit, and Proprietary General Hospitals

Olfson M, Mechanic D (Columbia Univ/New York State Psychiatric Inst; Rutgers Univ, New Brunswick, NJ)

Am J Psychiatry 153:1613–1619, 1996 7–17

Introduction.—The primary source of acute inpatient psychiatric care falls on general hospitals, with the reduction in the number of public mental hospital beds. Investor-owned psychiatric facilities have expanded in recent years, although nonprofit general hospitals continue to represent the largest component of the psychiatric in-patient system. Knowing the performance of different providers would be helpful in evaluating who receives care at which types of hospital and what types of services are received. To examine the sociodemographic and diagnostic composition of psychiatric inpatients in public, private nonprofit, and proprietary general hospitals, data from a large, nationally representative sample of hospital discharges were analyzed.

Methods.—There were 1.83 million patients with a primary mental disorder diagnosis who were discharged from general hospitals, and 13,086 were discharged with first-listed mental disorder diagnoses in the National Hospital Discharge Survey. The data were analyzed to determine discharge diagnoses, hospital ownership, hospital procedures, sociodemographic composition, and treatment characteristics of the patients.

Results.—The patients were distributed unevenly into proprietary hospitals (11.7%), private nonprofit hospitals (78.9%), and public hospitals (9.4%). Public and private nonprofit hospitals were more likely than proprietary hospitals to have psychiatric patients diagnosed with a comorbid substance-related disorder (public, 29.9%; nonprofit, 31%, proprietary, 17.4%), schizophrenia (public, 23.4%; nonprofit, 18.8%; proprietary, 12.6%), a general medical disorder (public, 62.4%; nonprofit, 57.4%; proprietary, 41.1%), or a personality disorder (public, 11.6%, nonprofit, 11.3%; proprietary, 4.7%). Public hospitals had far more uninsured psychiatric patients than the other types of hospitals (public, 17%; nonprofit, 9.9%; proprietary, 6.4%).

Conclusions .—In caring for patients who are uninsured and have severe mental illness, public general hospitals play an important role. It is critical that policy makers identify and develop resources to replace the care that the public general hospitals currently provide to poor patients with severe psychiatric disorders. A framework of insurance coverage should be created to cover individuals who are now uninsured or underinsured if the hospital sector is to be reconfigured.

► I am afraid that the authors' caution that policy makers should not shut down more beds in public hospitals because it will imperil uninsured patients will go unheard. There are several reasons. First, there is no policy being made at a macro level concerning such issues. Second, both private and public leaders are forcing cost-cutting regardless of its impact. And third, we do not have a "system" anyway. I suspect we will only realize some of the consequences of marketplace forces way after the fact, just as happened with deinstitutionalization.

J.A. Talbott, M.D.

Differences in the Use of Psychiatric Outpatient Services Between the United States and Ontario

Kessler RC, Frank RG, Edlund M, et al (Harvard Med School, Boston; Univ of Michigan, Ann Arbor; Univ of Toronto; et al)
N Engl J Med 336:551–557, 1997 7–18

Introduction.—There is debate over whether uninsured people have access to mental health care, with some saying that too many mental health care resources are devoted to people with low levels of need. This trend would expand if access were increased. Although Canadians have universal health care, the Canadian government spends a lower percentage of the gross national product on health care. The use of outpatient services for psychiatric problems among young and middle-aged adults in the United States was compared with use in Ontario, Canada. Self-reports of use of services and disorders that were listed in the *Diagnostic and Statistical Manual of Mental Disorders*, (ed. 3, revised) were used.

Methods.—Two surveys were analyzed, with 1 survey having been conducted in Ontario and the other in the United States. Both had identical assessments of needs for services and their use among a population of 15–54 years of age. The U.S. survey was administered to 8,098 respondents and had a response rate of 82.4%, and the Ontario survey was administered to 9,953 respondents and had a response rate of 76.5%.

Results.—Psychiatric disorders, poor mental health, or workdays lost or cut short because of psychiatric problems in the previous year were significantly more likely to have been reported by respondents in the United

States than in Ontario. Outpatient treatment for psychiatric problems in the previous 12 months was obtained by 13.3% of respondents in the United States and by 8% of respondents in Ontario. People with less severe mental illness had a higher probability of the use of services in the United States, according to an analysis of subgroups. Among patients who had similar numbers of psychiatric disorders over the same time periods, the average number of visits did not differ significantly between the 2 countries. The use of services and the measures of perceived need were more strongly matched in Ontario than in the United States.

Conclusion.—The match between some measures of need and treatment is not as strong in the United States as in Ontario; however, the mental health care system in the United States provides treatment to a larger proportion of the population than in Ontario. The problem of having a demand for psychiatric services by people with a low level of need should be addressed in any plan that would expand coverage for psychiatric disorders in the United States.

► This study will not be welcomed by those who are arguing against the perceived strictness of the "medical necessity" guidelines of managed care companies. The interesting question for me is to what extent society and individuals suffering from "lower need" disorders value treatment of these conditions.

J.A. Talbott, M.D.

An Integrated Regional Emergency Psychiatry Service

Kates N, Eaman S, Santone J, et al (McMaster Univ, Hamilton, Ont)

Gen Hosp Psychiatry 18:251–256, 1996 7–19

Objective.—De-institutionalization, inadequate housing, and shorter inpatient stays all have contributed to the increased need for and use of Psychiatry Emergency Services (PES). Integration of PES into traditional hospital services can reduce costs and duplication of services. The goals, mandate, and evolution of emergency psychiatry teams (EPT) services developed in 1 Canadian program and the advantages and shortcomings of the model were reviewed.

The Clinical Location.—A psychiatric hospital near 5 general hospitals in the downtown area was selected. It has approximately 16 beds per 100,000 population.

Goals.—The regional EPT acts as a gatekeeper facility that provides assessment, provides access to community resources, and acts as a training facility.

How It Functions.—Walk-in or referred patients are assessed by a nurse or social worker and then by a psychiatrist who oversees the development of a treatment plan. Patients may be admitted, discharged to their family physician, or referred to a community agency.

Other Roles for EPT.—The EPT can provide short-term care, triage for inpatients, and after-hours intervention for registered patients as well as training for psychiatry, emergency medicine, or family practice medicine residents.

Advantages.—The PES provides "hassle free" admissions, skilled staff, liaison with community groups, a backup protocol in case of patient overload, and regular meetings with emergency department staffs. It concentrates psychiatric staff in 1 location, making delivery of services cost-effective and relieves pressure on community hospitals with a decreasing number of beds.

Obstacles.—The host hospital often does not have enough beds and is responsible for reminding other services of their role in the region. Psychiatric patients requiring medical treatment sometimes are shuttled back and forth between facilities.

Summary.—An experienced, sensitive, and responsive staff with access to sufficient numbers of beds and outpatients and community support is necessary to provide PES. Collaboration between facilities and cooperation between staffs are necessary to make this system work.

► This presents an interesting dilemma for those of us in the currently very competitive American system: if we consolidate emergency services, which may be more efficient, will we lose our inpatient admitting edge? The Canadian authors have exactly the opposite problem—they found an excess of admissions to their "home service." I guess it all depends on where the economic incentive lies.

J.A. Talbott, M.D.

Team for the Assessment of Psychiatric Services (TAPS) Project 33: Prospective Follow-up Study of Long-stay Patients Discharged From Two Psychiatric Hospitals

Leff J, Trieman N, Gooch C (TAPS Research Unit, London)

Am J Psychiatry 153:1318–1324, 1996 7–20

Objective.—In England, the money saved by closing psychiatric hospitals is re-invested in community services to treat the mentally ill. An evaluation of this policy was conducted by studying several closure schedules for 2 English long-term hospitals for nondemented patients.

Methods.—Demographic, medical, psychiatric, social behavior, and living skills data were collected for 737 patients, hospitalized continuously for more than 1 year, who were placed in staffed community housing in their districts, averaging 9 patients per house (78%), or with relatives (31%). Approximately one fourth attended outpatient clinics, and the others had medication provided by family physicians. Half attended day care, and all were expected to participate in the maintenance of the home. Patient attitudes were assessed by questionnaire, and the amount of care they required was recorded by professional caregivers. Data were analyzed statistically.

Results.—There were 24 patients who died, 3 who moved away, 23 who refused follow-up, and 7 who were lost to follow-up. A total of 671 patients (52.8% men), with an average age of 53.9 years, were followed up for a year. Of the deaths, 2 were by suicide. Two patients were imprisoned, 5 were sent to psychiatric institutions because of violent behavior, 7 were presumed to be homeless, and 102 were re-admitted to a psychiatric ward. Of re-admitted patients, 78% were discharged to their community homes. Re-admission risk was lower for older and for long-stay patients. Negative psychiatric symptoms decreased over time, but other psychiatric symptoms and social behavior problems remained unchanged. Patients had greater freedom, and their living skills increased significantly. Significantly more patients viewed their medication as helpful, although compliance problems did not change. Most patients wanted to remain in the community homes. Their medical conditions and care requirements did not change, and their number of social contacts did not increase, although they had more individuals they considered as friends and acquaintances. Contacts with relatives decreased significantly.

Conclusions.—Carefully planned closures of psychiatric hospitals can be accomplished with few significant disadvantages to long-stay patients. The patients prefer community living, although there will continue to be those whose disabilities will require significantly more services than are usually found in community homes.

► The Team for the Assessment of Psychiatric Services Program, or TAPS, is now up to its 33rd chapter; not as long-running as *The Mousetrap,* but pretty good. Each chapter represents a piece of the puzzle, which when fitted together seems to firmly document the effectiveness of hospital closure, with complete re-investment in good community care. Obviously, the toughest to place and handle patients were dealt with last,[1] had to have special consideration, and still may have been "trans-" instead of de-institutionalized.[2] But in general, the lack of our problems of homelessness and crime in their affected population is heartening.

J.A. Talbott, M.D.

References

1. Trieman N, Leff J: The TAPS Project 36: The most difficult to place long stay psychiatric in-patients outcome one year after relocation. *Brit J Psych* 169:289–292, 1996.
2. Trieman N, Leff J: Difficult to place patients in a psychiatric hospital closure programme: the TAPS project 24. *Psychol Med* 26:765–774, 1996.

Effects of Mental Health Services Reform on Clinical Practice in the United Kingdom

Shepherd G, Muijen M, Hadley TR, et al (Sainsbury Centre for Mental Health, London; Univ of Pennsylvania, Philadelphia; Univ of Maryland, Baltimore)

Psychiatric Serv 47:1351–1355, 1996 7–21

Background.—The British National Health Service, local government social services departments, the welfare benefits system, and the organization of primary health care have undergone major reform in the past few years. The impact of these reforms on the management and clinical practice of mental health care was discussed.

Impact of Reform.—The shortage of acute psychiatric beds in London and other inner cities has led to the premature discharge of psychiatric patients to inadequate community supports. The effects of contracting and the introduction of the purchaser–provider split has resulted in a climate of competition and rivalry among provider units that once functioned in an environment of collaboration and cooperation. There has been a rapid erosion of the tradition of public spirit that motivated many clinicians and other mental health care staff. The widespread feeling that the new trusts are more interested in making money than providing services has lowered morale. Many believe that managers are cost-conscious but not necessarily cost-effective.

Conclusions.—Although the health care reforms in the United Kingdom have had some positive effects, there have been many negative effects, especially on morale. Many clinicians and other staff members feel that the reform has been an assault on the underlying values of the National Health Service.

► What I found interesting in this report of the recent changes in the British system was that despite the very different histories, political background, funding, and administration of our 2 nations' mental health "systems," so much seems to be coming together. Now in the United Kingdom, there is a perceived shortage of acute beds and the impression of premature discharge, a climate of rivalry and competition, an "erosion of the tradition of public spirit," and the accusation that managers are cost-conscious without being conscious of cost-effectiveness.

J.A. Talbott, M.D.

Mental Health Reform in Georgia, 1992 to 1996

Elliott RL (Mercer Univ, Macon, Ga)

Psychiatric Serv 47:1205–1211, 1996 7–22

Background.—Public mental health systems have experienced many serious problems, including fragmentation of services, funding, and administration; inflexibility leading to a lack of innovation; lack of responsiveness to consumers and families; and chronic underfunding. During a

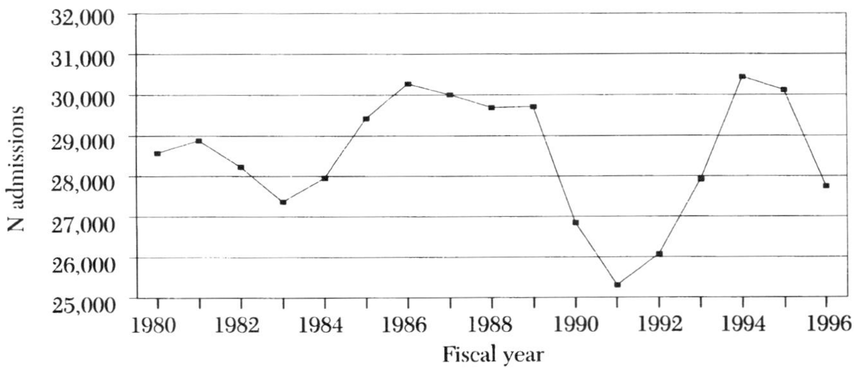

FIGURE 1.—Admissions to Georgia state hospitals, fiscal years 1980–1996. (Courtesy of Elliott RL: Mental health reform in Georgia, 1992 to 1996. *Psychiatric Serv* 47:1205–1211, 1996. Copyright 1996, the American Psychiatric Association, Reprinted by permission.)

time when some public mental health systems are embarking on structural reform, consumer and family advocacy and privatization have become important trends. These 3 movements—the development of mental health authorities, consumerism, and privatization—are reflected in Georgia's program of reform.

Mental Health Reform in Georgia.—A 1990 report ranked Georgia 26th among state mental health systems in both funding and performance. Hospital admissions had declined, however (Fig 1), during the period from 1987 to 1991, a result of additional money provided for community services. A commission created to evaluate the state's public mental health system proposed 14 principles to guide the reform. Among key recommendations was the creation of regional boards, with at least half of the board members required to be consumers or consumers' families. Hospital and community funds were to be combined, providing for flexible shifting of funds as use of state hospitals decreased.

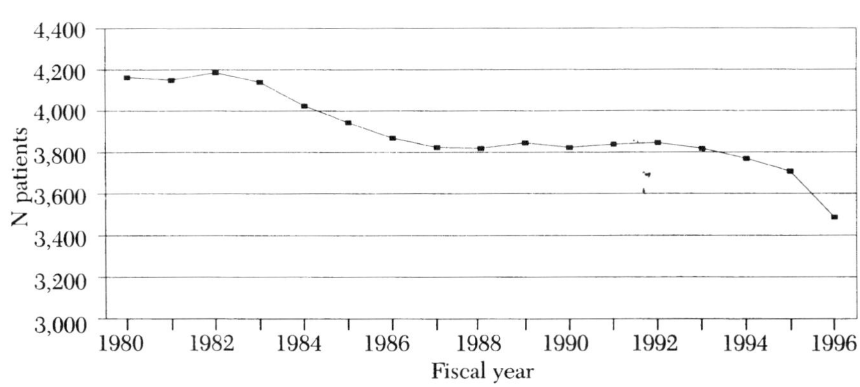

FIGURE 2.—Average annual census in Georgia state hospitals, fiscal years 1980–1996. (Courtesy of Elliott RL: Mental health reform in Georgia, 1992 to 1996. *Psychiatric Serv* 47:1205–1211, 1996. Copyright 1996, the American Psychiatric Association. Reprinted by permission.)

Implementation.—Early reform implementation began in the years 1992–1994, and regional boards were staffed by August 1993. At this time, there are few objective, systemwide data by which the progress of reform can be judged, but admission rates for state hospitals show an increase whereas average length of stay (Fig 2) has decreased. Failure to reduce hospital use can be attributed to various causes, including senior administrators' loss of focus, lack of funding to operate regional boards, and minimal staffing of boards. And the decision-making authority of regional mental health authorities may be undermined by a Medicaid section 1115 waiver that would permit managed care organizations to assume responsibility for key decisions.

Future Prospects.—Four years of mental health reform in Georgia have cost almost $15 million but produced few documented systemwide benefits. Several proposed solutions will be considered by the Georgia general assembly in 1999, but the most important lesson to be learned is the need to maintain focus on the original goals of reform.

► The issue of how well states are managing the shift to managed care of their "traditional public populations" is a critical one these days. Almost all states are in transition to this next phase, and those not fully involved are watching those states, such as Massachusetts, Tennessee, and Pennsylvania, that have been "at it" longer. Georgia attempted a reform in 1992 that gave more power to consumers, a trend many believe may help check some of the excesses of managed care. Ironically, the author believes that "managed care-ization" will actually undermine the current reform. We will keep watching!

J.A. Talbott, M.D.

Inpatient Hospitalization

Sunny Hospital Rooms Expedite Recovery From Severe and Refractory Depressions

Beauchemin KM, Hays P (Univ of Alberta, Edmonton)
J Affect Disord 40:49–51, 1996 7–23

Objective.—Light therapy is known to ameliorate symptoms of seasonal affective disorder, a mild winter depression that affects women more than men. The effect of light on hospital stays of depressed patients was studied in a psychiatric inpatient unit. Half of the rooms were bright and sunny; half were not.

Methods.—Duration of stay between October 1993 and September 1995 was determined for 174 patients with depression or bipolar disorder who had spent their entire stay in either a bright or a dim room. Random admissions and diagnoses were assumed.

Results.—Patients in brightly lit rooms stayed an average of 16.9 days, whereas patients in dimly lit rooms stayed significantly longer (19.5 days). For males, the durations were 15.3 days for brightly lit rooms and 22.1

days for dimly lit rooms; for females, 17.9 days vs. 18.6 days. The sex differences were not significant.

Conclusion.—Patients with depression hospitalized in bright, sunny rooms had significantly shorter stays than those hospitalized in dimly lit rooms.

▶ I think this study is nifty: simple, clear, and prompting the query, "Why didn't we think of it before?" The only quibble I have with it is that there is no comparison with other quality-of-life–enhancing environmental changes, for example, changing the color of the paint or adding flowers; there is not even a mention of the Hawthorne effect.

J.A. Talbott, M.D.

Trends in State and County Mental Hospitals in the U.S. From 1970 to 1992

Witkin MJ, Atay J, Manderscheid RW (Ctr for Mental Health Services, Rockville, Md)

Psychiatric Serv 47:1079–1081, 1996 7–24

Background.—Despite the closing of a number of state mental hospitals, these institutions still consume a lot of financial resources. The decrease in the number of state mental hospitals, average daily patient use, and number of full-time staff is documented.

Methods.—Data presented were obtained from the Inventory of Mental Health Organizations, General Hospital Mental Health Services, the Cen-

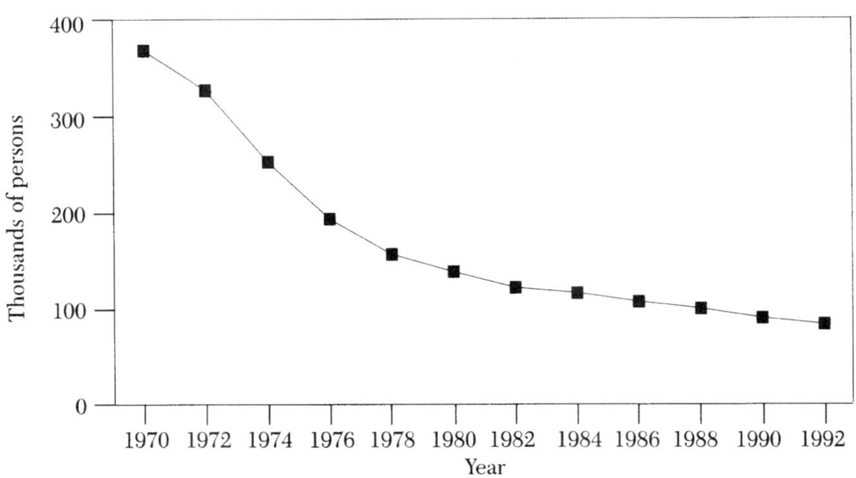

FIGURE 1.—Average daily census of state and county mental hospitals, 1970–1992. (From Witkin MJ, Atay J, Manderscheid RW: Trends in state and county mental hospitals in the U.S. from 1970 to 1992. *Psychiatric Serv* 47:1079–1081, 1996. Copyright 1996, the American Psychiatric Association. Reprinted by permission.)

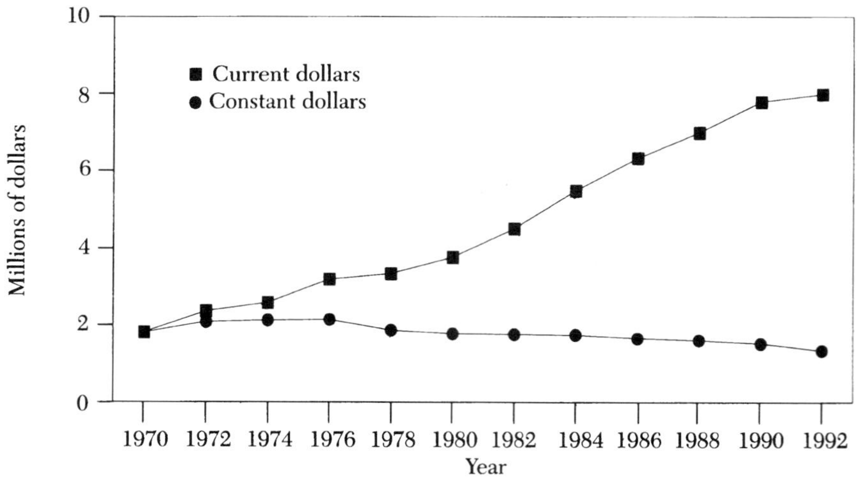

FIGURE 2.—Expenditures of state and county mental hospitals, 1970–1992. (From the Witkin MJ, Atay J, Manderscheid RW: Trends in state and county mental hospitals in the U.S. from 1970 to 1992. *Psychiatric Serv* 47:1079–1081, 1996. Copyright 1996, the American Psychiatric Association. Reprinted by permission.)

ter for Mental Health Services in 1992, and the National Institute of Mental Health.

Results.—The number of mental hospitals declined from 310 to 273 as a result of ward, building, and unit closings or conversions. County mental hospitals also have declined. Only Wisconsin and New Jersey operated county facilities in 1992. Newly opened facilities had fewer beds. State resources were redirected to community services. Mental hospitals house 84,000 patients daily and employ 120,000 individuals. Daily inpatient populations have declined from 367,629 to 83,693 during the period of study as a result of the use of psychoactive drugs, deinstitutionalization, reduced stays, alternative community-based programs, and changing laws on commitment and retention (Fig 1). Approximately 84% of the inpatient population decline is attributed to downsizing. Although expenditures have increased from $1.8 to $8 billion, the rate of expenditure is tapering off and has actually declined if adjusted for inflation (Fig 2). Whereas the number of professional staff has increased, other staff has decreased by 55% as a result of state requirements for more treatment services rather than simply custodial services, the opening of new hospitals for children, the requirement to hire more specialists, and downsizing.

Conclusion.—The number of state mental health patients has declined dramatically over the period of study primarily because of hospital closings or conversions and the emphasis on shifting funds to community-based programs, changes in the laws, improved psychotropic medications, and decreased hospital stays as a result of managed care. The number of state mental hospitals will continue to decline.

► I am concerned that the actual decrease in constant dollars expended in state hospitals portends a return to warehouse-type care. Downsizing and redeployment is one thing; depriving patients of barely adequate care, quite another.

J.A. Talbott, M.D.

The State of the State Mental Hospital in 1996
Bachrach LL (Univ of Maryland, Gaithersburg)
Psychiatric Serv 47:1071–1078, 1996 7–25

Objective.—Since de-institutionalization of mentally ill patients began in the 1970s, functions and funds of state mental hospitals have increasingly been transferred to community programs. Yet state mental hospitals remain an important part of the care of long-stay mentally ill patients. This study presents a perspective of state mental hospitals in the care of long-stay mentally ill patients.

The Prevailing View of State Mental Hospitals Today.—There are no standard criteria for evaluating state mental hospitals today. Some facilities provide care and rehabilitation, others serve as gateways into integrated health care systems, and still others offer little. Some facilities have been accused of neglect or abuse or having incompetent staff or inhumane living conditions. Funding is declining.

Who Is Being Served Today?—"Old" long-stay patients (those residing in such facilities for 5 to 10 years), new long-stay patients, and short-stay patients who often return make up the population in most mental hospitals today. The number of short-stay patients using state mental health facilities is determined by the makeup of the community served by the hospital, the laws and regulations governing commitment, the types of services available in the community, and the commitment of the community to serve the mentally ill.

The Fate of Mentally Ill Individuals No Longer Served in State Hospitals.—Community care has improved the lot of many patients who were formerly in institutions. Others are underserved or unserved. Between one third and one half of homeless individuals probably have long-term mental illness. Other individuals with long-term mental illness are in jail or prison.

What is the Appropriate Role of State Mental Hospitals Today?—Instead of determining by geography where a state mental hospital should be located, the types of services provided should be evaluated in terms of the needs of both patients and their families.

Unified Systems of Care.—A unified system may be the answer to service planning endeavors. Mental hospitals should offer the types of services they are best at providing, and duplication of services should be avoided. Interagency cooperation, including community agencies, must be fostered.

Conclusion.—State mental hospitals vary in the quality and types of services they provide. Resident populations differ from community to community. Unified care systems should be developed to included state mental hospitals and community-based service organizations.

▶ Because the author quotes me in this contribution as visionary in 1983 about the future of state hospitals, I cannot pretend to be unbiased. However, as I visit public facilities today, I am struck by the concern about what their role will be in our 1990s world of rapid competitive managed care. Fortunately, I think we have got enough smart individuals in the field to come up with different creative solutions for different public facilities.

J.A. Talbott, M.D.

The Evolving Role of the State Hospital in the Care and Treatment of Older Adults: State Trends, 1984 to 1993

Semke J, Fisher WH, Goldman HH, et al (Univ of Washington, Seattle; Univ of Massachusetts, Worcester)

Psychiatric Serv 47:1082–1087, 1996 7–26

Objective.—There is little information about the use of state mental hospital facilities by severely and chronically mentally ill geriatric patients. Although there is a relatively high prevalence of severe mental illness and neuropsychiatric disorders among older individuals, the number of older adults in these facilities is declining. Use trends of state mental hospitals by older adults were studied.

Methods.—Statistics on state mental hospital use between 1984 and 1993 by individuals aged 65 years and older by age and diagnosis were obtained from the Center for Mental Health Services for the United States Department of Health and Human Services.

Results.—Although 10 states had increased populations of older adults in mental health facilities, the use of state mental hospitals decreased nationwide during the study years for all age groups, but more so for older adults. The number of older adults hospitalized for dementia, delirium, and amnesia or schizophrenia also declined. State mental hospitals serve multiple populations, including those with schizophrenia, mood disorders, and more frequently today, those with Alzheimer's disease.

Conclusion.—Although there is a trend today toward declining populations of older adults in state mental hospitals, needs of aging baby boomers and successful medical efforts at prolonging life may spark a resurgence of interest in the use of state mental hospitals to care for this large population.

▶ One of the groups most affected by the onset of de-institutionalization in 1955 was the elderly population. The changes were twofold; a diminution in the state hospital population resulting from death of elderly patients living their lives out in state facilities, and a decrease in the number of admissions of older individuals with organic conditions or those who had long-standing schizophrenia and lacked housing/care. Nursing homes and other "alternatives" have clearly picked up the slack; but given what we know about the amount of psychosocial care provided in most such homes, I am not convinced we have done our elderly patients any favors.

J.A. Talbott, M.D.

The Benefits of Psychiatric Hospitalization for Older Nursing Home Residents

Kunik ME, Ponce H, Molinari V, et al (Baylor College of Medicine, Houston; Texas Southern Univ, Houston)

J Am Geriatr Soc 44:1062–1065, 1996 7–27

Objective.—A high prevalence of dementia, sleep disorders, adjustment disorders, schizophrenia, anxiety, agitation, social withdrawal, and depression is found in older nursing home residents that could possibly be better treated in a psychiatric hospital. Although there is a low rate of hospitalization for mental disorders, sex, severity of cognitive impairment, and behavioral problems were associated with admission. Demographics and treatment outcomes of nursing home residents admitted to the geropsychiatric unit of 1 hospital were studied.

Methods.—A retrospective cohort study of 53 admissions of 43 patients to the geropsychiatric unit from a nursing home between November 1993 and May 1995 examined and scored cognitive impairments, behavioral symptoms, and contributory medical conditions at admission and discharge using the Mini-Mental State Examination, the Brief Psychiatric Rating Scale, the Hamilton Rating Scale for Depression, the Cohen-Mansfield Agitation Inventory, the Rating Scale for Side Effects, and the Global Assessment of Functioning. Reasons for admission included violent behavior, psychosis, depression, and sexual inappropriateness. Scores were compared statistically.

Results.—From admission to discharge, a significant decrease was found in levels of general psychiatric symptoms, depression, and agitation. Global functioning improved significantly. Cognitive status and medication side effects remained unchanged. For patients admitted for specific reasons, there were significant decreases in violence, psychosis, depression, and hostility but none for inappropriate sexual behavior. Of the 41 patients with complete data, 33 were returned to the nursing home, 2 were discharged to a personal care home, 2 were discharged home under supervision, 1 required long-term hospitalization, and 3 were referred for medical treatment. Seventeen of 19 patients with dementia were returned to the nursing home, and 16 of 22 patients without dementia were returned to the nursing home. Four patients with chronic mental illnesses were discharged to a less restrictive environment.

Conclusion.—Some patients with mental problems who are in nursing homes benefit from admission to a psychiatric hospital. In this study, 10% of such patients were discharged to a less restrictive environment.

► This is another side of the coin described by Semke (Abstract 7–26). Here we see that patients in nursing homes benefit greatly from admission, in this case to a Veterans Affairs hospital. The good news is that 10% were found to be able to be discharged to a lesser restrictive environment; the bad is that the authors conclude that maybe it was the lack of psychosocial services in the nursing homes that prompted their admission in the first place.

J.A. Talbott, M.D.

A Two-Year Follow-up on the Effects of a Smoking Ban in an Inpatient Psychiatric Service

Velasco J, Eells TD, Anderson R, et al (Univ of Louisville, Ky)

Psychiatric Serv 47:869–871, 1996 7–28

Objective.—Behavioral disruptions among patients in psychiatric units were evaluated 2 years after a smoking ban was implemented.

Background.—Concern about tobacco-related diseases has led to smoking restrictions in hospitals and other medical facilities. Many psychiatric facilities have banned smoking despite concern that individuals with mental illness would not be able to tolerate such a ban and that it would interfere with their ability to cope with treatment. The prevalence of cigarette smoking among patients in psychiatric units is estimated at 52% to 88%, compared with about 33% in the general population. Studies of these patients' ability to avoid smoking have reported inconsistent findings. In 1991, behavior in patients in psychiatric units was evaluated before and immediately after a smoking ban was instituted. No behavioral disruptions were seen, except for an increase in p.r.n. medication for anxiety. Follow-up data at 2 years were described.

Methods.—During a 1-month period, 96 patients were admitted to a locked, inpatient psychiatric unit 2 years after a nonsmoking policy was implemented. About 40% of the patients had psychoses, 40% had an affective disorder, and 20% had chemical dependence or personality or organic mental disorders. Patient behavior was observed and recorded during the 1-month period by nursing staff. Nicotine gum was available for the first assessment period 2 years before, and this and a transdermal skin patch were available for the follow-up period.

Results.—During both assessment periods, the average length of stay was 9 days. The number of verbal assaults increased significantly immediately after the smoking ban was begun but was similar to the number of verbal assaults in the follow-up period 2 years later. The use of soft restraints was similar before and immediately after the smoking ban but increased significantly 2 years later. Use of replacement nicotine was significantly higher immediately after and 2 years after the smoking ban. The use of p.r.n. medication for anxiety was significantly higher immediately after the smoking ban than before.

Conclusions.—Dangerous behavior did not occur in patients admitted to a locked psychiatric service after the institution of a smoking ban. Minor difficulties did occur but did not disrupt the treatment environment. Individuals in psychiatric units who are acutely disturbed can tolerate abstinence from smoking.

► We have now had almost 10 years of studies on smoke-free psychiatric wards/hospitals. Despite all the staff fears of problems with a ban,[1] this study confirms that immediate problems are no longer found 2 years later. Maybe it is time for a moratorium on such articles; the evidence does seem "in."

J.A. Talbott, M.D.

Reference

1. Haller E, McNeil DE, Binder RL: Impact of a smoking ban on a locked psychiatric unit. *J Clin Psych* 57:329–332, 1996.

Predicting Readmission to the Psychiatric Hospital in a Managed Care Environment: Implications for Quality Indicators

Lyons JS, O'Mahoney MT, Miller SI, et al (Northwestern Univ, Chicago)

Am J Psychiatry 154:337–340, 1997 7–29

Introduction.—Psychiatric hospital readmission, particularly when it occurs relatively soon after a previous discharge, may indicate failure of the earlier inpatient care. However, little documentation exists on the significance of readmission rates. A series of patients was followed for 6 months after discharge to determine the relationship between hospital readmission and the quality of inpatient psychiatric services.

Methods.—The 225 patients in the series were consecutively admitted to 7 hospitals within a large regional managed care program during the period July 1994 to February 1995. Each patient was assessed by a case manager using both the Severity of Psychiatric Illness Scale and the Acuity of Psychiatric Illness Scale. Data collected included reasons for admission, complications to the psychiatric disorder, complications to treatment, severity and persistence of illness, clinical status, and nursing status.

Results.—The study group had an average age of 30.8 years and was predominantly female (60.7%). The most common admission diagnosis (63.5%) was major affective disorder. Length of hospital stay averaged 6.7 days. During the 6-month follow-up period, 45 (17.6%) patients were readmitted to a hospital, 18 of them within 30 days of discharge from the index admission. No associations were found between readmissions and age, gender, or diagnostic group. Patients readmitted within 30 days had a higher level of self-care impairment and tended to have more medical complications. Those readmitted within 6 months had more symptom severity and less family involvement and tended to have more substance abuse complications. Significant predictors of readmission within 1 year were impairment in self-care, severity of symptoms, and a premorbid level of dysfunction. The potential for suicide was significantly but negatively associated with readmission. There was no evidence that early readmission was related to poor hospital outcome or premature discharge.

Conclusion.—Patients at risk for psychiatric readmission have impaired self-care and more severe and persistent difficulties than nonreadmitted patients, yet readmission does not appear to indicate a poor outcome from the index hospitalization. Thus readmission rates are not an accurate indicator of the quality of inpatient psychiatric services.

▶ This study presents an interesting conclusion because for years we have assumed that by figuring out why patients are readmitted we can decrease readmissions by intervening more effectively. I agree with the authors that the use of readmission rates would be inappropriate if it were assumed that they measured quality. However, they do represent something, for example, community support or responsiveness to treatment—factors which must be addressed.

J.A. Talbott, M.D.

Outpatient/Community Care

A Home-based Program for the Treatment of Acute Psychosis
Wasylenki D, Gehrs M, Goering P, et al (Univ of Toronto)
Community Ment Health J 33:151–162, 1997 7–30

Introduction.—Traditionally, seriously ill psychiatric patients could be treated only in hospitals; however, recent studies have shown that acutely ill patients could be treated at home and that about 75% of patients could be kept out of the hospital. Processes necessary to establish and disseminate home treatment programs were described, as well as assessments of the impact and comparative cost of a home treatment program developed in metropolitan Toronto.

Methods.—The Clarke Institute of Psychiatry and the Home Care Program for Metropolitan Toronto joined hands to develop the Home Treatment Program for Acute Psychosis. Training sessions for nurses, homemakers, and social workers were implemented and covered mental disorders, psychiatric medications, and crisis intervention. Clients treated at home were excluded if they were judged to be imminently dangerous to themselves or others. About 80% of eligible patients were schizophrenic, and 40% had co-existing substance use disorder. Clients were assessed regarding their attitudes toward home treatment by way of a questionnaire. There were 3-month follow-up measures, which included attitudes, family impact, and treatment comparison and satisfaction. Organizational adjustment necessary to implement the program were evaluated, as were costs.

TABLE 2.—Treatment Comparison Questionnaire

Advantages for Home Treatment
- More communication with staff
- Provided help more readily
- Opportunity to plan and make decisions
- Less anxious and stressed
- Relationships less disrupted
- Daily routine less disrupted
- People expressed fewer negative attitudes
- Treated with more dignity and respect
- Provided more support

Advantages for Hospital Treatment
- Felt more safe
- Less difficult to separate emotionally

(Courtesy of Wasylenki D, Gehrs M, Goering P, et al: A home-based program for the treatment of acute psychosis. *Community Ment Health J* 33:151–162, 1997.)

Results.—There were 34 episodes of home treatment completed that involved 27 different patients in the 18-month period. The mean length of episodes was 28 days, with 30.8% of patients having affective disorders, 57.7% having schizophrenia and 7.7% having anorexia nervosa. Community-based providers were found to be more positive than hospital providers. Clients and family members maintained positive attitudes toward home treatment after episodes of care. There was a clear preference for home treatment over inpatient hospitalization on 9 of 11 points (Table 2). To facilitate smooth functioning of home treatment programs, some structural modifications were necessary, together with interactions among the several agencies involved, according to the organizational analysis.

Conclusion.—Symptoms were reduced, family burden decreased, satisfaction was high, and participants preferred home treatment to hospital admission. Home treatment is less costly than hospitalization, according to the economic data.

▶ Since the Program of Assertive Community Treatment (PACT) study was published in 1978,[1] the field has used it as a model or standard for many community programs. It is refreshing to see the Clarke group come at the issue slightly differently than the Wisconsin group (PACT), while demonstrating many of the same clinical and economic effects. The cost differential (if one pretends that there are no longer any hospitals for which we must pay fixed costs) is striking indeed.

J.A. Talbott, M.D.

Reference

1. Stein LI, Test MA: Alternative to mental hospital treatment. *Arch Gen Psychiatry* 37:392–405, 1980.

Client Outcomes in a Three-Year Controlled Study of an Integrated Service Agency Model

Chandler D, Meisel J, Hu T-w, et al (Univ of California, Berkeley)
Psychiatric Serv 47:1337–1343, 1996 7–31

Background.—There are few long-term, controlled studies in the mental health services research. A 3-year controlled study of an integrated service agency model in California was reported.

Methods.—To determine whether they improved outcomes for a cross-section of clients with severe and persistent mental illness, 2 integrated service agency demonstration programs combining structural and program reforms were investigated. At 1 urban and 1 rural site, clients were randomly assigned to an integrated service agency program or a comparison group receiving standard services.

Findings.—Clients in the integrated service agencies had less hospital care, greater workforce participation, and fewer group and institutional living arrangements. They also had a lower use of conservatorship, more social support, more leisure activity, less family burden, and higher client and family satisfaction. The urban clients but not the rural ones did better on measures of financial stability, personal well-being, and friendship. Among the urban clients, 72.6% in the integrated services group were in the workforce during the 3-year study, compared with 14.6% in the standard treatment group. Arrest and conviction rates, self-reported ratings of self-esteem, symptoms, medication compliance, homelessness, and criminal victimization were similar in the 2 groups at both sites. The capitated costs were much higher in the integrated services group than in the control group.

Conclusions.—The 3-year outcomes for clients with severe mental illness in integrated service agencies were broadly favorable. However, the cost of such services was higher than that of standard care.

▶ Although the authors say that the State of California has made a decision to support a higher-cost but better-outcome treatment system for high users, I am less than convinced that this can occur widely with larger populations. Although cost-benefit analyses are essential for our arguments to policy markers, I fear that whether capitation rates will continue at adequate rates or "racheting down" will occur here as it has elsewhere remains to be seen.

J.A. Talbott, M.D.

Mental Health, 'Burnout' and Job Satisfaction Among Hospital and Community-based Mental Health Staff

Prosser D, Johnson S, Kuipers E, et al (Inst of Psychiatry, London; Univ College London)

Br J Psychiatry 169:334–337, 1996 7–32

Objective.—Stress and job satisfaction were evaluated in community-based and hospital-based mental health care workers.

Background.—With the move to community care for individuals who are mentally ill, mental health workers have experienced much change and had to adapt to new roles and responsibilities. Mental health workers in any setting are subject to stress, but those in community settings may experience exceptionally intense pressure. It is unclear whether community mental health services have enough staff to provide care for all the individuals with severe mental illness in the community. There is concern that staff burnout may make it difficult for community programs to provide high-quality care for long periods.

Methods.—The 12-item version of the General Health Questionnaire, the Maslach Burnout Inventory, and the job satisfaction section of the Job Diagnostic Survey were sent to 160 community-based and hospital-based mental health care workers.

Results.—Of the 160 workers, 121 responded. Respondents consisted of 71 nurses, 23 psychiatrists, 9 occupational therapists, 9 nursing assistants, 6 social workers, and 3 psychologists. Of these, 29 were mainly community-based, 50 worked in wards, and 42 worked in hospital day care or outpatient settings; 66% of respondents had been in their current job for less than 2 years. Community-based mental health staff scored significantly higher on the 12-item version of the General Health Questionnaire and the emotional exhaustion component of the Maslach Burnout Inventory than hospital-based inpatient, day care, and outpatient staff. Job satisfaction was similar for all settings.

Conclusions.—Community-based work in the mental health fields may be more stressful than hospital-based work, or it may be more stressful because of inadequate resources. The community services in this study were newly established, and higher stress may have been a consequence of change. These findings are limited by the small sample size.

► I found this fascinating because I and others[1] have been more impressed that, at least among psychiatrists, burnout on our vastly decreased length-of-stay inpatient units is a bigger problem than in community settings. Burnout was a subject much written about in the early days of deinstitutionalization and community mental health centers; perhaps it is time to go back to it given our newer tools and knowledge. Certainly all the workplace changes, for example, more acute care patients, "downsizing," and greater competition, must have some adverse staff consequences.

J.A. Talbott, M.D.

Reference

1. Lebenluft E, Summergrad P, Tasman A: The academic dilemma of the inpatient unit director. *Am J Psychiatry* 146:73–76, 1989.

Clinicians' Judgment of Capacity of Nursing Home Patients to Give Informed Consent

Barton CD Jr, Mallik HS, Orr WB, et al (Univ of Maryland, Baltimore; Johns Hopkins Univ, Baltimore, Md; Tulane Univ, New Orleans, La; et al)
Psychiatric Serv 47:956–960, 1996 7–33

Objectives.—The ability of nursing home staff to recognize clinical competency in patients was studied, as well as how informed consent for medical treatment is obtained for such patients.

Background.—When a patient gives informed consent to medical treatment, it means that the patient is knowing, competent, and voluntary. The physician must explain the treatment so that the patient understands its indications, risks, benefits, and alternative treatment. It is presumed that adult patients are competent to make such decisions for themselves. Although only a judge can declare a patient incompetent, physicians often assess a patient's ability to make informed decisions about health care. This capacity is termed clinical competency or medical capacity. The process of obtaining informed consent for clinically incompetent individuals in nursing homes may not be well established or well followed. In nonemergency situations, physicians must choose an alternative means of obtaining informed consent when it is believed that a patient is not clinically competent.

Methods.—Forty-four individuals were admitted to a nursing home associated with a major teaching hospital. The individuals who participated were evaluated for clinical competency and completed the Hopkins Competency Assessment Test and the Mini Mental State Examination. A researcher blind to the test results reviewed each participant's chart to determine how the staff had viewed the participants' clinical competency.

Results.—Of 44 participants, 20 were identified by the Hopkins Competency Assessment Test as incompetent to give informed consent for medical treatment. Staff had identified 13 of those same individuals as clinically incompetent. None of the individuals identified as clinically incompetent by staff were provided with health care representatives in accordance with state statutes.

Discussion.—The prevalence of clinical incompetency to give informed consent to medical treatment in these nursing home residents was high. The clinicians identified only 65% of individuals judged to be clinically incompetent by the Hopkins Competency Assessment Test. As a result, patients who did not have the capacity to make decisions about their health care were allowed to do so. It was surprising to learn that no steps were taken to use alternative means of obtaining informed consent for individuals who were judged to be clinically incompetent, although the reasons for this were not investigated in this study. One limitation of this study is the ability of the Hopkins Competency Assessment Test to determine clinical competency.

► This is kind of scary. I just wish I knew more about whether the patients had worse outcomes as the result of the misdetection or lack of follow-up of competency status. Maybe the authors' surmise that surrogates helped make decisions is correct; maybe even clinicians were acting for the best outcomes.

J.A. Talbott, M.D.

Risk-adjusted Outcome Measures and Quality of Care in Nursing Homes

Mukamel DB (Univ of Rochester, NY)

Med Care 35:367–385, 1997 7–34

Introduction.—Although cost is an important factor in assessing health care, the quality of the health care is also important. The Committee on Nursing Home Regulation of the Institute of Medicine in 1986 recommended that nursing home quality of care regulations for Medicare and Medicaid certification be reoriented to a more resident-centered and outcome-oriented evaluation as opposed to an assessment of the process of care. To assess quality of care based on risk-adjusted outcomes, the use of the patient review instrument—a reimbursement reporting system used by the New York State Department of Health—was evaluated.

Methods.—To develop 5 risk-adjusted outcome measures, data for all residents in approximately 550 nursing homes in up-state New York were used. The 5 measures were rates of major accidents, dehydration, physical restraints, increases in severity of decubitus ulcers, and decline in functional status activities of daily living. To adjust for individual patient's risk factors, logistic models were used. The face validity, content, construct, and criterion validity of these measures was examined.

Results.—Deficiency citations were significantly correlated with measures based on activities of daily living decline, deterioration in decubiti, and physical restraints rates. Performance was not as good for measures based on accident rates and rates of dehydration. Across regions and between for-profit and nonprofit nursing homes, there was significant variation in these quality measures.

Conclusion.—The average number of deficiency citations per annual survey is 1 benchmark of quality. Information regarding quality of care is important for the efficient operation of competitive market. Individual patients, however, do not often have access to such information. Based on data collected for reimbursement purposes, valid risk-adjusted outcome measures of quality can be developed.

► Care in nursing homes is of special importance for us in psychiatry; both because so many of our chronic patients have been "transinstitutionalized" to them and because nursing home quality is so variable. This study focuses on the physical rather than the mental and psychosocial aspects of standardizing care evaluations. However, it must be extended to those areas.

J.A. Talbott, M.D.

Mentally Disordered Women in Jail: Who Receives Services?

Teplin LA, Abram KM, McClelland GM (Northwestern Univ, Chicago)

Am J Public Health 87:604–609, 1997 7–35

Introduction.—Severe psychiatric disorders are found among many jail inmates. In a previous study of male inmates, it was found that 37% of those with a severe mental disorder received mental health services while in jail. A similar study for women has not been conducted, yet women comprise 10% of the jail population. This study evaluated the proportion of female jail detainees with severe mental disorders, who needed mental health services, and what proportion received services.

Methods.—Trained interviewers administered a psychiatric evaluation to 1,272 randomly selected female jail detainees in a large Midwestern city. Using records and case files, researchers ascertained whether the women received services.

Results.—Of the 955 women who were selected for the study, it was found that 116, or 10.4% of the female jail population, needed mental health services. Of these, 23.5% ultimately received these services. The odds of a mentally ill woman's receiving services depended on the type of disorder, treatment history, and sociodemographic variables. Those with schizophrenia were 65 times more likely to receive services than the reference group (persons with none of the disorders, in the final model). Those who had had psychiatric treatment previously increased the odds of receiving services more than 80 times. The odds of receiving services was reduced by having had 2 or more prior arrests. White high school graduates with a major depressive episode were 15 times more likely to receive services compared with the reference group.

Conclusion.—The magnitude of mental health service needs in correctional facilities far exceeds the current resources. Screening techniques must be improved and more liaisons, must be formed between the criminal justice and mental health systems.

▶ Together with nursing homes (see Abstract 7–34), the other site that has become the recipient of "transinstitutionalization" has been the correctional system. Although we know from the epidemiologic catchment area study that only 20% or so of the population with psychiatric illnesses receives treatment (not too different from the 23.5% rate in this study), here we have a captive, stable population, not a community sample; therefore, they should be getting treatment at a much higher rate.

J.A. Talbott, M.D.

The Effectiveness of Outpatient Civil Commitment

Munetz MR, Grande T, Kleist J, et al (Summit County Alcohol, Drug Addiction, and Mental Health Services Board, Cuyahoga Falls, Ohio; Northeastern Ohio Universities, Beachwood; Community Support Services Inc, Akron, Ohio)

Psychiatric Serv 47:1251–1253, 1996 7–36

Background.—Outpatient civil commitment is proposed as a means to reduce rehospitalization rates among recidivists with severe mental illness, yet the effectiveness of such placement has not been shown. To assess the effects of outpatient civil commitment on community tenure and functioning, outcome was reviewed for 20 patients maintained for at least 12 months on an outpatient commitment order.

Methods.—The patients were committed to the Summit County (Ohio) Alcohol, Drug Addiction, and Mental Health Services Board between January 1992 and November 1993. All had a history of recurrent hospitalizations, noncompliance with outpatient treatment, and good response to treatment. Data were recorded on hospital use, criminal arrests and convictions, drug and alcohol abuse, use of various services, and residential and employment status during the 12-month periods before and after commitment.

Results.—The patient group included 11 men and 9 women with a mean age of 41.4 years; 8 were white and 12 were nonwhite (predominantly black). Most (18 of 20) were unmarried. Diagnoses were schizophrenia in 15, schizoaffective disorder in 2, and bipolar disorder in 3. The mean number of lifetime hospitalizations (most involuntary) was 12.9. Compared with the 12 months before the outpatient civil commitment, patients maintained on outpatient commitment had significantly fewer and shorter admissions to the state hospital. In 4 patients, however, there was a lack of improvement in medication compliance and an increase in hospital use. The group as a whole showed a statistically significant increase in the number of psychiatric appointments kept. Employment status, independent living, and substance abuse showed little change during outpatient commitment.

Discussion.—In this small series of patients with severe mental illness, outpatient civil commitment reduced hospital use and improved treatment compliance. When specific clinical and system guidelines are followed, outpatient civil commitment may help to reduce the tendency toward hospital recidivism and reintegrate patients into the community.

► One of the most controversial issues in our field in recent years has been that of outpatient commitment. On the one hand, many individuals favoring community care thought that such provisions would lead to better treatment. However, opponents felt that no new legislation was needed and that early experiences showed problems and low utilization in those states making such efforts. There are lots of caveats to this study (the lack of controls, sample size, retrospective design, etc.), but these early results support those who advocate the use of outpatient commitment.

J.A. Talbott, M.D.

A Model for Evaluating Intensive Outpatient Behavioral Health Care Programs

Raskin R, Novacek J, Bahlinger D, et al (Tulsa Inst of Behavioral Sciences, Oklahoma; Univ of Oklahoma, Tulsa)

Psychiatric Serv 47:1227–1232, 1996 7–37

Background.—Considerable evidence shows that partial hospitalization is an effective treatment modality for the mentally ill. There is no consensus, however, about which program components are most beneficial or about the best way to evaluate and compare such programs. A model for evaluating the effectiveness of intensive outpatient behavioral health care programs in a managed care environment was proposed and applied to a brief partial hospital–crisis stabilization program.

Methods.—The model specifies 5 criteria to be used in the evaluation: client selection, program attendance, service use and focus of treatment, client improvement, and cost-effectiveness. This model was tested with a sample of 285 adults, 200 with severe mental illness who were admitted for outpatient treatment or 85 who were receiving outpatient treatment at a state-funded community mental health center. Diagnoses included major depression in 52% and schizophrenia in 22%; 39% had a coexisting substance abuse disorder and 68% were indigent. Data evaluated were pre- and postprogram ratings of symptoms, level of functioning and treatment readiness; current and retrospective reports of symptoms based on client interviews; and clients' service and financial records.

Results.—Ninety-eight of 200 new admissions were assigned to a partial hospital–crisis stabilization program and 102 to regular outpatient counseling. Ratings by the intake staff indicated significantly more symptom severity, poorer daily functioning, poorer quality of life, and less treatment readiness in clients assigned to the partial hospital program. The program was completed by 60 of 98 clients. No-shows and dropouts accumulated $15,272 in service costs—a figure that, projected onto the total number of individuals assigned to such a program at the community mental health center during 1994, would represent 23% of its fully allocated operating costs. Clients who participated in the partial hospital program had reduced symptoms, improved daily functioning, and improved treatment readiness. Thus, treatment costs were lower for clients who showed more improvement.

Discussion.—The evaluation model proposed here yielded data required to show program effectiveness. Results are specific to short-term hospital programs of 1–30 days that focus on crisis stabilization—programs that represent about one third of the partial hospital programs currently operating in the behavioral health care industry. Findings support a positive relationship between clinical effectiveness and cost-effectiveness.

► Now here is a result that should please everyone: *both* increased clinical effectiveness and cost-effectiveness. After a burst of enthusiasm for partial hospital programs in the 1960s, many insurance companies withdrew support in the 1980s; now perhaps we will see a rekindling of interest in what most of us believe in our gut is better care—but only because we can prove its efficacy.

J.A. Talbott, M.D.

Predictors of Missed Appointments for Psychiatric Consultations in a Primary Care Clinic

Grunebaum M, Luber P, Callahan M, et al (New York Hosp–Cornell Med Ctr; Cornell Univ, New York; Columbia Univ, New York; et al)

Psychiatric Serv 47:848–852, 1996 7–38

Introduction.—Little is known about the demographic and clinical factors that increase the likelihood of a patient becoming a no-show, missing appointments at general medical and psychiatric clinics. A study conducted at a primary care medicine clinic sought to determine predictors of missed appointments for psychiatric consultations.

Methods.—During 1994, the clinic recorded 39,600 patient visits. Patients receiving Medicaid and Medicare accounted for 65% of the primary-payer mix. The mean patient age was 45 years; 67% of patients were female and 55% were black or Hispanic. Of 281 patients referred for psychiatric consultations, 175 kept the appointments and 106 did not. Each sample was reduced to 90 patients, and the 2 groups were compared for demographic and clinical variables and assessed for interaction between the patient and the primary care clinician.

Results.—Patients who kept their appointments did not differ significantly from no-shows in demographic characteristics, including mean age. In univariate analysis, patients with cognitive impairment other than psychosis were significantly less likely to miss their psychiatric consultation. Except for this variable, however, the 2 groups did not differ significantly in type of medications prescribed or symptoms prompting referral. The no-show rate was similar in patients with and without a history of substance abuse. Three of 8 variables related to interaction between patient and primary care clinician were significant predictors of missed appointments in logistic regression analysis: a mild degree of observed patient distress, significant resistance to seeing a psychiatrist, and a longer wait between the referral and appointment date.

Discussion.—Demographic variables did not predict which patients attending a primary care clinic would keep their appointment for a psychiatric consultation. Significant predictors of no-show status were less distress, resistance to seeing a psychiatrist, and a longer wait for the consultation appointment. Limiting referrals to those with moderate or severe distress, reducing patient resistance to the consultation, and shortening the wait for an appointment might reduce the no-show rate.

▶ There is sparse and unfortunately old literature on ways of increasing outpatient department treatment compliance. The findings in this study of primary care patients are consistent with that work. Now, however, as we assume new and expanded roles in primary care, we have to bring our knowledge of how to improve treatment continuance to these patients.

J.A. Talbott, M.D.

The Homeless Mentally Ill

An Experimental Comparison of Three Types of Case Management for Homeless Mentally Ill Persons

Morse GA, Calsyn RJ, Klinkenberg WD, et al (Univ of Missouri, St Louis; Wright Inst, Berkeley, Calif)
Psychiatric Serv 48:497–503, 1997 7–39

Introduction.—At some point during their lifetime, about 14 million Americans have been homeless, and more than a third have severe mental illness. Mental illness precedes homelessness in most cases, with those being discharged from psychiatric inpatient facilities being at high risk of becoming homeless within 6 months. Few studies have evaluated the effectiveness of programs available for the homeless, such as assertive community treatment, in which comprehensive services were provided for an unlimited period; broker case management, in which brokers arrange for services from a variety of providers; and assertive community treatment augmented by community workers, paraprofessionals who assist clients with recreational and other activities of daily living. The 3 methods were compared for effectiveness in treating homeless clients.

Methods.—There were 135 individuals recruited from psychiatric emergency room and inpatient units randomly assigned to assertive community treatment only; broker case management only; or assertive community treatment augmented by support from community workers only.

Results.—Superior outcomes were found among clients assigned to assertive community treatment only and assertive community treatment with community workers, when compared with those assigned to broker case management. The variables that had better outcomes in the assertive community treatment programs were number of contacts with the treatment program, use of resources, severity of thought disorder, client satisfaction, and activity levels. About 33% of clients assigned to the broker management program did not attend the program. In many instances, the broker program had waiting lists of 3 to 4 months. More days in stable housing were achieved by clients in the assertive community treatment only condition than in the other 2 treatment modalities. Income, self-esteem, and substance abuse were not affected by any of the treatment methods.

Conclusion.—In assisting individuals with serious mental illness who are at risk of homelessness, assertive community treatment is superior to broker case management. More intensive and comprehensive services were provided by the assertive community treatment programs to people with serious mental illness than by the broker case management program.

► It has always seemed obvious to me that case managers who broker services are less effective than case managers who themselves provide some of the services needed by patients. This is certainly true here in the case of the homeless or those at risk for homelessness. Because these authors (in Abstract 5–62) showed that the most effective programs are no more costly, translating these results into action should not be difficult.

J.A. Talbott, M.D.

An Examination of the Relationship of Homelessness to Mental Disorder, Criminal Behaviour, and Health Care in a Pretrial Jail Population

Zapf PA, Roesch R, Hart SD (Simon Fraser Univ, Burnaby, BC)

Can J Psychiatry 41:435–440, 1996 7–40

Objective.—The prevalence of homelessness and its relation to mental illness, criminal behavior, and health care was investigated.

Background.—Research has shown that a substantial number of individuals in jail are mentally ill. Many of these individuals also may have been homeless at the time of their arrest. Martell conducted a study of New York City's primary forensic evaluation and treatment center and concluded that among criminal offenders, homeless individuals have a significantly higher risk of indictment for violent crimes. Other studies have shown a relation between homelessness, criminal activity, and mental disorder.

Methods.—Adult males were selected from admissions to a facility for pretrial defendants in a large metropolitan area. Data were obtained from interviews for 684 men and from health care files and institutional progress logs for 106 men. Information was collected on living conditions, employment status, psychosocial functioning, substance use, and use of health care services.

Results.—A significant relation was found between homelessness and severe mental disorder, and between homelessness and previous psychiatric history. There were no significant differences between homeless and nonhomeless individuals for type of crime for which the individual was incarcerated and for contact with health care services during the previous year.

Conclusions.—Although a significant relation was found between homelessness and mental disorder, most individuals who are homeless do not have a mental disorder. There is a need for a stronger link between the mental health and legal systems so that individuals who are mentally ill receive help rather than end up in the prison system. The jail often is not seen as part of the community and is isolated from other community services. To treat these individuals more effectively, social service, housing, mental health, and substance abuse service providers must combine their efforts.

► Seems obvious, doesn't it? OK, then why are we not doing it on a universal basis? Here is another example of a finding/fact that we have known about since at least 1978, about which systematically we have done little.

J.A. Talbott, M.D.

Housing Outcomes for Homeless Adults With Mental Illness: Results From the Second-round McKinney Program

Shern DL, Felton CJ, Hough RL, et al (Univ of South Florida, Tampa; New York State Office of Mental Health, Albany; San Diego State Univ, Calif; et al)

Psychiatric Serv 48:239–241, 1997 7–41

Background.—The best epidemiologic estimates indicate that about one third of homeless Americans have a mental illness. In the early 1990s, the National Institute of Mental Health sponsored projects in 4 cities (known as the second-round McKinney research demonstration program) to determine the efficacy of various housing, support, and rehabilitative services for decreasing homelessness. The overall success of these projects in attaining this goal was reported.

Methods and Outcomes.—The projects were conducted in Baltimore, Boston, San Diego, and New York City. A total of 896 homeless mentally ill persons were included. Although different case management models were used in the different cities, all involved assertive outreach and case management teams as the primary service vehicle. After the intervention, most of the subjects were living in community housing. The increase in community housing was 47.5% for those in active treatment conditions. At the final follow-up, 78% of the community housing participants were stably housed.

Conclusion.—Offering a range of acceptable housing alternatives, coupled with case management, treatment, and rehabilitative services, can effectively engage and stably house homeless persons with severe mental illness. The challenge now is to develop the political will and financing strategies to support these proven methods for reducing homelessness.

► The McKinney Program was a massive project to measure the impact of multiple interventions with the homeless mentally ill. The "success rate" of 80% is striking as it is the similarity among very different cities. The authors' caution that its replication on a wider scale depends on political will and resources is a caution I would echo. I wish there were an opportunity on our

Internal Revenue Service tax form to indicate, just as we do concerning political contributions, what we would support.

J.A. Talbott, M.D.

Preventing Recurrent Homelessness Among Mentally Ill Men: A "Critical Time" Intervention After Discharge From a Shelter

Susser E, Valencia E, Conover S, et al (Columbia Univ, New York; New York State Psychiatric Inst; Natl Inst of Mental Health, Bethesda, Md)

Am J Public Health 87:256–262, 1997 7–42

Introduction.—Compared with the general population of the United States, individuals with chronic mental illness are at significantly increased risk of becoming homeless. This risk may be reduced by health care intervention because homelessness among the mentally ill is attributed in part to discontinuity in mental health services. A randomized study tested the value of critical time intervention (CTI) in preventing homelessness after transition from institutional to community living.

Methods.—The study participants comprised 96 men with severe mental illness who were going to community housing from a shelter. Most were

TABLE 1.—Services Received by Mentally Ill Men in the Critical Time Intervention (CTI) and Usual Services Only (USO) Groups During the 18 Months After Discharge From Shelter to Community Living

	CTI Group	USO Group
1–3 months	Accommodation phase: CTI workers Make home visits Accompany patients to appointments Meet with caregivers Substitute for caregivers when necessary Give support and advice to patient and caregivers Mediate conflicts between patient and caregivers Help negotiate ground rules for relationships	Transition services: shelter staff Assist patients and caregivers upon request Substitute for caregivers when necessary
4–7 months	Tryout phase: CTI workers Observe trial of ground rules Help to modify ground rules as necessary	Usual services: Services provided by community formal and informal supports Patient and caregivers can phone for advice
8–9 months	Termination phase: CTI workers Reaffirm ground rules Hold parties/meetings to symbolize transfer of care	
10–18 months	Usual services	

(Courtesy of Susser E, Valencia E, Conover S, et al: Preventing recurrent homelessness among mentally ill men: A "critical time" intervention after discharge from a shelter. *Am J Public Health* 87:256–262, 1997. Copyright American Public Health Association.)

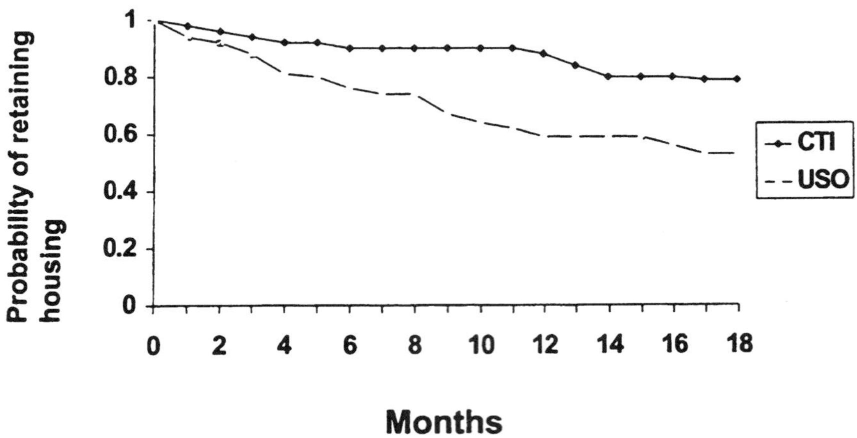

FIGURE 1.—Survival from homeless episodes lasting 30 nights or more over 18 months of follow-up of mentally ill men in the critical time intervention (CTI) and usual services only (USO) groups. (Courtesy of Susser E, Valencia E, Conover S, et al: Preventing recurrent homelessness among mentally ill men: A "critical time" intervention after discharge from a shelter. *Am J Public Health* 87:256–262, 1997.)

African-American or Latino and all suffered from severe mental illness, usually schizophrenia or some other psychotic disorder. The men were randomly assigned either to CTI or usual services only (USO) groups. Over an 18-month period, the CTI group received CTI plus usual services for 9 months, then USO for the following 9 months (Table 1). Those in the USO group received usual services for the entire period. Men in both groups underwent diagnostic as well as other types of assessment before randomization and face-to-face evaluation every 30 days. The 2 groups were compared for the mean number of homeless nights during the 18-month follow-up period.

Results.—The CTI group was at higher risk of homelessness than the USO group because men in the CTI group reported cocaine dependence and long-term homelessness more often. Follow-up revealed that the average number of homeless nights was 30 for the CTI group and 91 for the USO group, a statistically significant difference. The differences between the 2 groups did not diminish after the final 9 months of the study, when both CTI and USO groups received only usual services (Fig 1).

Conclusion.—Critical time intervention was an effective means of reducing homelessness among men with severe mental illness who were moving from institutional to community care. Even in this difficult population of inner-city men, many of whom were substance abusers, the active interventions of CTI produced long-term benefits.

► This study should help support the provision of services to persons in transition between hospital and community care. Table 1 demonstrates the services provided and Fig 1 shows the divergent rates of survival in community housing. Coupled with another article in the same issue of this journal (Bassuk EL, Buckner JC, Weinreb LF, et al: Homelessness in female-headed families: Childhood and adult risk and protective factors. *Am J Public Health* 87:241–248, 1997), which demonstrates both protective and risk factors to becoming homeless, we have more data to use as a basis for intervention.

J.A. Talbott, M.D.

Posttraumatic Stress Disorder

PTSD Symptoms and Comorbid Mental Disorders in Israeli War Veterans

Skodol AE, Schwartz S, Dohrenwend BP, et al (Columbia Univ, New York; New York State Psychiatric Inst, New York; New York Univ)
Br J Psychiatry 169:717–725, 1996 7–43

Background.—Posttraumatic stress disorder (PTSD) often is accompanied by mood disorders, psychoactive substance use, personality disorder, and other anxiety disorders. Patterns of mental disorders co-morbid with PTSD symptoms were studied in young Israeli men exposed to combat.

Methods.—Six hundred seventeen men were chosen through a general population sampling. The participants were assessed using a 2-phase case-identification procedure. Psychiatrists administered a modified lifetime version of the Schedule for Affective Disorders and Schizophrenia.

Clinical implications

- All patients with symptoms of PTSD should be thoroughly assessed for the presence of other mental disorders.
- Patients with PTSD symptoms and one or more comorbid mental disorders are more likely to seek treatment than are patients with PTSD or a mental disorder alone.
- Treatment plans for patients with PTSD may need to be individually tailored to take into account comorbidity with other mental disorders.

Limitations

- The assessment of PTSD was not made using a structured clinical interview method.
- The dating of combat experiences was approximate, and precise connections between the onsets of PTSD symptoms and particular combat experiences could not be made.
- The power to detect differences in rates of disorders with low prevalence in relation to combat exposure was limited.

BOX.—Clinical implications. (Courtesy of Skodol AE, Schwartz S, Dohrenwend BP, et al: PTSD symptoms and comorbid mental disorders in Israeli war veterans. *Br J Psychiatry* 169:717–725, 1996.)

Findings.—Men reporting PTSD symptoms more frequently reported major depressive disorder, substance use disorders, and personality disorders than men who had been in combat but had no symptoms. Among the former group, the odds ratios were 3.2 for major depressive disorder, 1.9 for substance use disorders, and 3.0 for personality disorders. Co-morbid disorders were not risk factors for PTSD, with the possible exception of personality disorders. Increased help-seeking was associated with co-morbid PTSD and RDC disorders.

Conclusions.—Individuals with PTSD are at risk for other mental disorders. These findings may be useful in understanding the risk factors associated with such co-morbidity and in guiding treatment and prevention efforts (Box).

► I included in this article as a reminder that there is universality to the occurrence of some disorders and co-morbid disorders. I also included it to highlight the figure, which shows a new trend in journal reader-friendliness; for example, showing what is clinically relevant in an easily comprehensible manner.

J.A. Talbott, M.D.

Consistency of Memory for Combat-related Traumatic Events in Veterans of Operation Desert Storm

Southwick SM, Morgan CA III, Nicolaou AL, et al (Yale Univ, New Haven, Conn; VA Med Ctr, West Haven, Conn)

Am J Psychiatry 154:173–177, 1997 7–44

Introduction.—Whether memory for combat-related traumatic events is fixed and indelible or malleable and subject to substantial distortion has been questioned. In veterans of Operation Desert Storm, a prospective investigation of memory for serious combat-related traumatic events was conducted.

Methods.—There were 62 veterans who were exposed to a variety of stressors, including bizarre disfigurement of dead bodies, the death of several unit members, and subsonic unarmed cruise decoy missile attacks. Fifty-nine veterans (46 men and 13 women) completed questionnaires about their experiences 1 month after the war and 2 years later. A comparison of the questionnaire responses was made to determine their consistency between the time lapse.

Results.—For events that were objective and highly traumatic in nature, there were many instances of inconsistent recall. On at least 1 of 19 items, 88% of participants changed their responses; 61% changed their responses on 2 or more items. Forty veterans (70%) recalled an item at 2 years that they did not recall at 1 month, whereas 27 (46%) did not recall an event at 2 years that they had recalled at 1 month. The number of responses on the trauma questionnaire that changed from no at 1 month to yes at 2 years was significantly related to the score on the Mississippi Scale for Combat-Related Posttraumatic Stress Disorder.

Conclusion.—The position that traumatic memories are fixed or indelible was not supported by this study. Amplification of memory for posttraumatic stress disorder symptoms occurs with an increase in posttraumatic stress disorder symptoms. The accuracy of recall for traumatic events is questioned, as is the relationship between the degree of posttraumatic stress disorder symptoms and the level of exposure to trauma.

▶ This research offers an interesting addition to the debate about false memories. The fact that as symptoms increase, so does the amplification of traumatic events, should lend an air of caution to those so certain that patients' recollections are accurate. Unfortunately, as the authors point out, most trauma studies rely on self-reports *after the fact;* although it would be a methodological nightmare, clearly knowing the exact nature of the stressor and conducting studies prospectively, would be far superior.

J.A. Talbott, M.D.

Posttraumatic Stress Disorder Associated With Peacekeeping Duty in Somalia for U.S Military Personnel

Litz BT, Orsillo SM, Friedman M, et al (Natl Ctr for Post-Traumatic Stress Disorder, Boston; Tufts Univ, Boston)

Am J Psychiatry 154:178–184, 1997 7–45

Background.—The United States military is currently asked to secure peace in dangerous places. Combat-trained soldiers in these situations are very visible and exposed to serious threats, yet must exhibit restraint and neutrality. To better understand the psychiatric consequences of peacekeeping duty in volatile situations, the prevalence of posttrauamtic stress disorder (PTSD) among soldiers on peacekeeping duty in Somalia was investigated.

Methods and Findings.—A cohort of 3,461 active duty personnel deployed to Somalia were surveyed approximately 5 months after returning to the United States. Ninety percent were men. Approximately 17.8% had previously served during a conflict, primarily in a combat or combat-support role in the Persian Gulf War. Eight percent met diagnostic criteria for PTSD. The rewards of military service, war zone stress, and frustrations with peacekeeping (i.e., restrictive rules of engagement) best predicted PTSD symptom severity.

Conclusion.—Missions such as that in Somalia probably represent a new paradigm of dangerous military operations for United States soldiers. For some combat-trained soldiers, restrictive rules of engagement may be difficult to reconcile and may place these soldiers at risk for PTSD.

▶ Soldiers, we were taught in the Army, are trained to fight, not to perform other activities. Certainly, following World War II, many in the military continued on in Europe to provide civilian re-stabilization. Now it appears that the United States military will be called upon more and more to perform peace-keeping roles. This report highlights the need to be alert to prevention, recognition and treatment of PTSD in these soldiers, just as in their combat-exposed counterparts.

J.A. Talbott, M.D.

Rape-related Psychotraumatic Syndromes

Darves-Bornoz J-M (Universitaire de Tours, France)

Eur J Obstet Gynecol Reprod Biol 71:59–65, 1997 7–46

Background.—In France, victims of sexual abuse are referred to designated forensic centers but receive no psychological treatment. Such patients are hypothesized to have severe psychopathology, mainly chronic posttraumatic stress disorder (PTSD). The longitudinal course of PTSD and the prevalence of disorders during the 6 months after rape was investigated. In addition, the disorders were grouped into syndromes related to chronic PTSD while remaining distinct from it. Predictive factors for chronic PTSD were also sought.

Methods and Findings.—Ninety-two rape victims consecutively admitted to a special forensic center were interviewed regularly by a psychiatrist during the 6 months after the rape. The prevalence of chronic PTSD was found to be high. Incest was a predictive factor for chronic PTSD. By 6 months, these victims commonly exhibited phobic and dissociative or borderline-like features.

Conclusion.—Rape victims need specialized psychiatric care at an early stage. The current data call into question the classification of many victims as personality disordered. It may be more helpful to view some of these victims' clinical signs as part of the clinical description of a post-traumatic disorder.

▶ Several things about this study are noteworthy: the high numbers of persons raped in 1 city in 1 year, the involvement of men as victims, the severity of PTSD after rape, and the chronicity of PTSD with incestuous rape. I sometimes worry that we do not take rape seriously enough—as a society or as members of the medical profession. I hope this article will be heard as a "wake-up call."

J.A. Talbott, M.D.

Psychiatric Sequelae of Posttraumatic Stress Disorder in Women

Breslau N, Davis GC, Peterson EL, et al (Henry Ford Health Sciences Ctr, Detroit; Case Western Reserve Univ, Cleveland, Ohio; Univ of Michigan, Ann Arbor)

Arch Gen Psychiatry 54:81–87, 1997 7–47

Background.—Posttraumatic stress disorder (PTSD) has been found to be highly co-morbid with other psychiatric disorders. Epidemiologic data also show that PTSD is more likely to occur in women than in men. Little is known about the temporal order of PTSD and the co-morbid disorders with strong lifetime associations—depression, anxiety, and substance use disorders. The psychiatric sequelae of PTSD were therefore studied in a large sample of women.

Methods.—Eight hundred one women with children participating in a study of cognitive and psychiatric outcomes by birth-weight level were included. The National Institute of Mental Health Diagnostic Interview Schedule, revised according to *Diagnostic and Statistical Manual of Mental Disorders,* (ed. 3, revised) was administered to determine lifetime psychiatric disorders.

Findings.—The lifetime prevalence of traumatic events was 40%. Fourteen percent of the women had PTSD. Increased risks for first-onset major depression and alcohol use disorder were associated with PTSD, with hazards ratios of 2.1 and 3.0, respectively. The risk of major depression after PTSD was as high as that after other anxiety disorders. The risk of first-onset major depression was significantly increased among women with pre-existing anxiety and PTSD. Pre-existing major depression increased women's vulnerability to the PTSD-inducing effects of traumatic events and risk of exposure to traumatic events.

Conclusions.—The risk of first-onset major depression and alcohol use disorder is increased by PTSD. The causes of these temporally secondary disorders is not clear. The effect of PTSD or underlying vulnerabilities exposed by the traumatic experience may be involved.

► As with Abstract 7–43, the intertwining of PTSD and co-morbid affective and addictive disorders is troubling and still not clear. A question prompted by this study is what "protects" the two thirds of women who experience "trauma" but in whom PTSD does not develop. Forty percent is a very high incidence for any environmental event.

J.A. Talbott, M.D.

Posttraumatic Stress Disorder Among Female Vietnam Veterans: A Causal Model of Etiology

Fontana A, Schwartz LS, Rosenheck R (Yale Univ, New Haven, Conn; Vietnam Veterans of America Inc, Washington, DC)

Am J Public Health 87:169–175, 1997 7–48

Introduction.—Studies of posttraumatic stress disorder among veterans of the Vietnam and Persian Gulf wars reveal that military service can be traumatizing for women as well as men. Using the National Vietnam Veterans Readjustment Study database, investigators examined both war and sexual trauma for their role in chronic posttraumatic stress disorder among female veterans of Vietnam. Only in recent years has sexual trauma been recognized for its importance in the development of the disorder.

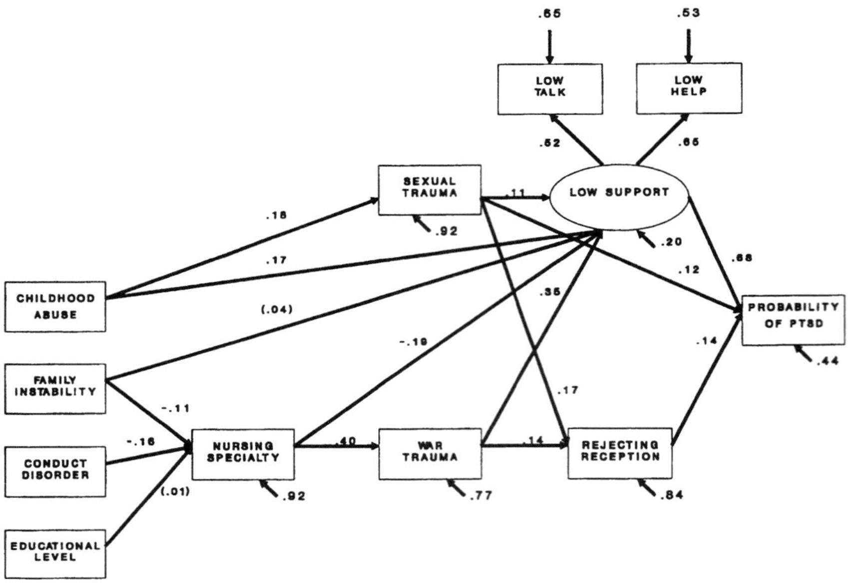

FIGURE 1.—Etiologic model for the probability of posttraumatic stress disorder among Vietnam theater women. (Courtesy of Fontana A, Schwartz LS, Rosenheck R: Posttraumatic stress disorder among female Vietnam veterans: A causal model of etiology. *Am J Public Health* 87:169–175, 1997. Copyright American Public Health Association.)

Methods.—National samples of 433 women who served in the Vietnam theater and 300 female Vietnam Era veterans were included in the database. Because of small numbers, ethnic minority subjects and Vietnam era women who served in a war zone at some other time were eliminated. The final sample consisted of 396 Vietnam theater women whose average age was 46.8 years and 250 Vietnam Era women whose average age was 44.99 years. Approximately half of the theater women and two thirds of the era women were married. At the time of the survey, conducted from 1986 to 1988, 8% of the Vietnam theater women and 2% of the Vietnam Era women were estimated to have posttraumatic stress disorder. Data were analyzed using the following measures: premilitary risk factors and traumas, service as a nurse and traumatic exposure while in the military, homecoming reception, postmilitary trauma, and posttraumatic stress disorder.

Results.—Structural equation modeling yielded an etiologic model (Fig 1) with highly satisfactory fit and parsimony. The reduced model consisted of paths that were common to both samples or that were noteworthy for one. Low support from family and friends at homecoming was an important contributor to the development of posttraumatic stress disorder, accounting for 63.6% of the effects for Vietnam theater women and 63% of the effects for Vietnam Era women. Trauma during military service accounted for 22.7% of the effects for Vietnam theater women and for 29.3% of the effects for Vietnam Era women. For the Vietnam theater women, the effects of sexual (10.4%) and war (12.3%) trauma were divided about equally.

Discussion.—Although sexual trauma was far less common than war trauma, it was nearly as important in terms of the development of posttraumatic stress disorder in these female Vietnam veterans. With an unsupportive homecoming reception, women were left to cope with such traumatic experiences alone and placed at increased risk for the disorder.

► This study targets sexual abuse among the etiologic elements of posttraumatic stress disorder in military women. It is a shocking commentary that sexual abuse, albeit less common than war trauma, was "nearly as influential" as war trauma in contributing to later posttraumatic stress disorder. We may not be able to control the elements that contribute to armed conflicts, but we can certainly affect the amount of sexual trauma in our society.

J.A. Talbott, M.D.

Social Network Disturbances and Psychological Distress Following Earthquake Evacuation

Bland SH, O'Leary ES, Farinaro E, et al (State Univ of New York, Buffalo; Univ Federico II, Naples, Italy)

J Nerv Ment Dis 1845:188–194, 1997 7–49

Introduction.—Although exposure to natural disasters is known to be associated with increased psychological distress, some disaster-exposed individuals appear to escape without psychological consequences. A study of male factory workers in a suburb of Naples, Italy tested the hypothesis that psychological distress after disaster evacuation is related to disruption of social networks.

Methods.—Residents of Pozzuoli, a coastal town affected by gradual shifting of the land (bradyseism), experienced numerous tremors and shocks during September and October of 1983. A national disaster was declared, and approximately 25,000 of the town's 70,000 inhabitants were evacuated. Among those affected were men who worked at the Olivetti Factory in Naples and were members of the Olivetti Heart Study. Data gathered after the earthquake provided assessment of psychological distress symptomatology for 817 men. Questions related to relocation and disruption of social networks were included in the screening.

Results.—Study participants ranged in age from 21.6 years to 70.1 years (mean 46.8). Most of the men were married (95.8%) and had less than a high school education (81.2%). After the earthquake, 550 were not evacuated, 142 were evacuated and then returned to their original homes, and 125 were permanently relocated. Across all dimensions of distress, those permanently relocated reported significantly higher distress symptoms. Evacuated men who returned to their original homes did not differ in distress scores from those who were spared evacuation. Distress was greater with increasing distance from the preearthquake residence but did not appear to be related to decreases in visits to family and friends.

Discussion.—Permanent relocation after an earthquake led to levels of distress that were significantly higher than those experienced by individuals who returned to their homes after the disaster. Despite the fact that all the men kept their jobs at the factory, the social network disruption caused by relocation caused considerable distress.

▶ Here is another hint about the etiological factors behind stress disorders, which indicts the disruption of social networks, following a catastrophic civilian event. One article[1] demonstrates that limited social networks contribute to earlier death in the old-old group of women. Clearly, social networks are highly influential in human lives.

J.A. Talbott, M.D.

Reference

1. Yasuda N, Zimmerman SI, Hawkes W, et al: Relation of social network characteristics to 5-year mortality amoung young-old versus old-old white women in an urban community. *Am J Epidemiol* 145:516–553, 1997.

Dissociation, Somatization, and Affect Dysregulation: The Complexity of Adaptation to Trauma

van der Kolk BA, Pelcovitz D, Roth S, et al (Harvard Med School, Boston; Duke Univ, Durham, NC; North Shore Univ/Cornell Med Ctr, Manhasset, NY; et al)

Am J Psychiatry 153:83–93, 1996 7–50

Objective.—The relation between the current diagnostic formulation of posttraumatic stress disorder and associated feature of dissociation, somatization, and affect dysregulation was studied.

Background.—The diagnostic criteria for posttraumatic stress disorder in the *Diagnostic and Statistical Manual of Mental Disorders (DSM)* of the American Psychiatric Association focus on intrusive memories and disordered arousal. Other symptoms of posttraumatic stress disorder are viewed as strategies to block emotions and somatic sensations associated with the trauma. A century of clinical observation and research has shown that individuals experience other symptoms that cannot be explained by this model of alternating intrusion and numbing. It is becoming clear that severe or prolonged trauma can result in complex characterological adaptations, problems with affect regulation, impaired capacity for cognitive integration of experience, and impaired capacity to differentiate relevant from irrelevant information. The *DSM-IV* lists dissociation, somatization, and affect dysregulation as associated features of posttraumatic stress disorder and as separate diagnoses.

Methods.—The participants were 395 adolescents older than 15 years, adults seeking psychiatric treatment, and 125 individuals not seeking psychiatric treatment. All had been exposed to psychological trauma. Information on posttraumatic stress disorder, symptoms of dissociation, somatization affect dysregulation, nature of the trauma, and age of onset was collected.

Results.—Participants were divided into 3 groups: those with current posttraumatic stress disorder; those with lifetime posttraumatic stress disorder but not currently meeting criteria; and those who never had posttraumatic stress disorder. High interrelations were seen among posttraumatic stress disorder, dissociation, somatization, and affect dysregulation. Participants who met the criteria for lifetime posttraumatic stress disorder scored significantly lower on these disorders than those with current posttraumatic stress disorder, but they had significantly higher scores than those who never had posttraumatic stress disorder. Significantly fewer symptoms were noted in participants whose posttraumatic stress disorder developed after psychological trauma as adults than in those who experienced the trauma in childhood. Participants who had posttraumatic stress disorder after experiencing trauma as adults had significantly more symptoms than victims of disaster.

Discussion.—The idea that there is closer association between posttraumatic stress disorder, dissociation, somatization, and affect dysregulation than is currently suggested by the *DSM-IV* is supported. These features of posttraumatic stress disorder often occur together in the same individual. This co-occurrence is partly a function of the nature of the trauma and the age when it occurred. The diagnosis of posttraumatic stress disorder does not fully describe the extent of the suffering of these individuals.

► It is very difficult to provide terse, facile comments on this article. It is complex and careful, as befits an article dedicated to the work of John Nemiah. The idea, however, that posttraumatic stress disorder, dissociation, somatization, and affect regulation are a spectrum phenomenon makes sense, and the treatment implications (psychotherapeutic) are sensible.

J.A. Talbott, M.D.

Behavioral and Neuroendocrine Responses to Sodium Lactate Infusion in Subjects With Posttraumatic Stress Disorder

Jensen CF, Keller TW, Peskind ER, et al (Va Puget Sound Health Care System; Seattle; Univ of Washington, Seattle)

Am J Psychiatry 154:266–268, 1997 7–51

Background.—Research has shown that sodium lactate infusion induces flashbacks and panic attacks in male combat veterans with concurrent posttraumatic stress disorder (PTSD) and panic disorder. The effects of sodium lactate in persons with PTSD but not panic disorder were investigated.

Methods.—The subjects were 7 patients with PTSD without panic disorder, 7 with panic disorder only, and 7 healthy persons. Behavioral, cardiovascular, catecholamine, and cortisol responses to infusion of 0.5-M sodium lactate were compared.

Findings.—Six of the 7 patients with PTSD reported flashbacks or other intrusive PTSD symptoms during lactate infusion. Substantial anxiety symptoms accompanied the flashbacks. None of the subjects in the other 2 groups experienced such symptoms. The patients with PTSD were found to have low cortisol levels.

Conclusion.—Sodium lactate infusion induces flashbacks in patients with PTSD without co-morbid panic disorder. The relation between anxiety responses that accompany a flashback in PTSD and those experienced during a panic attack is still not clear.

► So it is not panic disorder that is the essential ingredient in lactate-provoked flashbacks. In an accompanying editorial,[1] the authors point out that many patients with PTSD are, and will be, seen in primary care clinics. I just hope that we can find a way to transfer the rich research in psychiatry on PTSD to those working in primary care, if that is where the patients will be seen and treated.

J.A. Talbott, M.D.

Reference

1. Hales RE, Zatzick DF: What is PTSD? *Am J Psychiatry* 154:143–145, 1997.

Magnetic Resonance Imaging Study of Hippocampal Volume in Chronic, Combat-related Posttraumatic Stress Disorder

Gurvits TV, Shenton ME, Hokama H, et al (VA Med Ctr, Manchester, NH; Brigham and Women's Hosp, Boston; Harvard Med School, Boston)

Biol Psychiatry 40:1091–1099, 1996 7–52

Introduction.—Evidence from animal studies suggests a relation between sustained stress and hippocampal degeneration. This relation was subsequently explored in studies of patients in whom posttraumatic stress disorder (PTSD) developed after combat or childhood physical or sexual abuse. Hippocampal atrophy was shown at MRI in all of these groups. A study of Vietnam veterans used quantitative volumetric MRI techniques to explore the anatomical substrate of functional neurologic compromise in PTSD.

Methods.—The study participants, all male, were 14 Vietnam combat veterans, 7 with a diagnosis of PTSD and 7 with no lifetime PTSD. None had a current organic mental, bipolar, or psychotic disorder, a neurologic disorder, or a history of major head trauma. Some veterans in each group had past dependence or abuse of alcohol or other substances. Co-morbid current or past lifetime Axis I disorders were common in the PTSD group. In addition to MRI volumetric analyses, veterans underwent psychometric

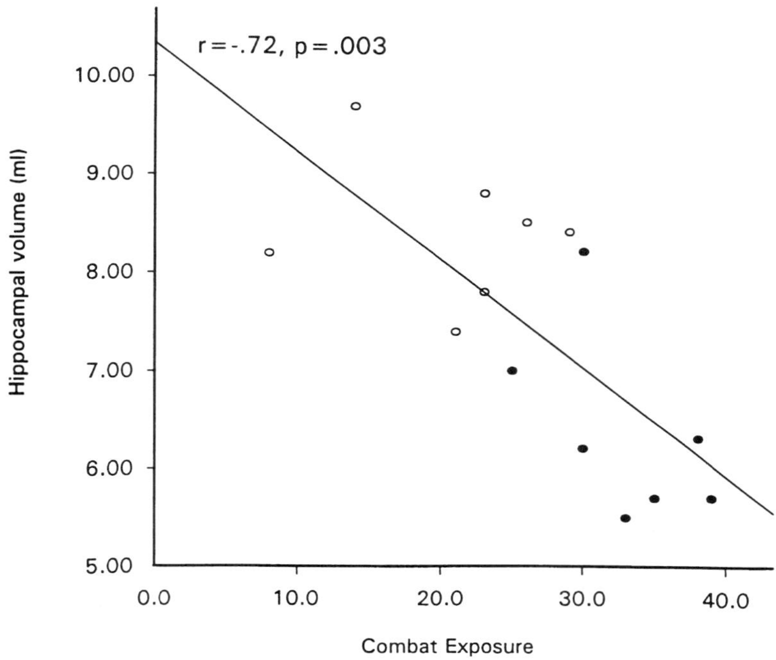

FIGURE 2.—Total hippocampal volume as a function of combat exposure scale score. *Closed circles* participants with posttraumatic stress disorder (PTSD); *open circles*, participants without PTSD. (Reprinted by permission of Elsevier Science Inc. from Magnetic resonance imaging study of hippocampal volume in chronic, combat-related posttraumatic stress disorder, by Guruits TV, Shenton ME, Hokama H, et al, *Biological Psychiatry*, Vol. 40, 1091–1099, Copyright 1996 by Elsevier Science, Inc.)

and neuropsychological testing and neurologic/neuropsychiatric evaluations. Volumetric MRI data also were obtained for 8 normal nonveterans.

Results.—Compared with combat controls and nonveteran controls, the veterans with PTSD had significantly smaller left and right hippocampi. The difference in hippocampal volume remained significant after adjusting for age, whole brain volume, and lifetime alcohol consumption. No statistically significant differences were observed in intracranial cavity, whole brain, ventricles, ventricle:brain ratio, or amygdala in the 3 groups. Both veteran groups had an increase in subarachnoidal CSF. Among PTSD and non-PTSD veteran groups, a partial correlation between Combat Exposure Score and total hippocampal volume remained significant (Fig 2) after adjusting for age, whole brain volume, and lifetime months of abusive drinking.

Discussion.—Combat veterans with PTSD had diminished left and right hippocampal volume in comparison with both combat and noncombat controls. Total hippocampal diminution was 26% relative to controls. Low hippocampal volume may be a result of PTSD, a risk factor for a greater likelihood of exposure to combat, or a precombat vulnerability factor for the development of PTSD upon combat exposure.

► As I have noted in previous volumes of this YEAR BOOK, I have always been struck by the essentially "organic" nature of PTSD symptoms, both acutely and chronically. The almost-linear relation between hippocampal size and combat exposure is pretty convincing (see Fig 2). How this fits together with other biological markers of PTSD is unclear, but we are closer to understanding this very puzzling illness.

J.A. Talbott, M.D.

Event-related Potentials in Post-traumatic Stress Disorder of Combat Origin

Attias J, Bleich A, Furman V, et al (Sheba-Med Ctr, Israel; IDF, Med Corps, Israel; Hebrew Univ, Jerusalem)

Biol Psychiatry 40:373–381, 1996 7–53

Introduction.—Patients with posttraumatic stress disorder (PTSD) re-experience the traumatic event and also avoid situations or stimuli resembling the event. When exposed to simulated combat noise or hypnotically induced imagery of traumatic events, these patients have increased physiologic responses, compared with combat veterans without PTSD. Visual stimuli were used to examine the event-related potential (ERP) patterns of combat veterans with and without PTSD.

Methods.—Study participants were 40 Israeli combat veterans, 20 with a diagnosis of PTSD and 20 without PTSD. The groups were age-matched and had a similar military history. None of the veterans had received pharmacologic treatment during the 12 months before the study, and all were free of alcohol or drug abuse. Both groups completed 3 self-reporting psychological questionnaires. Veterans were told that the ERP recordings were part of their neurologic evaluation and follow-up. The ERPs were recorded with scalp electrodes and in response to 3 sets of computer-generated visual stimuli, presented in the form of a modified oddball paradigm. Veterans were asked to press a button in response to target stimuli only. Of primary interest were the N1, N2, P2, and P3 components of ERPs.

Results.—Stimuli included domestic animal pictures (targets), emotionally neutral pictures of furnishings and flowers (nontargets), and combat-related pictures (nontarget probes). In each stimulus set, the reaction time was significantly delayed for patients with PTSD, compared with controls. Target stimuli, as expected, evoked accentuated P3 amplitudes in both controls and patients. Nontarget combat-related pictures elicited enhanced P3 and N1 amplitudes in patients with PTSD but not in controls. Patients with PTSD also had prolonged P3 latencies and reaction times to target stimuli, and N2 amplitudes were accentuated for both targets and combat-related pictures. The N1 latencies for probe stimuli did not differ significantly between patients and controls, but the N1 component was significantly prolonged in the PTSD group in response to target stimuli.

Conclusions.—Veterans with PTSD differed from veterans without PTSD in ERPs for picture stimuli with varying emotional content. Patients with PTSD may have an altered state of early and late cognitive selective attention processing. Responses in patients with PTSD also differ from those associated with various psychiatric and brain disorders.

► Here is more evidence for the "differentness" of PTSD from psychiatric illnesses such as schizophrenia and depression that are less "organic-looking." The authors note that these responses are "unique" to PTSD; clinically, it certainly seems self-evident that processing and attention are quite impaired in patients with PTSD, especially immediately after the trauma.

J.A. Talbott, M.D.

Linking Combat and Physical Health: The Legacy of World War II in Men's Lives

Elder GH Jr, Shanahan MJ, Clipp EC (Univ of North Carolina, Chapel Hill)

Am J Psychiatry 154:330–336, 1997 7–54

Introduction.—The legacy of war reverberates for many decades through social institutions and individual lives. The psychosocial effects of war on veterans are thought to vary according to past experience. A longitudinal study was designed to investigate the effects of World War II experiences on health by examining the well-being of veterans throughout life.

Methods.—The subjects were men from the Stanford-Terman archives. Data collection began in 1922, and four questionnaires were administered on family, education, and work before the war. The questionnaires were administered in 1922, 1928, 1936, and 1940. Questionnaires sent in 1945 and 1950 were mainly concerned with military experience. Survey data continued to be collected for 69 years. Of the 328 World War II veterans who were born before 1925, 236 were sent overseas, and 204 experienced combat. Life history records were reviewed to construct variables that described physical and emotional health. Efforts were made to depict combatants' war experiences and to examine these experiences in terms of a range of prewar characteristics.

Results.—No selective forces were found that determined which members of the Stanford-Terman cohort experienced combat. Approximately half the men entered the war as officers, and three fourths were officers by the end of the war. After the war, most had moved up in occupational status and were married at least once. War experiences, however, did have an impact on subsequent health. During the years between 1945 and 1960, significantly more of those who were sent overseas and those exposed to combat experienced a physical decline (n = 69) or death (n = 19). This finding did not vary according to the theater of engagement or military rank. A combatant's self-worth before the war did not moderate the risk of physical decline or death.

Discussion.—Men who were engaged in combat during World War II had significantly increased odds of experiencing physical decline or death between 1945 and 1960 (odds ratio = 2.85). The effects of combat were not altered by military rank, theater of engagement, or prewar level of self-worth. Suggested causes of physical decline after combat include an increased involvement in high-risk behaviors, feelings of helplessness, and adaptive mechanisms.

► This is an impressive and disturbing finding, one that has not been stressed much, as far as I'm aware. The ability of combat to affect physical decline and death is great, and research needs to be done to find the reasons for this and to ameliorate them.

J.A. Talbott, M.D.

Postdisaster Psychosocial Intervention: A Field Study of the Impact of Debriefing on Psychological Distress

Chemtob CM, Tomas S, Law W, et al (Univ of Hawaii, Manoa; Hôpital Henri Mondor, Crèteil, France)

Am J Psychiatry 154:415–417, 1997 7–55

Introduction.—Studies of debriefing as a postdisaster psychosocial intervention have yielded equivocal outcomes. Some authors report that debriefing is well accepted but has no differential impact on psychometric measures. Research completed after Hurricane Iniki, which struck the Hawaiian island of Kauai on September 11, 1992, sought to determine whether disaster-related psychological distress is reduced by debriefing.

Methods.—Two groups of residents who were exposed to the hurricane were debriefed at separate times. Group 1 was debriefed 6 months after the disaster. Before and approximately 90 days after the debriefing, participants completed the Impact of Event Scale. Group 2 was debriefed during the week when group 1 was retested and was then retested 90 days later. Twenty-five group 1 and 18 group 2 participants were available for follow-up. The debriefing intervention required about 5 hours, including 3 hours of group processing and 2 hours of lecture. Its aim was to provide ventilation of feelings, normalization of responses, and education about normal psychological reactions.

Results.—The Impact of Event Scale scores decreased from before to after treatment in both study groups, suggesting that debriefing contributed to a substantial reduction in hurricane-related distress. Neither the degree of property damage nor the participant's level of education significantly affected the treatment outcome. Some research participants were regular staff members of a local mental health center, and others had no previous experience in the mental health field; the treatment was effective for both clinicians and nonclinicians.

Discussion.—Debriefing is a psychosocial intervention, which can contribute to lowered levels of distress after a disaster. Despite the length of time that had passed since the hurricane, the experience was still quite vivid to study participants. This timing might be more effective than an immediate debriefing and allows for screening of continued distress.

► Debriefing is a common mechanism for dealing with mass casualties and civilian accidents. To date, however, such efforts have been based on logical and theoretical grounds. Now we have a controlled study supporting its efficacy.

J.A. Talbott, M.D.

Trauma Management Therapy: A Preliminary Evaluation of a Multicomponent Behavioral Treatment for Chronic Combat-related PTSD

Frueh BC, Turner SM, Beidel DC, et al (Ralph H Johnson Veterans Affairs Med Ctr, Charleston, SC; Univ of South Carolina, Charleston; Johns Hopkins Med Ctr, Baltimore, Md; et al)

Behav Res Ther 34:533–543, 1996 7–56

Introduction.—Trauma Management Therapy (TMT) is a new, comprehensive and multicomponent behavioral treatment for chronic combat-related post-traumatic stress disorder (PTSD). Modeled after an effective method for treating social phobia, TMT is designed to reduce the symptoms characteristic of PTSD and improve social and occupational adjustment. A sample of patients with chronic combat PTSD took part in an initial evaluation of TMT.

Methods.—Study participants, 15 male veterans of combat in Vietnam, met the *Diagnostic and Statistical Manual of Mental Disorders*, ed 3, revised criteria for PTSD. Excluded were veterans with a history of heart disease and those who met criteria for Axis I thought disorder or current substance abuse/dependence or for Axis II Antisocial Personality Disorder. Nine of the 15 who entered treatment were white; 6 were black. All had a concomitant Axis I disorder and 11 had a concomitant Axis II disorder. All underwent a comprehensive battery of measures before and after TMT. The TMT consisted of 29 treatment sessions administered over 17 weeks and using elements of intensive exposure therapy, programmed practice, and structured social and emotional skills training. Exposure was individualized to the specific features considered to be the primary basis of the fear. Other treatment components were social skills training, anger management, and veterans' issues management.

Results.—Four patients dropped out, leaving 11 for analysis. Both the Clinical Global Impressions severity-of-illness rating and the Hamilton Rating Scale for Anxiety showed significant improvement from pretreatment to posttreatment. In addition, patients reported a significant increase in total hours of sleep and number of social activities and a decrease in the frequency of nightmares. All felt they had achieved some degree of improvement, and 10 of 11 would encourage other veterans with PTSD to participate in TMT.

Discussion.—Initial findings in this small patient sample suggest that TMT is an effective treatment for combat-related PTSD. Most of the critical features of PTSD showed significant improvement over a relatively short period (4 months). Without follow-up, however, it is uncertain whether the treatment gains will persist.

► As promising as this study is, it suffers from so much else that appears in the literature—a lack of controls or comparison treatments, a very small sample size, and a high dropout rate. The positive element was that these patients had very chronic, persistent symptoms. Promising, but it's only a start.

J.A. Talbott, M.D.

Epidemiology, Morbidity, and Mortality

Long-term Morbidity Associated With Delayed Treatment of First Admission Schizophrenic Patients: A Re-analysis of the Camarillo State Hospital Data

Wyatt RJ, Green MF, Tuma AH (Natl Inst of Mental Health, Washington, DC; Western Los Angeles Veterans Affairs Med Ctr, Camarillo, Calif; Univ of Pittsburgh, Pa)

Psychol Med 27:261–268, 1997 7–57

Introduction.—Despite the prevailing attitude that schizophrenic patients can be greatly helped by antipsychotic medication, there may be a subgroup of schizophrenic patients who benefit more from no medication. To test this hypothesis, a comparison was made of schizophrenic patients treated with medication upon admission to a hospital and schizophrenic patients who were not treated with medication.

Methods.—A retrospective review was conducted of patients admitted to Camarillo State Hospital in the late 1950s and early 1960s. Random assignments were made of patients to be treated with or without antipsychotic drugs. For the 2 years after discharge, the number of rehospitalization days and total prescribed chlorpromazine equivalents were calculated. A comparison was made to other patients who matched criteria for schizophrenia for age, educational status at first admission, race, and gender to assess the patients' continuing ability to function. Across a period of 6–7 years after discharge, their Global Assessment of Functional Scale score was estimated.

Results.—Fewer rehospitalization days were required for patients initially treated with antipsychotic medications than for nonmedicated patients during the second year after discharge. Those patients initially treated with medication were functioning at a higher level, as measured by Global Assesment of Functional Scale scores at 6–7 years after initial discharge when compared to patients who were not initially treated with antipsychotic medications (Fig 1).

NO POSTAGE
NECESSARY
IF MAILED
IN THE
UNITED STATES

BUSINESS REPLY MAIL
FIRST-CLASS MAIL PERMIT NO 135 ST LOUIS MO

POSTAGE WILL BE PAID BY ADDRESSEE

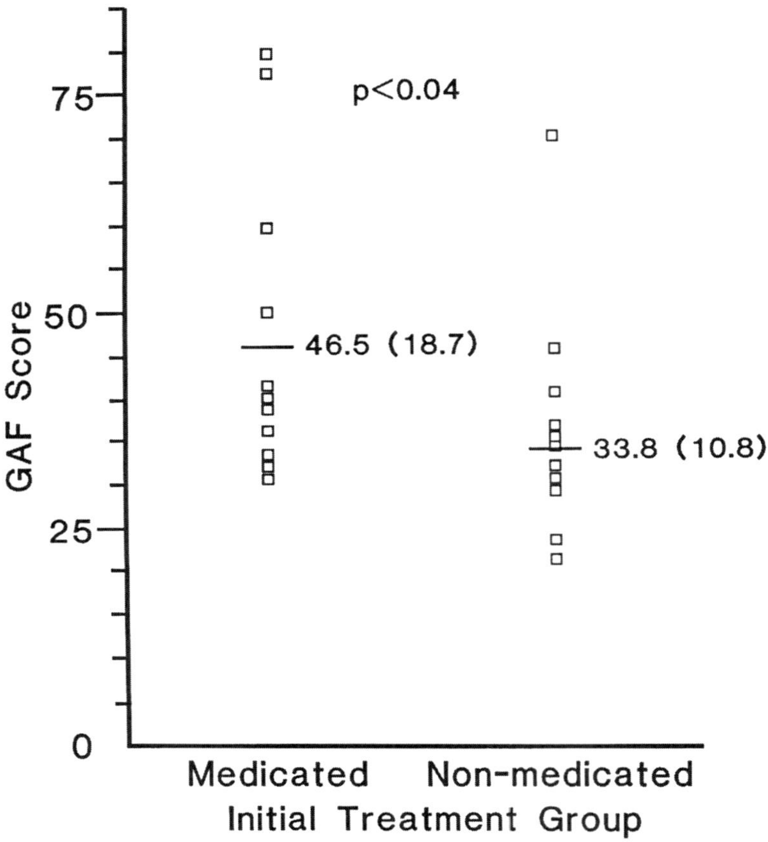

FIGURE 1.—Global Assessment of Functional Scale (GAF) scores 6–7 years after discharge for 11 initially medicated patients meeting DSM-IV criteria for schizophrenia, closely matched with 11 patients initially not treated with antipsychotic medications. Patients were matched for age, educational level at first admission, race, and gender. All patients were discharged from the hospital within 6 months of their first admission. Statistics: paired 2-tailed *t* test. (Reprinted with the permission of Cambridge University Press, from Wyatt RJ, Green MF, Tuma AH: Long-term morbidity associated with delayed treatment of first admission schizophrenic patients: A re-analysis of the Camarillo State Hospital data. *Psychol Med* 27:261–268, 1997. Reprinted with the permission of the Cambridge University Press.)

Conclusion.—The immediate morbidity associated with schizophrenia and detrimental changes possibly related to prolonged untreated psychosis are decreased by early treatment with antipsychotic medications for schizophrenic patients.

► This is powerful documentation of the necessity for very prompt recognition, intervention, and psychopharmacologic treatment of patients having their first break of schizophrenia. Perhaps I am wrong, but I think there is still some pessimism about the relentlessness of the course of schizophrenia, leading some to feel "so what" if the person is recognized and treated as soon as possible. To get at the recognition issue, we need more public education, such as that advocated by Mr. Jack Hinkley a few years ago.

J.A. Talbott, M.D.

Mortality and Medical Comorbidity Among Psychiatric Patients: A Review

Felker B, Yazel JJ, Short D (Univ of Washington, Seattle; Veterans Affairs Med Ctr, Salem, Va; Univ of Virginia, Charlottesville)

Psychiatric Serv 47:1356–1363, 1996 7–58

Background.—Mentally ill individuals have long comprised a disenfranchised minority with limited access to general medical care. Such individuals are at increased risk of death and medical co-morbidity. To advocate for improved health care for individuals with mental illness, the current literature on excess mortality and the underrecognition and undertreatment of co-morbid medical illnesses in this population were reviewed.

Methods and Findings.—Sixty-six studies published between 1934 and 1996 and a German paper from 1912 were reviewed. Standardized mortality ratios for psychiatric patients, derived from comparisons with the general population and matched control groups, repeatedly showed excess mortality from natural and unnatural causes. No single diagnostic group appears to be at particularly high risk. However, substance abuse disorders alone or combined with other psychiatric disorders have consistently been associated with increased mortality. Fifty percent of individuals with mental illness have known medical disorders, and 35% have undiagnosed medical conditions. One fifth have a medical problem that may cause or exacerbate their psychiatric conditions. Atypical presentations of medical illnesses are common. Changes in vision best predict the presence of medical illness. Elderly patients and those with organic brain syndromes are most likely to have co-morbid medical conditions.

Conclusions.—Individuals with mental illnesses have difficulty receiving adequate medical care. This has been attributed to the psychiatric disorder, to the patient, and most important, to deficiencies in physician assessment of such patients. Both political advocacy and the development of primary care programs that can efficiently meet the needs of mentally ill patients with medical problems are needed.

▶ The high rate of substance abuse–related deaths is not suprising; indeed, it is an intuitive finding. However, I do not recall seeing anyone argue for increased treatment of these disorders to reduce mortality. I wonder how much underfunding of treatment for both "mental" and "addictive" disorders is because of stigma, a perception that its sufferers are lost to the workforce anyway, or ignorance/indifference.

J.A. Talbott, M.D.

Long-term Mortality After First Psychiatric Admission

Naik PC, Davies S, Buckley AM, et al (Univ of Birmingham, Solihull, England; Towers Hosp, Leicester, England; Leicester Gen Hosp, England; et al)

Br J Psychiatry 170:43–46, 1997 7–59

Background.—The long-term mortality rate and causes of death after a first psychiatric admission are not well understood. The results of a 16-year follow-up of a cohort discharged from their first admission to 1 center between 1974 and 1975 were reported.

Methods and Findings.—Eighty-seven consecutive patients were traced in 1992 to their general practitioner or until they died. The causes of death were documented, and observed mortality was compared with that expected. Eight men and 4 women had died. None had committed suicide. In addition, none of the deaths were open verdicts or accidental. The causes of death included bronchopneumonia, cerebral thrombosis, cerebral hemorrhage, myocardial infarction, pulmonary embolus, carcinoma, Alzheimer's disease, and gastrointestinal bleeding from a peptic ulcer. Ages ranged from 41 to 64 years. The mortality rate was higher than that expected, but the excess was not significant (Fig 1).

Conclusion.—Targeting patients discharged from their first psychiatric admission for careful follow-up may not be useful for reducing suicide rates. More research on long-term mortality after first psychiatric admission is warranted before expensive interventions are planned.

► I am concerned that this study could (1) lull professionals into not taking monitoring and follow-up of persons making suicide attempts seriously

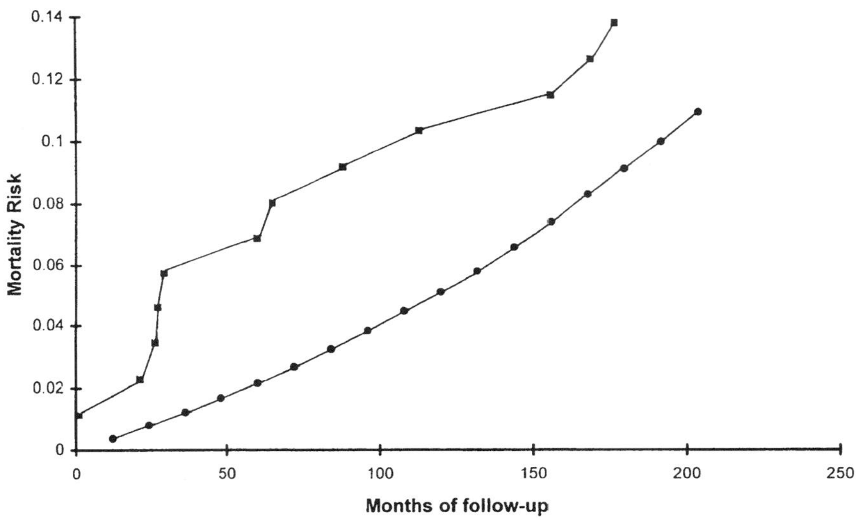

FIGURE 1.—Expected and observed cumulative mortality risk. *Circle* indicates expected; *square* indicates observed. (Courtesy of Naik PC, Davies S, Buckley AM, et al: Long-term mortality after first psychiatric admission. *Br J Psychiatry* 170:43–46, 1997.)

enough and (2) give policy makers more ammunition to reduce funds for community follow-up and care. Either would be disastrous. The figure, although demonstrating "statistically significant" results, surely shows a finding in the "wrong" direction.

J.A. Talbott, M.D.

Total Mortality in People Admitted to a Psychiatric Hospital

Hansen V, Arnesen E, Jacobsen BK (Univ of Tromsø, Norway)

Br J Psychiatry 170:186–190, 1997 7–60

Introduction.—In the old, hospital-based system of psychiatric care, mortality was higher for psychiatric patients than it was for the general population. It is uncertain if this remains true with the expansion of outpatient services in recent years. A study conducted at a psychiatric hospital in Norway sought to document the mortality of psychiatric patients within a system characterized by a low beds–population ratio.

Methods.—The hospital opened in 1961 with 500 beds. By 1980, the number of beds had been reduced by 50%, yielding a beds–population ratio of 4 per 10,000 inhabitants. The hospital admission register was checked for the period from August 1980 to December 1992. Linkage of the patients admitted during these years with the Norwegian Central Register of Persons revealed that 328 individuals had died. Data were used to calculate age-adjusted total mortality rates and standardized mortality ratios (SMRs) for psychiatric inpatients, compared with the general population.

Results.—Patients were divided according to gender and age. In all age-groups, men had the highest mortality rates, and mortality increased with age for both sexes. Compared with the mortality of the general population, however, the ratio of observed to expected deaths (O–E ratio) was highest in psychiatric patients aged 20 to 29 years. Above that age-group, the O–E ratios for women decreased faster than they did for men. Ninety-nine, or nearly one third (30%), of deaths in the study sample were the result of accident or suicide. Even after these 99 deaths were excluded, both sexes showed excess mortality, compared with the general population (SMR = 2.6 [men], SMR = 2.0 [women]). For both men and women, the mortality rates and SMRs were highest in the first year after a first-ever admission. Mortality was significantly higher for patients with a diagnosis of organic psychosis than it was for those in other diagnostic groups, even with adjustments for age, gender, and commitment (observation or treatment) status.

Conclusion.—There are fewer patients hospitalized today for psychiatric disorders than there were in the past, but mortality remains high in this population. Men are at particularly high risk and appear to die at rates similar to those reported 50 years ago. This finding is remarkable, given improvements in treatment, institutional standards, and living conditions in the society at large.

▶ I've included this article as a reminder that it is not just suicide for which the mentally ill are at increased risk. They are also at increased risk for severe medical illnesses.

J.A. Talbott, M.D.

Gender Differences in the Onset of Depression Following a Shared Life Event: A Study of Couples

Nazroo JY, Edwards AC, Brown GW (Royal Holloway Univ, London)
Psychol Med 27:9–19, 1997 7–61

Background.—Clinically relevant depressive disorders are known to be more prevalent among women than among men. Several explanations for this difference have been proposed. One is that this difference, which appears to be greatest during the childbearing years, may be the result of differences in social roles. This possible explanation was investigated.

Methods.—A community sample of 100 couples was studied. All had recently had at least one threatening life event that was potentially depressogenic for both partners. Interviews were conducted using a semistructured form. Depression onset was assessed using the Present State Examination. Data were collected to characterize each partner's actual role activity and commitment, rather than assuming that a gender difference in roles existed uniformly among all couples.

Findings.—Women had a greater risk of a depressive episode after the life event than did men. The magnitude of this difference was similar to that in previous reports of gender differences in depression. Women's increased risk was entirely limited to depressive episodes after events involving children, housing, or reproductive problems and was present only among couples with clear gender differences in associated roles. Role differences seemed to result in the women being more likely to take responsibility for such events and in the men distancing themselves from the events.

Conclusion.—Gender differences in the rates of depression in the general population appear to be largely attributable to the differences in women's and men's roles. Further research on this issue is warranted.

▶ For quite a while we have been aware of the difference in the rates of depression between men and women. The authors' idea that women's roles are connected to "caring" rings true as does the finding that men are more distant from family/home issues, which were the origin, in this study, of the threatening life events.

J.A. Talbott, M.D.

Lifetime Axis I and II Comorbidity and Childhood Trauma History in Dissociative Identity Disorder

Ellason JW, Ross CA, Fuchs DL (Richardson, Tex; Charter Health System of Dallas)

Psychiatry 59:255–266, 1996 7–62

Introduction.—Patients with dissociative identity disorder have 2 or more distinct identities or personality states that take control from time to time. This disorder has been likened to severe childhood trauma. No previous studies of the co-morbidity of dissociative identity disorder have used comprehensive structured interviews in a large clinical sample. To gain further insight into the effects of childhood trauma, Axis I and II co-morbidity was evaluated in patients with dissociative identity disorder.

Methods.—The study included 135 inpatients with a clinical diagnosis of dissociative identity disorder. Dissociation and childhood trauma were evaluated with the Dissociative Experiences Scale and the Dissociative Disorders Interview Schedule. The Structured Clinical Interview for Diagnostic and Statistical Manual of Mental Disorders, (ed. 3, revised) (SCID) was used to determine the lifetime prevalence of Axis I and II disorders.

Results.—Ninety-six percent of patients reported childhood physical or sexual abuse or both. Eighty-two percent of patients met the criteria for a severe mental disorder on the SCID. The modal diagnoses included major depression, posttraumatic stress disorder, panic disorder, obsessive-compulsive disorder, social phobia, simple phobia, and somatization disorder. Mood disorders were the most frequent type of co-morbidity. Anxiety, somatoform, and eating disorders were common as well. Borderline, avoidant, and self-defeating personality disorders were the most frequent co-morbid Axis II diagnoses. There was some overlap of schizotypal and borderline criteria.

Conclusions.—Patients with dissociative identity disorder meet the criteria for many other diagnoses as well. This co-morbidity should be borne in mind for treatment planning and outcomes research. Psychotic disorders diagnosed on the SCID in these patients may represent false positives, resulting from the inability of the available instruments to differentiate between psychosis and dissociation.

▶ I have included this article because it represents a diagnostic entity much in dispute these days. The article was written by 3 individuals who are in private practice or employed by the private hospital "chain" that funded the work; it was published in the journal *Psychiatry*, not known for publishing major epidemiologic research such as the ECA Study; it assumes that patients' memories of childhood abuse are accurate *without corroboration*; and it reaches the conclusion that dissociative disorders "may be more prevalent" than once believed. I think we need a bit more than this.

J.A. Talbott, M.D.

Suicide and Violence

Accuracy of 3 Brief Screening Questions for Detecting Partner Violence in the Emergency Department

Feldhaus KM, Koziol-McLain J, Amsbury HL, et al (Denver Health Med Ctr; Colorado Emergency Medicine Research Ctr; Univ of Colorado, Denver)

JAMA 277:1357–1361, 1997 7–63

Introduction.—For many women, partner violence is an important health risk. A recent national household survey showed that each year, 1 million women and about 150,000 men were victims of partner violence, and in any given year, up to 12% of women experience partner violence. It has been recommended that routine screening be conducted of all women seen in physicians' offices, emergency departments, and prenatal clinics. Physicians seldom detect partner violence in their patients because of time constraints and the lack of accurate, proven screening tools. A brief screening instrument was devised for use in the emergency department or other urgent care setting.

Methods.—There were 322 women included in the study, with a median age of 36 years. Of these, 54% were uninsured, 45% were white, 30% were Hispanic, and 19% were black. A partner violence screen was developed which had 3 questions regarding perceived personal safety and past physical violence. The questions were: "Have you been hit, kicked, punched, or otherwise hurt by someone within the past year? If so by whom?"; "Do you feel safe in your current relationship?"; and "Is there a partner from a previous relationship who is making you feel unsafe now?" This screen was compared with the Index of Spouse Abuse and the Conflict Tactics Scale.

Results.—There was a 29.5% prevalence rate of partner violence according to this partner violence screen. In comparison, the prevalence rate was 24.3% for the Index of Spouse Abuse and 27.4% for the Conflict Tactics Scale. The sensitivity in detecting partner abuse in the partner violence screen was 64.5% when compared with the Index of Spouse Abuse, and the specificity was 80.3%. The sensitivity of the partner violence screen was 71.4% when compared to the Conflict Tactics Scale, and the specificity was 84.4%. Negative predictive values ranged from 87.6% to 88.7%, and positive predictive values ranged from 51.3% to 63.4%. Acute episodes of partner violence were found in 13.7% of the visits.

Conclusion.—A history of physical or nonphysical partner violence was found in 1 of every 4 women using emergency departments within the previous year. Up to 71% of women with such a history can be detected with the partner violence screen. A large number of women who have a history of partner violence can be detected with 3 brief questions.

► This procedure is so simple that there must be a trick to it. Just ask 3 questions and you uncover 60% to 70% of the 27% of women (incredible!) presenting to an emergency service with a history of domestic violence!

Of course there is. The trick is, you have to care about uncovering the problem rather than focusing on the host of other problems and symptoms that patients present with, and you have to *ask*. But if you do both, there it is.

J.A. Talbott, M.D.

The Impact of Hospitalization on Clinical Assessments of Suicide Risk

McNiel DE, Binder RL (Univ of California, San Francisco)

Psychiatric Serv 48:204–208, 1997 7–64

Background.—Patients with major mental illness frequently need evaluation of their potential for suicide. There is little information regarding how these routine assessments are carried out in clinical practice, however. There have been no studies of factors associated with the potential for suicide at discharge vs. admission. Changes in evaluated suicide risk during psychiatric hospitalization were evaluated, including an assessment of demographic and clinical characteristics associated with higher risk estimates.

Methods.—The study included 241 patients hospitalized on a locked, short-term inpatient psychiatric unit. The patients' mean stay on the unit was 17 days. A total of 71 treating physicians assessed the patients' risk of self-harm at admission and again at discharge. The physicians also estimated the risk of self-harm in the short- and long-term, i.e., within the next week and within the next year. Symptoms at admission and discharge were rated using the Brief Psychiatric Rating Scale. Self-directed aggression during hospitalization was rated using the Overt Aggression Scale.

Results.—The physicians' mean estimates of short-term risk declined, from admission to discharge, from 42% to 21%. However, estimates of long-term risk showed a lesser change during hospitalization, from 40% to 29.5%. Factors associated with risk estimate at both admission and discharge included history of suicidal behavior and current symptoms, including depression, anxiety, and emotional withdrawal. Other factors associated with risk estimate at discharge included substance abuse, psychosocial stressors, and living alone.

Conclusion.—This study shows a reduction in patients' estimated short-term risk of self-harm during psychiatric hospitalization. There is no significant reduction in estimated long-term risk, however. Risk estimates at discharge are influenced by variables that do not change during hospitalization, such as psychosocial stressors, substance abuse history, and living alone. Further research is needed to find out how to improve valid predictors of self-harm in clinical assessments. Such studies would also be useful in establishing a prevailing standard of care for medicolegal purposes.

► To me, as a clinician, this is certainly an intuitive finding. Two studies must follow to really help us. First, we need to determine whether what we *believe* is true, i.e., Is hospital care better in the short run than in the long run? Second, what interventions in the community can make long-term survival better?

J.A. Talbott, M.D.

Media Violence, Gun Control, and Public Policy
Zuckerman DM (Washington, DC)
Am J Orthopsychiatry 66:378–389, 1996 7–65

Objective.—Violence is increasingly viewed as a public health problem as well as a social one. Studies consistently link violence in the media to violent behavior in childhood and adulthood. The availability of guns in the United States may be a major reason why media violence translates into violent behavior more here than in other countries. Media violence and gun control have been 2 key targets for policy makers. Current knowledge about media violence and gun control was reviewed, with an analysis of the implications for public policy.

Media Violence.—There is a long history of concern about the effects of violence on television. Laboratory studies, field studies, and natural experiments all suggest that violence on television leads to aggressive behavior in children and teenagers. The impact of other sources of exposure to violence, such as video games, remains to be determined. The United States lacks a clear policy on television, and little has been done to prevent or reduce television violence. One legislative proposal is the so-called "V-chip" or "C-chip," which would allow parents to block certain types of television programs. This approach relies heavily on the rating system with which it is used. However, it is unclear whether the children whose exposure to violence would be reduced by this approach are the ones who need protection most. In any case, the chips would be available on new television sets only.

Guns and Gun Control.—Guns are widely available in the United States, and most gun murders are committed by individuals known to the victim. Thus, the availability of a gun can quickly turn an argument into a homicide. Murders are more likely to occur in households with a history of violence. Most of the guns involved in homicide are handguns. The available evidence on the effectiveness of gun control is inconclusive. It seems that the only way to reduce access to guns is through national restrictions. Policy recommendations have included restrictions on gun ownership, reduced availability of guns or the most lethal types of guns, and increased information on gun injuries.

Implications.—There is growing support for the idea that reducing levels of violence requires a change in attitudes toward guns and violence. The C-chip has a good chance of becoming a reality, but it will take some time to have a substantial impact. Efforts should be made to increase prosocial messages on television. Video and other media should be used in well-designed school-based programs to change attitudes toward guns and violence. These efforts would only be enhanced by state or national laws to reduce the availability of guns. Research support for the effectiveness of gun control in reducing crime may help to marshal public support for reasonable gun control measures.

► There is precious little written in the literature about successful preventive programs. Considering the preoccupation of the American public and press with violence in our society, this article marshals much of the data and arguments for policy changes. Short of gun control, which seems ever less likely given our current Congressional makeup, and installation of "V-chips" in television sets, a much-touted panacea, though, I am concerned whether the public is convinced of the need to implement actual educational interventions based on controlled research.

J.A. Talbott, M.D.

Using Qualitative Data to Inform Public Policy: Evaluating "Choose to De-Fuse"

Levine IS, Zimmerman JD (Nathan Kline Inst for Psychiatric Research, Orangeburg, NY; New York City Health and Hosps Corp)

Am J Orthopsychiatry 66:363–377, 1996 7–66

Purpose.—A great deal of attention has focused on the problem of youth violence, including its causes and the need for preventive programs. However, there has been little research into the effectiveness of such programs. One such program, called "Choose to De-Fuse" was evaluated.

Methods.—The program was the "Youth Against Violence: Choose to De-Fuse," initiative of the New York City Department of Mental Health, Mental Retardation, and Alcoholism Services. The exploratory evaluative study, done at the request of the Department, was designed to refine the themes and messages of the campaign. The research design included focus groups with subsets of urban youth. Seventy-three youths at risk for violence participated, including 1 group of homeless youths with a history of being victims of violence. The focus groups were asked about their perspectives regarding youth violence; the program's public service announcements (PSAs); the campaign materials, that is, shirts and hats; the campaign slogan and theme; and measures to reduce youth violence.

Findings.—Violence was a pervasive influence in the participants' lives. They reported seeing it everywhere they went and believed that social institutions did little to protect them from it. They believed that youths acted violently to belong, to get attention, to feel protected, or to earn respect. In evaluating the PSAs, the youths preferred messages that were concrete rather than abstract and included familiar individuals, places, and events. Although they recognized the representations of violent scenarios depicted, they doubted their own power to defuse such situations in reality. The importance of clothes to self-esteem and perceived image in the at-risk group was confirmed. The youngsters liked the styles and colors of the campaign shirts and hats, and believed that seeing these items would remind them of the program's messages.

The participants found the "Choose to De-Fuse" theme a unifying one and were familiar with it from television PSAs and subway posters. They made several suggestions for improving and scheduling the PSAs for maximum impact. They suggested several interventions for violence prevention, including more positive portrayals of youths on television and school-based violence prevention programs. They emphasized the importance of early intervention with very young children, particularly the children of teenaged parents. They also said that interventions should be brought directly to the neighborhoods where violence occurs.

Discussion.—A city violence prevention program that was evaluated shows how researchers and policy makers can work together in an effort to prevent youth violence. Such evaluations can aid in finding ways of using television and other media to prevent youth violence.

▶ Here is a program that does attempt to reduce teen violence, but much more support, research, and alternative programs need to be provided.

J.A. Talbott, M.D.

Work and Rehabilitation

Quality of Life and Self-esteem in Working and Nonworking Persons With Mental Illness

van Dongen CJ (Univ of Wisconsin, Oshkosh)

Community Ment Health J 32:535–548, 1996 7–67

Background.—Work is important to mental health and may be particularly beneficial for those with severe mental illness. Patients with chronic mental illness generally have poor quality of life and self-esteem, which may be exacerbated by unemployment. Work may be associated with an improved quality of life, although the nature of this relation is unclear. Quality of life and self-esteem were compared in working and nonworking patients with severe mental illness. Factors affecting quality of life and self-esteem in these groups were evaluated as well.

Methods.—The study included 92 patients with severe and persistent mental illness. Fifty-one were workers, working at least 8 hr/week for at least 3 months, and 41 were nonworkers. They were assessed on the quality of life (QOL) interview, Rosenberg's Self-Esteem Inventory, and the Drug Attitude Inventory. A newly developed perception-of-work instrument was used as well. The 2 groups were compared for QOL and self-esteem. Also, relation between demographic characteristics, attitudes toward psychotropic medication, and perceptions of the meaning of work were assessed.

Results.—Self-esteem was significantly higher among the workers. Although there was no significant difference in overall QOL, the workers scored higher on all QOL subscales but 1. Demographic factors were unrelated to differences in self-esteem, QOL, or valuing of work. Also, working vs. nonworking status had no significant effect on attitudes toward psychotropic medications. Work was deemed more important by the workers, who found that working distracted them from their symptoms and helped improve their mental health. This was in contrast to the nonworkers' expressed fear that working would negatively affect their mental health.

Conclusions.—Individuals with severe mental illness who work appear to have better self-esteem and possibly better quality of life than those who do not work. Attitudes toward drug treatment are unrelated to quality of life or self-esteem and are no different for workers than for nonworkers. Whereas patients may fear that working will be detrimental to their mental health, it actually seems to promote better mental health. Positive work experience should be encouraged for individuals with severe and persistent mental illness.

► This is so intuitively obvious that you wonder why it has not been shown or published before. Although most of the positive effects were self-reported rather than objectively rated, knowing the power of a positive attitude to the ability of individuals with schizophrenia to manage, it is very heartening. Lower hospitalization rates should get insurers' attention!

J.A. Talbott, M.D.

Job Preferences of Clients With Severe Psychiatric Disorders Participating in Supported Employment Programs

Becker DR, Drake RE, Farabaugh A, et al (New Hampshire–Dartmouth Psychiatric Research Ctr, Concord; Dartmouth Med School, Hanover, NH; Indiana Univ–Purdue Univ at Indianapolis)

Psychiatric Serv 47:1223–1226, 1996 7–68

Introduction.—Job placement programs for patients with severe psychiatric disorders stress individualized placements, matched to the individual's strengths, weaknesses, and preferences. These patients may lack the experience needed to make work choices, so they often are helped to explore their job options in vocational training programs. In transitional employment programs, job slots often are designed without considering clients' specific preferences. Data on the job preferences of severely mentally ill adults were gathered.

Methods.—The study included 135 patients with severe mental disorders in 2 supported employment programs. The participants were followed up for 18 months. Every 6 months, they were asked about their job preferences, including job type, work hours, and wages. The realism of the job preferences and their stability over time were assessed. Job preferences and jobs were matched to see whether participants with jobs in their preferred areas were more satisfied and stayed on the job longer than other participants.

Results.—Eighty-one percent of the participants expressed 1 or more job preferences at baseline. The preferences were realistic, that is, in line with the types of jobs available in the program, and relatively stable over time. Twenty-five percent of the participants were working competitively at 6-month follow-up, and 64% of these were in jobs that matched 1 of their baseline preferences. These participants were more satisfied with their jobs and twice as likely to stay on the job as those who were not working in their preferred areas. New or changed preferences were more likely for participants who took part in a program emphasizing rapid job search, compared with those in a prevocational skills training program. Participants who got a competitive job were more likely to develop or change their preference.

Conclusions.—In supported employment programs for the mentally ill, matching the job to the client's job preferences increases job satisfaction and tenure. These individuals are more likely to develop explicit job preferences by actually looking for work or doing a job than by participating in a prevocational training program. Further studies should explore job preferences among various groups of individuals with psychiatric disabilities.

► This finding is obvious as well. However, if knowing what folks want and finding jobs they want will increase their satisfaction and tenure, it makes sense to do it.

J.A. Talbott, M.D.

Adding a Vocational Focus to Mental Health Rehabilitation

Blankertz L, Robinson S (Matrix Research Inst, Philadelphia)

Psychiatric Serv 47:1216–1222, 1996 7–69

Objective.—For patients with severe mental illness, the lack of vocational programs in community mental health centers is a substantial barrier to working. Attitudes toward or motivation to work is an important aspect of vocational rehabilitation. There are few data on developing the motivation to work. A community mental health center program was designed to increase work participation for clients with severe mental illness.

Methods.—One hundred twenty-two currently unemployed clients with severe mental illness were entered into the study. They were randomly assigned to experimental and control groups. Clients in the experimental group participated in a work-focused program conducted by 2 employment specialists. The specialists' sole function was to help them develop the skills and attitudes needed to enter the state vocational rehabilitation system or to look for work. The program included group and individual sessions and a trial work experience. Positive changes were rewarded. The control group received the usual services, with no specialized vocational services. After 9 months, the 2 groups were compared in terms of skills gained, changes in work attitudes, employment, and entry into the state vocational rehabilitation system.

Results.—Fifty-six percent of clients in the vocational services program showed positive changes in vocational status, such as a competitive job, participation in training and evaluation programs conducted by the state vocational system, and formal referral to the state program. In contrast, just 1 client in the control group entered a training program run by the state system. All clients in the program showed improvements in skills and work attitudes. On logistic regression analysis, positive outcomes were predicted by participating in the program, rather than by client characteristics.

Conclusions.—A targeted vocational program in a community mental health center can be a valuable aid to rehabilitation for clients with severe mental illness. Within a few months, this type of program can help clients to develop the skills and attitudes they need to get a job or enter the vocational rehabilitation system. Group participation and a system of rewards seem to play an important role in the success of such a program.

► This is another obvious conclusion, but one that should make the investment worthwhile. If only insurers valued work or return to work highly enough to fund these additional staff.

J.A. Talbott, M.D.

Rediscovering General Psychiatry: Creation of an Academic Division

Goldbloom DS, Buckingham RA, Voore P (Clarke Inst of Psychiatry, Toronto; Univ of Toronto)

Can J Psychiatry 42:58–62, 1997 7–70

Introduction.—There is an ongoing debate over the role of the general psychiatrist in an era of subspecialization. General psychiatry should emphasize multidisciplinary teamwork, management of cases that cross the line between medicine and psychiatry, service to the severely mentally ill, and the role and delivery of psychotherapy. In response to internal and external stimuli, and in keeping with developments in medicine and surgery, a university department of psychiatry recently formed a division of general psychiatry. The development and initial experience of this division are reviewed.

Experience.—The 2 main factors leading to the development of a division of general psychiatry were the trend toward increasing subspecialization and the public need for specific psychiatric services. In addition, research suggested that the general psychiatrist had become mainly a psychotherapist, with a lack of balance between the roles of direct patient care provider and consultant. The program sought to enhance the core of PGY2 training in general hospital psychiatry, in keeping with the stated expectations of the Royal College of Physicians and Surgeons of Canada. Other objectives included the creation of "career-track" and postresidency fellowship positions in general psychiatry; the provision of community-based experiences for residents, including work in underserved areas; and the creation of an academic role for the generalist psychiatrist.

In just 2 academic years, several important changes have occurred. The program has developed PGY2 training guidelines for general psychiatry, including specific knowledge, skill, and attitudinal objectives. Experiences have included increased training in emergency psychiatry and substance abuse and participation in an outreach program. Senior residents have filled career-track positions in general psychiatry at 4 teaching hospitals. These positions include teaching of junior residents and medical students, increased autonomy, and greater community involvement. The general psychiatry faculty have played major roles in education and educational scholarship, and lesser contributions to research. Important developments in undergraduate education have included promotion of the observed structured clinical examination format of student evaluation and provision of experiences for medical students.

Conclusions.—The success of the newly developed university division of general psychiatry must be evaluated by the academic and clinical careers of trainees, the first of whom completed their residency in 1997. The academic focus for general psychiatry remains to be seen; however, as in general medicine, the emphasis is likely to be on clinical epidemiology, ethics, and education.

▶ When residents ask me whether or not to subspecialize, I have a set answer. It is that they should not be just like every other psychiatrist but that they should have a special interest, which may include a specialty. However, I caution them against over-subspecialization. We never know where we'll wind up in life, and I think it is a grave mistake to limit one's experience so that you're not able to practice plain old general "psychiatry" if called upon to do so, regardless of your training.

J.A. Talbott, M.D.

Social Distance Towards the Mentally Ill: Results of Representative Surveys in the Federal Republic of Germany

Angermeyer MC, Matschinger H (Univ of Leipzig, Germany)

Psychol Med 27:131–141, 1997 7–71

Introduction.—In the mid-1970s in the old Federal Republic of Germany, psychiatric care was in a very poor state. Among the many reforms suggested at that time were steps to better integrate the mentally ill into society and to reduce existing prejudices against the mentally ill. Little is known about the public's attitudes toward the mentally ill now, 20 years after the first reforms were proposed. Integrating the mentally ill into society should bring people into closer contact with them, thus providing the chance to correct existing prejudices. Current public attitudes toward

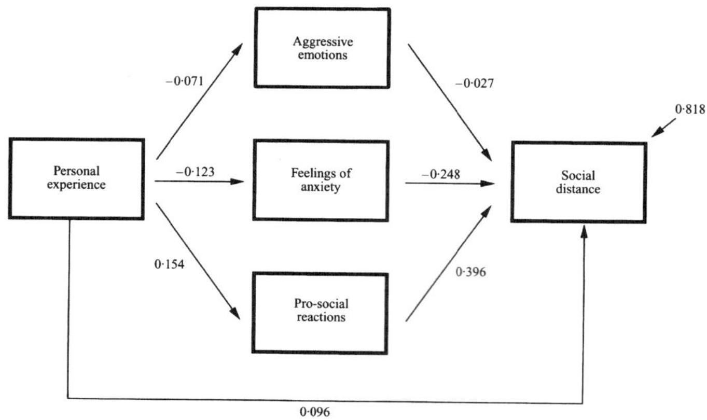

FIGURE 1.—Influence of personal experience with mental illness on social distance toward individuals with schizophrenia. (Courtesy of Angermeyer MC, Matschinger H: Social distance towards the mentally ill: Results of representative surveys in the Federal Republic of Germany. *Psychol Med* 27:131–141, 1997. Reprinted with permission of Cambridge University Press.)

the mentally ill in Germany were studied, with a focus on the concept of social distance.

Methods.—A total of 11 representative surveys regarding attitudes toward the mentally ill were performed in Germany during the early 1990s. Eight of these surveys were performed in areas formerly in the Federal Republic of Germany. The study included measures of social distance, emotional reactions toward the mentally ill, personal experience with the mentally ill, and personal values.

Results.—The public showed high levels of rejection toward the mentally ill. The amount of social distance desired increased with the degree of intimacy implied by the suggested relationship—for example, patients

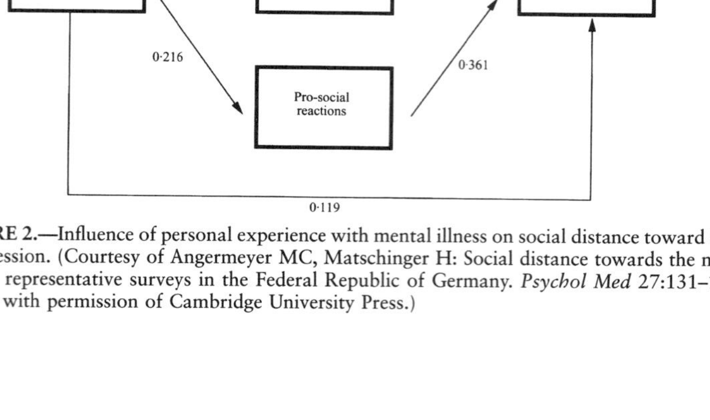

FIGURE 2.—Influence of personal experience with mental illness on social distance toward individuals with depression. (Courtesy of Angermeyer MC, Matschinger H: Social distance towards the mentally ill: Results of representative surveys in the Federal Republic of Germany. *Psychol Med* 27:131–141, 1997. Reprinted with permission of Cambridge University Press.)

might be accepted as neighbors or coworkers but would not be accepted into the respondents' circle of friends. The type of disorder had a strong effect on the extent of social distance. Rejection was greatest for patients dependent on alcohol, even more so than for those with schizophrenia (Fig 1). Rejection was least for patients with major depression or panic disorder with agoraphobia (Fig 2). Respondents who had personal experience with mental illness expressed less of a need for social distance; this may be attributed to increased positive emotional reactions and reduced anxiety toward the mentally ill. People who endorsed more "liberal" or "modern" values tended to express greater acceptance of the mentally ill.

Conclusion.—The German public continues to show a great deal of social distance toward the mentally ill. The results suggest that personal contact with the mentally ill may help to reduce feelings of resentment and prejudice against this minority group. Public attitudes toward the mentally ill vary among the different disorders. Alcoholics are met with the greatest level of rejection, followed by schizophrenia, and then the depressed.

► We know that in the United States, although the problem of stigma of the mentally ill has been getting better since World War II, we are still a long way from its elimination. Many have argued that deinstitutionalization has worsened the situation by exposing citizens to the most visibly disturbed, drug-abusing and homeless of those deinstitutionalized. However, the German groups' finding of the difference between keeping greatest distance from those with alcohol abuse, than those suffering from schizophrenia, and least from those suffering from depression, demonstrates a sophistication on the part of the public that I did not expect.

J.A. Talbott, M.D.

Issues in the Treatment of Lesbian Women and Gay Men With Chronic Mental Illness

Hellman RE (South Beach Psychiatric Ctr, Brooklyn, NY)
Psychiatric Serv 47:1093–1098, 1996 7–72

Purpose.—Some patients with chronic mental illness are gay or lesbian. Affirmative models of psychosocial rehabilitation for individuals with lesbian or gay sexual orientation have not been widely disseminated into care for those with chronic mental illness. A clinical context for inpatient and outpatient treatment of chronic mental illness in gay men and lesbian women was described.

Mental Illness in Lesbians and Gays.—There are up to 500,000 gay men and lesbian women with severe psychiatric disorders in the U.S. population. The issues facing homosexuals as a social minority are relevant to their clinical assessment but are frequently ignored. Lesbians and gays with mental illness face dual stigmata, which poses difficult developmental issues. Many will have their first episode of psychiatric decompensation in adolescence, during their "coming-out" process—this may further reinforce their already marginalized identity. In treatment, patients may suppress their sexual identity so as to preserve some sense of belonging. Given their experience with heterosexism and homophobia, these patients may enter treatment with guarded expectations. They are alienated from the gay community because of their psychiatric disability, and so they lack even that alternative for development. As individuals with chronic mental disease, they are dependent on families and psychiatric settings. Their inability to become individuated from a heterosexist and homophobic environment makes them all the more dependent on the role models around them

Treatment.—Affirmative treatment models provide the conceptual framework for mental health treatment of lesbians and gays. Although sexual orientation is not a central issue during inpatient assessment, it may be important for clients who have attempted suicide, are victims of physical or emotional abuse, or are in a drug abuse crisis. Hospitalization can provide the foundation for affirmative psychosocial growth. The clinician should assess the patient's sexual identity, although the patient may be reluctant to provide information. Patients should be assured that disclosure facilitates the treatment process. The staff must follow a supportive approach to ensure that hospitalization permits personal healing rather than reinforcing the social isolation and stigma of homosexuality.

The issue of disclosure is a central one for gay and lesbian patients in partial hospitalization settings. These patients should be helped to feel that disclosure is safe and acceptable in the therapeutic environment. A lesbian and gay support group can permit clients to share their concerns and experiences. For some, it may be the first time that they are able to be open with others. Higher-functioning patients in the outpatient setting may be able to take part in community-based support groups. However, the dual stigma faced by these patients suggests the need for special focus groups. Efforts are needed to improve acceptance of the mentally ill within the lesbian and gay community.

Discussion.—There are several issues involved in the clinical management of mental illness in gay men and lesbian women. The information provides a framework for affirmative inclusion of these patients in treatment programs for chronic mental illness. Although more research is needed to define the challenges faced by these clients, services must be established without waiting for study results.

▶ This article deals with a little-discussed but common issue. I have included it because as mental health systems take responsibility for diverse patient populations, "cultural competence" is needed to deal with all those enrolled, including those who are gay or lesbian. This is a good starting point to a better understanding of their particular issues.

J.A. Talbott, M.D.

Homesickness: A Review of the Literature

van Tilburg MAL, Vingherhoets AJJM, van Heck GL (Univ of Tilburg, The Netherlands)

Psychol Med 26:899–912, 1996 7–73

Introduction.—Those who have left their house and home to find themselves in a new and unfamiliar environment may experience homesickness, represented by an intense longing for home followed by depression, distress, and even negative health effects, such as deficiencies in the immune system, diabetes mellitus, and leukemia. Among refugees, homesickness can interfere with their integration into a new society. A review of recent psychological literature on homesickness, along with its symptoms and interventions, was conducted. One conceptual analysis shows that homesickness happens to all age groups, that it is frequently not acknowledged or experienced with embarrassment or denial, that it reflects a feeling of sadness about the place left. Behavior characteristics are apathy, lack of initiative, little interest in new environment, listlessness, fighting frequently, and not wanting to eat.

Models.—In 1 study of boarding-school students, it was found that up to 70% experienced homesickness and that up to 75% of the population has had at least 1 homesickness experience. There are 5 explanations for the distressing effects of leaving home, according to 1 study: loss, where the individual is separated from family, friends, and acquaintances; interruption of lifestyle, where a routine is discontinued; reduced control, where there is less control over the environment; role change and self-consciousness, because new tasks have to be fulfilled; and conflict, because the individual is torn between approach and avoidance tendencies toward the new environment. There is conflict between wishing to acquire new experiences and returning home. Generally, homesickness is more common among children than adults.

Interventions.—Real relief often is provided by returning home; however, other strategies also have been proposed. Stress management therapy is directed at expressing feelings and forming a commitment to the new environment. Telephone calls to parents for children were found to be effective. Exploring other problems and support in resolving them may reduce the need to cling to the old environment. Relief is provided by thought-stopping and time-outs for worry. Acceptance of homesickness feelings is necessary. Physical activities can take one's mind off the stress, whereas reading and other mental activities do not compete as well. Learning new social skills to attract more social support will help.

Conclusions.—Homesickness is a psychological state accompanied by specific emotional, behavioral, cognitive, and physical reactions. There are associations between homesickness and rigidity, lack of self-confidence, and neuroticism. A conceptual analysis of homesickness should be developed, and further research is needed on the association between homesickness and separation anxiety, adjustment disorder, nostalgia, and agoraphobia.

▶ Homesickness is a bit like the common cold—so ubiquitous we may trivialize its impact. Certainly, as the authors posit, we need more research. But it seems to me we already know what interventions can help its resolution, e.g., increased social supports, acceptant ventilation, new activities, etc.

J.A. Talbott, M.D.

Factors Affecting Medical Students' Selection of Canadian Psychiatric Residency Programs: Part I. A Comparison With American Peers

Leverette J, Massabki A, Peterson H (Queen's Univ, Kingston, Ont, Canada)

Can J Psychiatry 41:578–581, 1996 7–74

Objective.—The 13 English-speaking departments of psychiatry in Canada recently formed an intern matching service to match medical students to postgraduate year-1 positions in psychiatry. This provided a readily identifiable cohort in which to evaluate the choice of a particular training program. Factors affecting Canadian students' selection of a specific postgraduate psychiatry program were evaluated, including a comparison with factors identified in American studies.

Methods.—The study included 110 psychiatry trainees who started their training in the first year of the Canadian matching program. The trainees were sent a questionnaire regarding factors that affected their choice of a particular training program. The response rate was 60%.

Findings.—For the Canadian trainees, as in previous studies of American trainees, nonprogrammatic factors played an important role in program choice. The geographic location of the program was the most significant factor. Unlike their American counterparts, the Canadian trainees

TABLE 1.—A Comparison of Ranked Importance Factors in Program Choice Between Canadian and American Students

Factor	Canadian (1994)	American (1981)
Most important	• Geographic location	• Geographic location
	• Practice opportunities after training	• Clinical training available
	• Opportunities for clinical training	• Impression of faculty
	• Reputation of the program	• Intuitive feeling for program
Least important	• Linguistic and/or cultural issues	• Job opportunities after training
	• Government attitude to health care reform and Government attitude to psychiatric practice	• Research training
	• Licencing in province chosen for training	• Advice from mentor
	• Small number of residents in program and Education/job opportunities for partner	• Size of program

(Courtesy of Leverette J, Massabki A, Peterson H: Factors affecting medical students' selection of Canadian psychiatric residency programs: Part 1. A comparison with American peers. *Can J Psychiatry* 41:578–581, 1996.)

tended to emphasize the importance of job prospects after residency. The Canadian trainees attached more weight to the program's perceived reputation (Table 1).

Conclusion.—In deciding which psychiatric residency program to choose, students often attached great importance to nonprogrammatic factors. Many of the more important factors are not under the control of the training program. The choice may be geared more toward future employment opportunities during hard economic times.

► In both countries, the size of the residency program is unimportant but geography is. However, after that, there are no similarities. The fact that Americans go on their gut feelings, whereas Canadians rely more on a program's reputation perhaps fits the cultural stereotypes of both nations and, I guess, should tip us off as to how to pitch our interview days.

J.A. Talbott, M.D.

Family Members' Ratings of the Use and Value of Mental Health Services: Results of a National NAMI Survey

Hatfield AB, Gearon JS, Coursey RD (Univ of Maryland, College Park and Baltimore)

Psychiatric Serv 47:825–831, 1996 7–75

Objective.—Data collected in a 1993 survey of a large sample of families belonging to the National Alliance for the Mentally Ill (NAMI) were compared with findings of a 1976 NAMI survey to examine changes in service use as reported by the respondents' mentally ill relatives and the families' rating of service value. Studies published in the 1980s found significant discrepancies between families and providers in their perceptions of the adequacy of services for the mentally ill.

Methods.—The 1993 survey, distributed to all 1,008 local groups of NAMI, yielded a total of 3,099 responses from families in 50 states. The survey instrument was that used in the 1976 questionnaire, with some added questions. In the part of the survey reported here, families were asked to rate the value of 11 types of services that their relative might have used in the past 2 years. Responses were compared for the 2 surveys.

Results.—Compared with the general population, NAMI members have a higher educational level, a higher-than-average income, and a lower proportion of racial and ethnic minorities. Respondents had a mean age of 60 years; 83% were women. More than two thirds (68%) of the ill relatives were men, and their mean age was 36 years; most (83%) were adult children of the NAMI respondents. Common diagnoses were schizophrenia (57%) and bipolar disorder (21%). The most frequently used service was medication, followed by individual therapy, hospitalization, and case management. Families placed the highest value on medication (97%), hospitalization (90%), individual therapy (88%), case management (85%), residential care (82%), and crisis services (81%). Overall, community services were less valued than office-based services and medications. Those responding to the 1976 survey reported less use of medication and residential services, but more of hospitalization and of individual, group, and family therapies. All services were valued more highly in 1993 than in 1976.

Conclusions.—In contrast to expectations, services considered essential to the community service model—namely residential care, psychosocial rehabilitation, and crisis care—were used by only about one third of NAMI members' relatives and were rated moderately low in value. Hospital and office-based services received higher ratings. Services should be designed to accommodate the considerable diversity of needs among individuals with mental illness.

► There are some findings here that I and the authors found disturbing. The low value given community-based services, such as residential care, psychosocial rehabilitation, and critical care, things we have advocated for and moved toward for 25 years, coupled with the continuing high value of hospital and individual therapeutic elements, is most jarring. Maybe, as the authors suggest, this is because of the unavailability of good community services; I think it is more than that. I think the research, experience, training, and values that have been proven have neither reached the profession nor the public yet. After that, we would hope families and patients would join us.

J.A. Talbott, M.D.

8 Clinical Psychiatry

Introduction

As has become my tradition in the last few years, I have organized the contributions for this year from the most common psychiatric problems to the least. Therefore, I have begun with depression, anxiety, and substance abuse and moved to some of the less common conditions we treat, such as dissociative identity disorder and body dysmorphic disorder. In the second section, I have picked articles which return to some of the old themes in psychiatry with new evidence, and then I have selected a handful of articles in which new technology available to us is truly changing some of our ideas about the etiology, pathophysiology, and even treatments of our disorders. In the third section, I again close the year's review with a series of articles about our evolving interface with our primary care colleagues and other general physicians. As is the case each year, the amount of clinical psychiatric knowledge continues to explode, and therefore the task of choosing just some of the articles covering all of clinical psychiatry was a difficult one. I could have easily chosen three times the amount with no dropoff in quality or interest in the articles.

The first section contains articles in the area of depression, beginning with ones discussing more atypical and subsyndromal chronic depressions and their treatments. The next section of articles I have grouped together because they represent to me advances in our knowledge that we have needed as clinicians, including the first article to provide good information about the differences in depression in whites and blacks. The next group provides answers to a series of questions that we have sought, including the relative efficacy of tricyclics vs. selective serotonin reuptake inhibitors in melancholic depression, relapse after discontinuation, and a demonstration that antidepressants do, in fact, reduce suicide risk. These are followed by articles about new aspects of treatment for depression including complex phase advance sleep treatments and the P450 systems. The section closes with two interesting articles nailing down the observation that many people become seriously depressed after stopping smoking.

The next group of articles have to do with the anxiety disorders. They are significantly fewer this year, and I don't know what this represents. Many of us in the field have felt that there has been a plateauing of the growth of knowledge in the anxiety disorders field after an explosion over the last decade. In fact, I have only chosen five articles in this section this year, and all on panic disorder, which I admit may reflect my longstanding interest in this disorder. They begin with an article from Germany which adds to the growing amount of evidence that panic disorder is, in fact, a severe illness routinely complicated by co-morbidities with depression and other syndromes. This is followed by a review article by Barlow and colleagues reviewing the psychosocial treatments of panic disorder, an excellent review. The final two articles concern the efficacy of alprazolam in interfering with cortisol abnormalities in panic which may have important implications. The section ends with a review of cocaine-induced panic, unfortunately, a growing clinical problem.

The two articles I have chosen in the field of alcoholism have to do with the interaction of alcoholism and other issues that are important in our field, suicide and depression, and document how critical co-morbid alcoholism is to the outcome of depressed individuals.

The next section is a series of articles concerning schizophrenia. Although schizophrenia may be our most important condition, given the striking disability and health care costs associated with this illness, it is less common than the previous three. The first is a remarkable international 13-year study that provides a modern perspective on the prognosis for schizophrenia and turns some previous findings on their ears. Fortunately, they observed a more positive prognostic outlook for the person with this illness in modern times. The second study follows up on that with an important United States study of various aspects of maintenance treatment of schizophrenia. The last article in this section explores an increasingly prominent clinical issue of the occurrence of obsessive-compulsive disorder in patients with schizophrenia, truly a puzzling co-occurrence.

The next section combines a few articles away from the center of clinical psychiatry. The first two concern eating disorders, with the first taking advantage of scientific advances to further understand the serotonin abnormalities in anorexia nervosa. The second utilizes computers as part of the education of eating-disorder patients with good results. The remaining articles review areas of growing importance in psychiatry: adults with attention deficit hyperactivity disorder, the two-year outcome of inpatients with dissociative identity disorder, body dysmorphic disorder, and premenstrual dysphoric disorder, all of which are worth reading.

You can't pick up a newspaper or magazine without wrestling with the aging of our population. I have chosen just two articles concerning areas where problems of the elderly population are significantly impacting medicine, one concerning elderly home care and the second geriatric patients in primary care.

As promised, in the next section we revisit old theories in three articles. The first concerns a provocative animal model which may explain how early loss can lead to not only psychological but physiologic symptoms. If you have been a regular reader of this section, you know I believe it is of paramount importance for those in psychiatry to convey effectively our importance to our primary care and generalist colleagues. The second article provides an elegant theoretical basis of how our work connects to the somatic symptoms of our patients. This second article revisits the issues of sexual abuse in childhood, documenting the profound psychological and physical sequelae of these early wounds. In my opinion, this is one of the most important and rapidly growing areas in our field. In some ways, it returns us to the horrible secrets that Freud heard from his patients but did not believe. Perhaps it was not true in Victorian Vienna, but as many as 20% of women in modern U.S. times suffer these assaults. This section ends with an article that provides evidence of the kindling and sensitization phenomena in humans. This is a theory that has intrigued some of us for the last two decades and although provocative, evidence in humans has been slow in evolving. This is among the first.

The next section is a fascinating group of papers centering around new techniques which are telling us new things about clinical psychiatry, from etiology to pathophysiology to treatment. The first is a study of normals that made the front page of the *New York Times* because it demonstrated changes in simulated sadness and marked difference in the brain response to sadness and happiness in men and women. Despite the appeal of that to some, the real importance of this work will be illustrated as these techniques further illuminate the anatomy of depression and other psychiatric disorders and phenomena. The second reviews how MRIs may assist us in changing our diagnostic schema in psychiatry. Having tests which illustrate pathophysiology has been hard for us to reach in reality, but this article and others in this section illustrate how rapidly we are moving towards this end. For instance, the next article illustrates abnormalities in the prefrontal sulcus in depressed patients, and the next utilizes MRI evidence to show that the brain insult in schizophrenia occurred early in an individual's life. The next two use positron emission tomography scanning to provide evidence of an abnormal prefrontal thalamic cerebellar circuit in schizophrenia, and the next two provide evidence of increased dopamine receptors in schizophrenia as has been predicted by so many lines of evidence. The last two articles in this section illustrate how new techniques have improved our treatment capabilities. The first utilizes MRI imaging to guide in a more precise way stereotactic neurosurgery in obsessive-compulsive disorder. The last utilizes telemedicine to assess patients with schizophrenia in isolated areas and illustrates how reliable and acceptable this method is.

Few of us have applauded the changes managed care has brought to psychiatry, and the three articles in this section do not either. The first outlines that although physical and mental health outcomes were not different in fee-for-services systems versus HMOs, the physical health of elderly patients suffered in the HMO system. The next two articles deal with some of the issues that have been so important to psychiatry and concern the appropriate role of psychotherapy in a managed care system. They make a plea for seeking scientific evidence on which to base policies and present some of the arguments for and against the use of psychotherapy in psychiatry.

In articles more directly related to the primary care side of this issue, I have chosen a series that I hope will be educational. The first two have to do with the general issues of somatic symptoms rather than psychological symptoms, which is a serious problem for primary care physicians. The next articles review the development of screening instruments to detect psychiatric problems in primary care, an important step in beginning to tackle the huge set of issues presented by the 25% to 75% of patients in primary care who have generally unrecognized psychiatric problems. There is one article about how the general approach might help with some of the most bedeviling of patients—those with the so-called chronic fatigue syndrome. The section then goes on to review how patients treated for depression and anxiety fare in primary care, how lasting are the effects of intervention, and finally, how are interventions affect the high use of patient care services. The first has to do with depression and is more straightforward, and provides clear evidence that overutilization would be reduced with the proper treatment of depression. The last article in this section is one that has not been dealt with sufficiently, and that is the borderline personality disorder patient and health care utilization.

The next set of articles has to do with a set of observations of how psychiatric phenomena can affect a physical system, primarily the cardiovascular system. The first suggests that the long-term risks that we are observing in anxious individuals may be mediated through hypertension, and then others about the effects of mental stress, anger, and worry on the development of coronary artery disease. The last article in this group documents that despite how logical it would appear that we become more involved in the rehabilitation of coronary artery disease patients, it has to be done carefully. They illustrate that none of the psychosocial interventions had a positive effect.

In the continuing theme of how we might be helpful to our generalist colleagues, there are two articles about the relationship of psychiatric conditions and irritable bowel syndrome (IBS) and how IBS creates many difficulties for patients with it. The next article clearly documents that we can be helpful in the treatment of renal dialysis patients in that depression causes a primary interference in their quality of life. I close this section with how we can be of help in important ways to our generalist colleagues with the ultimate outcome measure—death. Dwight Evans and his group have demonstrated the first evidence that severe life event stress actually leads to earlier HIV disease progression and therefore death. Like the studies that David Spiegel[1] from Stanford provided in which group therapy elongated the life of breast cancer patients, this work should encourage our working with these and other patients in the primary care and general medicine settings.

I hope you enjoy the set of articles I have chosen this year. I did.

James C. Ballenger, M.D.

Reference

1. Spiegel D, Bloom JR, Kraemer HC, et al: Effect of psychosocial treatment on survival of patients with metastatic breast cancer. *Lancet* 2:888–891, 1989.

Depression

The Validity of Atypical Depression in DSM-IV

Lam RW, Stewart JN (Univ of British Columbia, Vancouver, Canada; Vancouver Hosp, and Health Sciences Centre, Canada)

Compr Psychiatry 37:375–383, 1996 8–1

Background.—Atypical depression has been defined in different ways over the past 4 decades. Specific manifestations of the illness were described in the 1940s through the 1970s, whereas *Diagnostic and Statistical Manual of Mental Disorders* (DSM), edition III defined atypical depression only as a depression that did not meet formal criteria for any depressive diagnostic category. All references to atypical depression were dropped in DSM-III, revised. In DSM-IV, atypical depression is included as a mood reactive depression with associated reverse vegetative symptoms or marked interpersonal rejection sensitivity. Using operational criteria for the validation of clinical syndromes, the authors of this study reviewed evidence for the clinical validity of atypical depression.

Methods.—A MEDLINE search was conducted for all English language articles published from 1969 through March 1966 having the words "atypical" and "depression" in the title or abstract. The references of these articles were reviewed for other relevant citations. Articles selected for analysis contained primary data-driven research, a definition of atypical depression that included depression and not anxiety alone, and data relevant to the validation of atypical depression (using Kendall's 6 criteria for establishing clinical validity).

Results.—Despite the relatively large number of studies that define clinical symptoms of atypical depression, interrelationships among the definitions are low. Few studies have examined clinical differences between atypical depression and other depressive subtypes, and little information is available on the prevalence of atypical depression in general or clinical populations. Also poorly defined is the course of atypical depression; studies of index episode duration have conflicting and inconsistent results. The criteria of clinical description and differential treatment response, however, provide supporting data for the diagnostic validity of atypical depression. Patients with this diagnosis have had a superior response to monoamine oxidase (MAO) inhibitors compared with tricyclic antidepressants. The few studies of newer antidepressant medications for atypical depression suggest that the disorder may respond better to selective MAO inhibitors. Only very limited data are available on family history or the genetics of atypical depression. Preliminary findings indicate that atypical depressives may have shortened rapid eye movement latency.

Discussion.—Current evidence supports the usefulness of atypical depression as a diagnostic concept, particularly for predicting differential drug response. Only marginal support, however, now exists for the establishment of atypical depression as a valid clinical syndrome.

▶ This article usefully reviews the issues surrrounding atypical depression and provides support for the validity and importance of this diagnosis. The authors also report the greater response of these patients to MAO inhibitors compared with other antidepressants, particularly the tricyclics.

J.C. Ballenger, M.D.

Socioeconomic Burden of Subsyndromal Depressive Symptoms and Major Depression in a Sample of the General Population

Judd LL, Paulus MP, Wells KB, et al (Univ of California, San Diego; San Diego VA Med Ctr, Calif; Univ of California, Los Angeles; et al)

Am J Psychiatry 153:1411–1417, 1996 8–2

Background.—Studies have shown that individuals with subthreshold depression have a higher rate of disability, workdays lost, greater use of mental health services, poor self-rated emotional health, and more lifetime suicide attempts than those without such depression. The association between impairment in daily living, subthreshold depressive symptoms, and major depression was evaluated.

Methods.—Using data from the National Institute of Mental Health Epidemiologic Catchment Area Program, 2,393 subjects from the Los Angeles Epidemiologic Catchment Area Site were divided into 3 groups: those with subsyndromal depressive symptoms, major depression, and no depression. Ten domains of functional outcome and well-being were evaluated among these groups.

Results.—High levels of household strain, social irritability, financial strain, limitations in physical or job functioning, restricted activity days, bed days, and poor health status were reported by significantly more subjects with depressive symptoms than by subjects with no depressive disorder or symptoms. Major financial losses, bed days, high levels of financial strain, limitations in physical or job functioning, and poor health status were reported by significantly more subjects with major depression than by those with no depressive symptoms. There were no significant differences between individuals with subsyndromal depressive symptoms and those with major depression, except for lower self-rated health status.

Discussion.—Subsyndromal depression is an important public health concern. One in 10 individuals in this study met criteria for subsyndromal depressive symptoms. Significantly more individuals with such symptoms reported impairment in 8 of 10 functional domains. Prospective, controlled studies are needed to determine effective treatment for these individuals because there is currently no information on treatment for subsyndromal depressive symptoms, or if individuals with such symptoms should be treated at all.

► Utilizing the large Epidemiologic Catchment Area study data, these authors have clearly demonstrated that what we have labelled as subsyndromal depressive symptoms are really quite a public health problem because of the significant impairments associated with this disorder. This is another example of how careful research leads to areas where our knowledge is too thin, and there is an immediate need for research in this area.

J.C. Ballenger, M.D.

Maintenance Therapy for Chronic Depression: A Controlled Clinical Trial of Desipramine

Kocsis JH, Friedman RA, Markowitz JC, et al (New York Hosp–Cornell Med Ctr)

Arch Gen Psychiatry 53:769–774, 1996 8–3

Introduction.—The efficacy of antidepressant drugs for chronic depression has been confirmed in previous studies. In the treatment of depression, several medications have been found to be effective, including tricyclic antidepressants, selective serotonin reuptake inhibitors, serotonin-2 receptor antagonists, and a reversible inhibitor of monoamine oxidase. Results of a long-term study comparing desipramine hydrochloride and placebo for maintenance therapy of remitted patients with chronic depression are compared.

Methods.—Patients were categorized into 3 groups: 51 met criteria for pure dysthmia, 64 for double depression, and 14 for chronic major depression. All were treated on an open basis with desipramine. After 10 weeks, full and partial remitters entered a continuation phase of open treatment with desipramine for 16 weeks. For the next 2 years, the remitted patients were randomized to continued desipramine treatment or placebo. Relapse rates were compared between the 2 groups.

Results.—According to the chronic depression subtype, acute-phase treatment results did not differ significantly. During the continuation phase, remission persisted with a high degree of stability. For the active desipramine group, the relapse rate was 11%, whereas for the placebo group, it was 52%. Most of the placebo relapses occurred during the first 6 months of therapy.

Conclusion.—In the prevention or postponement of relapse of depression in patients who responded to desipramine during the acute and continuation phases, long-term maintenance treatment with desipramine appeared to be more effective than placebo.

► Although this is a relatively simple study, actually an open trial, I chose it because it reflects real clinical practice and speaks to an important issue. The authors clearly demonstrate that continued treatment with desipramine maintained an antidepressant response, whereas substitution of placebo led to relapse rates 5 times as high. The rates were 11% with desipramine vs. 52% with placebo.

J.C. Ballenger, M.D.

Clinical Presentations of Major Depression by African Americans and Whites in Primary Medical Care Practice

Brown C, Schulberg HC, Madonia MJ (Univ of Pittsburgh, Pa)

J Affect Disord 41:181–191, 1996 8–4

Background.—Little is known regarding the influence of race on the clinical manifestations of major depression. The clinical presentations of this disorder among African-Americans and whites in primary medical care practice were described.

Methods.—One hundred nineteen African-Americans and 153 white Americans participating in a randomized control study of treatments for major depression were assessed. The psychiatric treatment histories, severity of depression, level of psychosocial functioning, and severity of medical illness were comparable in the 2 groups. However, there were differences in the co-morbidity of psychiatric disorders, severity of somatic symptoms, self-reported physical functioning, life stress, and health beliefs. The most striking difference was African-Americans' significantly poorer level of general health and greater impairment on the Medical Outcomes Scale physical functioning scales. Psychiatrist ratings showed that the African-Americans were significantly more impaired than the whites on 5 of the 10 Hamilton Depression Rating Scale somatic symptoms.

Conclusion.—Although African-American and white primary care patients with major depression are comparable in core mood symptoms and associated psychosocial impairment, cultural and perhaps biologic differences may mediate salient differences in symptom presentation, pattern of other Axis I psychiatric disorders, and physical disability. Because African-Americans are more likely to focus on physical symptoms and disability and may be guarded against some physicians, primary care physicians may less readily discern depression in these patients. Severity of sleep disturbance may be an important indicator of depression in African-American patients.

► This study examines the important issue of whether depression presents differently and, therefore, is recognized differently in African-Americans vs. whites in primary care practice. The authors find differences and report under-recognition of major depression in African-Americans. This depression is often related to increased reporting of physical symptoms. The authors observed that sleep disturbance may be a particularly valuable tipoff to depression in African-Americans in primary care.

J.C. Ballenger, M.D.

Pharmacotherapy for Major Depression With Melancholic Features: Relative Efficacy of Tricyclic Versus Selective Serotonin Reuptake Inhibitor Antidepressants

Perry PJ (Univ of Iowa, Iowa City)

J Affect Disord 39:1–6, 1996 8–5

Background.—Antidepressants are used to treat affective disorders with a depressive syndrome component. Because there are many variants of depressive syndromes, not all can be expected to respond to antidepressant drugs in the same way. The effectiveness of tricyclic antidepressants (TCAs) and selective serotonin reuptake inhibitors (SSRIs) were compared in 6 clinical trials of patients with endogenous/melancholic depression.

Study Results.—The first study to demonstrate a significant difference between the effectiveness of TCAs and SSRIs in the treatment of endogenous depression was the 1986 Danish University Antidepressant Group (DUAG) study. Tricyclic antidepressants were found to be more effective than SSRIs in treating this type of depression. Four other groups subsequently replicated these findings and the DUAG repeated their study in 1990 with the same results.

Conclusion.—Comparison of the Hamilton Depression Rating data from 6 controlled clinical trials shows that TCAs are more effective than SSRIs in the treatment of endogenous depression or major depression with melancholic features. These results suggest that health care providers should subtype depressed patients and treat melancholic patients with TCAs as a first-line treatment. For melancholic patients who have been treated with an SSRI and not responded, TCA treatment should be considered.

▶ Paul Perry reviews the evidence suggesting that TCAs are more effective than SSRIs in the treatment of melancholic or endogenously depressed patients. This remains a hotly contested issue, but much of the evidence suggests that TCAs are more effective in this subgroup of patients.

J.C. Ballenger, M.D.

High Relapse Rate After Discontinuaton of Adjunctive Medication for Elderly Patients With Recurrent Major Depression

Reynolds CF III, Frank E, Perel JM, et al (Univ of Pittsburgh, Pa)

Am J Psychiatry 153:1418–1422, 1996 8–6

Background.—Elderly patients may benefit as much from treatment with antidepressant medication as younger patients, although the response may be slower and there may be a tendency to relapse. This raises questions about the use of adjunctive or augmented pharmacotherapy to bring about remission in patients who respond slowly or partially to primary pharmacotherapy. Unanswered questions include what percentage of elderly patients with depression may need adjunctive medication, what will happen after adjunctive treatment, are patients given augmentation more or less likely to relapse than patients not given augmentation, and how long should adjunctive medication be used?

Methods.—The outcome of 158 elderly patients with late-life recurrent major depression was examined; 39 patients received adjunctive medication during acute-phase pharmacotherapy because of a slow or partial response to nortriptyline; 119 patients received no such adjunctive treatment. Adjunctive medication consisted of lithium, perphenazine, or paroxetine. Inpatient care was provided for 28 patients during acute-phase treatment.

Results.—The rate of response to acute therapy was lower in patients given adjunctive medication. Also in these patients, the relapse rate was higher during continuation therapy, and the rate of sustained remission was lower than for patients who did not receive augmented therapy.

Discussion.—In elderly patients with late-life recurrent major depression, augmentation therapy should be discontinued slowly to help prevent early relapse. These patients should also be monitored carefully. It is possible that the combination of medication is more important than the actual dose in maintaining mental health in these patients.

► The Pittsburgh group demonstrates definitively the value of augmentation therapy in elderly depressed patients, another of the facts we need to know in treating the full range of depressed patients.

J.C. Ballenger, M.D.

Epidemiological Data Suggest Antidepressants Reduce Suicide Risk Among Depressives

Isacsson G, Bergman U, Rich CL (Karolinska Inst, Huddinge, Sweden; Huddinge Univ, Sweden; Univ of South Alabama, Mobile)

J Affect Disord 41:1–8, 1996 8–7

Background.—Investigations of consecutive suicide victims from around the world have shown that 90% or more of all such individuals have mental disorders. Successful treatment of these individuals may lower the rate of suicide. Although antidepressant medication has been available for more than 30 years, no decrease in suicide associated with such medication has been reported. This may reflect a failure of these medications to prevent suicide, or limitations in the data or research. Research has shown that an individual with depression who is not treated is at a high risk of suicide, but it is not known if diagnosis and treatment of depression actually prevent suicide.

Methods.—Data on the rate of depression, the rate of treated and untreated individuals with depression, and the rate of suicide in Sweden were collected and analyzed. Data on the use of antidepressant medication in the population from 1990 to 1991 were obtained from the Swedish National Corporation of Pharmacies.

Results.—In Sweden, only 1 in 5 individuals with major depression was treated with antidepressants. The risk for suicide among individuals treated for depression with antidepressant medication was 141 per 100,000 person years. Among untreated individuals with depression, this risk was 259 per 100,000 person years.

Discussion.—These findings show that treatment of major depression with antidepressant medication can lower the rate of suicide among depressed individuals. Suicide prevention strategies should focus on recognizing and treating more individuals with depression. Improved models for evaluating the effects of current treatment methods would be valuable.

► Similar to the United States, only 20% of depressed patients in Sweden receive treatment with antidepressants. In this study, it is shown that treatment is associated with a lower risk of suicide and provides powerful data about the value of treatment of depression.

J.C. Ballenger, M.D.

Suicidal Risk During Controlled Clinical Investigations of Fluvoxamine

Letizia C, Kapik B, Flanders WD (Solvay Pharmaceuticals, Marietta, Ga; Ciba Vision Ophthalmics, Duluth, Ga; Emory Univ, Atlanta, Ga)

J Clin Psychiatry 57:415–421, 1996 8–8

Background.—Patients with major depressive disorder are at serious risk for suicide. Isolated case reports have described paradoxical suicidal ideation or behavior during antidepressant therapy. A meta-analysis was performed to further investigate the risk of suicide during fluvoxamine therapy.

Methods.—Data from double-blind, randomized, placebo-controlled, parallel-group clinical trials were pooled. The suicide item on the Hamilton Rating Scale for Depression was the main outcome measure. Emergence of substantial suicidal ideation and improvement or worsening in suicidal ideation were assessed using the Mantel-Haenszel adjusted incidence difference.

Findings.—Fluvoxamine was associated with a significantly greater improvement in suicidal ideation and significantly less worsening of suicidal ideation compared with placebo. There were no differences in the emergence of substantial suicidal ideation.

Conclusion.—Fluvoxamine therapy is not correlated with an increased risk of emergence of substantial suicidal thoughts in patients with depression. The meta-analysis suggests that fluvoxamine provides a protective effect on the risk of suicidal ideation.

► Obviously, one of the biggest controversies in our field in recent years has been whether selective serotonin reuptake inhibitors (SSRIs) can lead to greater suicidal ideation. Recent reviews of these data have indicated that use of all antidepressants, including SSRIs, leads to decreases in suicidal ideation in depressed patients. Here is another study demonstrating this fact.

J.C. Ballenger, M.D.

Birth Outcomes in Pregnant Women Taking Fluoxetine

Chambers CD, Johnson KA, Dick LM, et al (Univ of California-San Diego, La Jolla)

N Engl J Med 335:1010–1015, 1996 8–9

Introduction.—Fluoxetine is the most commonly used antidepressant drug in the United States. Its safety in pregnancy has not been fully determined, despite its widespread use in both sexes and all ages. The effects of treatment with fluoxetine during pregnancy were evaluated.

Methods.—Over a 6-year period, 228 pregnant women taking fluoxetine were prospectively identified. Pregnancy outcomes of these women were compared with those of 254 women who were not taking fluoxetine.

Results.—There were no significant differences between women taking fluoxetine and controls in spontaneous pregnancy loss or rate of major structural anomalies. There were 97 infants exposed to fluoxetine who were evaluated for minor anomalies. The frequency of 3 or more minor anomalies was significantly higher in the fluoxetine group, compared with 153 control infants who were evaluated similarly. A comparison between the 101 infants exposed to fluoxetine in the first and second trimester only and 73 infants exposed during the third trimester indicated that infants in the latter group had higher rates of premature delivery, more admissions to special-care nurseries, poor neonatal adaptation (including respiratory difficulty, cyanosis on feeding, and jitteriness), lower birth weight, and shorter birth length.

Conclusion.—Women who took fluoxetine during pregnancy did not have an increased risk of spontaneous pregnancy loss or major fetal anomalies. Infants of fluoxetine-treated mothers had an increased incidence of 3 or more minor anomalies, compared with controls. The combination of any 3 minor anomalies is considered rare. Perinatal complications are more frequent in women who take fluoxetine in the third trimester of pregnancy.

► With the increased use of medications, and particularly selective serotonin reuptake inhibitors, in the general population and therefore during pregnancy, we need more data regarding its use in pregnancy. In this study, 228 pregnant women taking fluoxetine were compared with 254 not taking fluoxetine. Although there were no more spontaneous pregnancy losses or major structural abnormalities in the pregnant group, there was a higher frequency of 3 or more minor anomalies, usually a rare event. Also there were more perinatal complications in patients who took fluoxetine during the third trimester, often considered a safe time to return to use of these psychotropics. This is an important article that all of us should read.

J.C. Ballenger, M.D.

Sleep Deprivation Combined With Consecutive Sleep Phase Advance as a Fast-acting Therapy in Depression: An Open Pilot Trial in Medicated and Unmedicated Patients

Berger M, Vollmann J, Hohagen F, et al (Klinikum der Albert-Ludwigs-Universität Freiburg, Germany)

Am J Psychiatry 154:870–872, 1997 8–10

Background.—Approximately 60% of all depressed patients respond to total sleep deprivation, but relapse after a night of sleep or a morning nap. These results suggest that early morning sleep may be more likely to restore depression. A strategy of total sleep deprivation followed by consecutive sleep phase advance therapy for 1 week was developed to prevent depression relapse. A group of 33 depressed patients were treated with this new regimen.

Study Design.—The study group consisted of 12 men and 21 women with an average age of 47 years, who were given a diagnosis according to DSM-III-R criteria of major depression, melancholic type. Their average

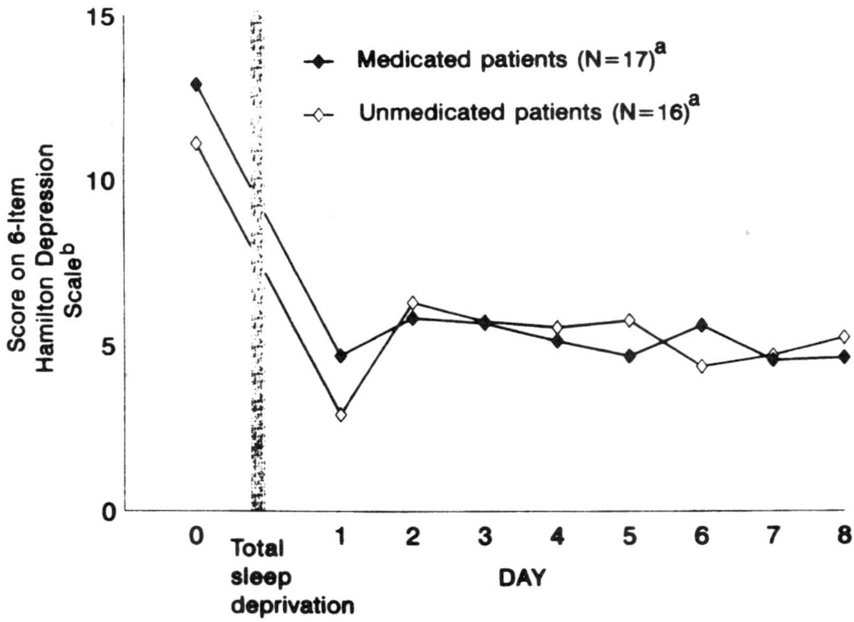

[a]Number of subjects varied.
[b]Average of morning (9:00 a.m.) and afternoon (4:00 p.m.) ratings.

FIGURE 1.—Impact of total sleep deprivation and consecutive sleep phase advance on depressed mood in 33 Inpatients. *Number of subjects varied. †Average of morning (9:00 AM) and afternoon (4:00 PM) ratings. (Courtesy of Berger M, Vollman J, Hohagen F, et al: Sleep deprivation combined with consecutive sleep phase advance as a fast-acting therapy in depression: An open pilot trial in medicated and unmedicated patients. *Am J Psychiatry* 154:870–872, 1997. Copyright 1997, the American Psychiatric Association. Reprinted by permission.)

depression rating on the 21-item Hamilton Depression Rating Scale before entrance into this study was 28.9. Sixteen of these patients were medication-free, while the rest continued to receive medication. After 2 baseline days, patients underwent total sleep deprivation. All 33 patients responded to this treatment with mood elevation. Phase advancement of the sleep period was immediately initiated, with an initial sleep period of 5:00 PM until midnight. Bedtime was delayed an hour each day for a week until a sleep period of 11:00 PM to 6:00 AM was achieved after 1 week. Patients were considered responsive if there was at least a 30% reduction in the averaged morning and afternoon value of the 6-item Hamilton depression scale after treatment.

Results.—Of these 33 depressed patients who responded to total sleep deprivation, 20 maintained their improved mood state during sleep phase advancement. There was no difference in response to therapy of patients with and without medications (Fig 1).

Conclusions.—The majority of patients with major depression who responded to total sleep deprivation were able to maintain their improved mood during sleep phase advancement therapy. This combination therapy has the potential for a rapid, sustained mood elevation response for patients with major depression.

▶ Fascinating phenomena in our field have been the rapid antidepressant response of total sleep deprivation but immediate relapse in these patients when they sleep again. This group has reported that when sleep deprivation is combined with a complex, but logical, phase advancement of the sleep period, the majority of these depressed patients maintain their antidepressant response.

J.C. Ballenger, M.D.

The P-450 System: Definition and Relevance to the Use of Antidepressants in Medical Practice

Goldberg RJ (Brown Univ, Providence, RI)
Arch Fam Med 5:406–412, 1996 8–11

Background.—In the liver, the oxidative metabolism of many compounds, both endogenous and exogenous, is conducted by a collection of isoenzymes called the cytochrome P-450 enzyme system. The activity of this system is inhibited by several widely used selective serotonin reuptake inhibitors. Medications that interfere with, or are normally metabolized by, this system were reviewed, and the clinical relevance of these interactions was addressed.

Findings.—Inhibiting medications compete with other substrates for the activity of 1 or more isoenzymes. Levels of substrates normally metabolized by these same enzymes, which may be coprescribed drugs, may, thus, be elevated. Hence, physicians should be aware that levels of some drugs may become elevated when coprescribed with an inhibitor. All substrates have the potential to be inhibitors, but all inhibitors are not substrates.

Discussion.—The therapeutic margin of a drug determines the significance of an elevated plasma level. When interactions are possible, special caution must be exercised with drugs that have narrow therapeutic margins, such as type 1C cardiac antiarrhythmics or terfenadine. Because metabolic clearance often involves multiple pathways, the potential drug interactions between drugs will not necessarily occur. Nevertheless, caution should always be exercised in the coprescription of drugs with possible interaction. Many enzyme systems have not yet been thoroughly investigated.

► There remains considerable controversy as to how important the interactions are among the antidepressants and the hepatic P-450 enzyme system. Opinion varies from considerable worry to a feeling that it is clinically a relatively rare event. This article reviews these data.

J.C. Ballenger, M.D.

The Dexamethasone Suppression Test in Patients With Mood Disorders

Rush AJ, Giles DE, Schlesser MA, et al (Univ of Texas, Dallas; Univ of Rochester, NY; Dallas Neuropsychiatry Associates; et al)

J Clin Psychiatry 57:470–484, 1996 8–12

Introduction.—There is controversy regarding the significance of the dexamethasone suppression test (DST). A comprehensive assessment of each area of major controversy was performed to (1) determine whether the endogenous/nonendogenous mood disorder dichotomy is validated by the DST; (2) determine whether other subtyping schemes relate to the DST; (3) assess the relative contributions of symptom severity, weight loss, and other factors to the DST; and (4) analyze the relative sensitivity of various postdexamethasone cortisol determinations in the detection of dexamethasone nonsuppression.

Methods.—The 1.0-mg overnight DST procedure was used to evaluate 131 consecutive adult inpatients and 356 consecutive adult outpatients. Of 487 patients, 422 had unipolar and 65 had bipolar disorder. Nonsuppression was defined as at least 1 postdexamethasone cortisol measurement greater than 4.0 μg/dL.

Results.—Nonsuppression was observed in 27% of all patients with major depression and 43% of all patients with bipolar illness. In outpatients, 35.2% of patients with endogenous and 9% of patients with nonendogenous depression were found to have nonsuppression. In inpatients, 61.5% of patients with endogenous and 18.5% of those with nonendogenous depression were found with nonsuppression. Sensitivities and specificities of the DST for the inpatient and outpatient group combined were 46.2% and 89.9%, respectively, in differentiating endogenous from nonendogenous major depressive episodes. Weight loss, gender, and symptom severity had little effect on the endogenous/nonendogenous dichotomy. The Research Diagnostic Criteria primary/secondary and Winokur and colleagues' family history subtypes for unipolar depression were not strongly validated by the DST. Combination of the 4 PM and 11 PM samples allowed detection of 91.0% of inpatients with abnormal 3-sample DST results. By themselves, the 8 AM sample detected 30%, the 4 PM sample detected 67%, and the 11 PM sample detected 62%.

Conclusion.—The endogenous/nonendogenous dichotomy was distinctly verified by DST response. The DST nonsuppression is increased in primary depression, compared with secondary depression. Familial pure depression and overall depressive severity were associated with a significant incidence of nonsuppression.

► Certainly the DST has been an important but controversial test in our field. John Rush and colleagues give us a good review and present new data for a large number of patients. Interestingly, they find support and validity for the use of the DST in certain areas, including the distinction between endogenous and nonendogenous depression, as well as the difference between primary and secondary depression.

J.C. Ballenger, M.D.

Development of Major Depressive Disorder During Smoking-cessation Treatment

Borrelli B, Niaura R, Keuthen NJ, et al (Brown Univ, Providence, RI; Massachusetts Gen Hosp, Boston)

J Clin Psychiatry 57:534–538, 1996 8–13

Background.—Although several studies have reported an association between smoking and major depressive disorder (MDD), few have prospectively assessed patients in whom MDD develops after smoking cessation. The development of MDD after smoking cessation was investigated in a descriptive study.

Methods.—One hundred fourteen nondepressed subjects participating in a study of the effect of fluoxetine on smoking cessation underwent the Structured Clinical Interview for Diagnostic and Statistical Manual of Mental Disorders, edition III, revised, before and after treatment. The Beck Inventory and the Hamilton Rating Scale for Depression were also administered to assess depressive symptoms.

Findings.—Thirty-two percent of the subjects reported a history of MDD before treatment. Seven percent met threshold criteria for MDD after treatment. None was taking the highest fluoxetine dose (60 mg), 4 were taking 30 mg, and 1 was taking placebo. All 5 subjects with MDD after treatment also had a history of it. Four also had a history of substance abuse and achieved at least 3 consecutive biochemically verified weeks of smoking abstinence. Subjects in whom MDD developed after treatment scored significantly higher on measures of depressed mood at baseline than those without MDD after smoking-cessation therapy.

Conclusion.—Some patients may be at risk for MDD after smoking cessation. Also, patients seen with MDD should be asked about their smoking status and recent attempts to quit. Large-scale epidemiologic studies may underestimate the rate of depression in the general population, as self-medication by cigarette smoking may mask it.

► Almost all of us encourage our friends and patients to discontinue smoking in a fairly aggressive and vigorous way. If we follow all these patients closely, however, we discover that some of them do poorly, in terms of psychiatric and physical difficulties, after stopping smoking. Increasingly we have recognized that some patients develop a major depression afterward. This depression is presumably related to the cessation of smoking. This article should help us balance our thinking and certainly encourage us to follow these patients more closely.

J.C. Ballenger, M.D.

Major Depression Following Smoking Cessation

Covey LS, Glassman AH, Stetner F (Columbia Univ, New York; New York State Psychiatric Inst, New York)

Am J Psychiatry 154:263–265, 1997 8–14

Background.—The link between cigarette smoking and certain psychiatric disorders raises questions about the emotional effects of quitting cigarette smoking. It is unclear whether individuals who stop smoking are vulnerable to major depression after the 2- to 4-week period of nicotine withdrawal.

Methods.—Three-month follow-up data were collected from a study of 126 individuals who successfully completed a smoking cessation program.

Results.—The incidence of new major depression at 3 months after the end of the program was 2% in individuals with no history of major depression, 17% in individuals with history of a single major depression, and 30% in individuals with recurrent major depression. A history of major depression and persistent withdrawal symptoms were independent predictors of major depression after smoking cessation treatment.

Discussion.—It is important to obtain information regarding a history of depression from individuals who enroll in smoking cessation programs. It is recommended that such individuals receive counseling beyond the 2- to 4-week period of nicotine withdrawal.

► Like the earlier article, the New York group of Glassman and colleagues document that individuals with a history of recurrent major depression are most at risk for having depression develop when they stop smoking.

J.C. Ballenger, M.D.

Anxiety Disorders

Predictors of Outcome in Panic Disorder: A 5-Year Prospective Follow-up Study

Scheibe G, Albus M (Univ of Düsseldorf, Germany; State Mental Hosp, Haar, Germany)

J Affect Disord 41:111–116, 1996 8–15

Background.—Until recently, little was known about the long-term course of panic disorder. In 1994, Shear and Maser advocated the use of a standardized assessment package for panic disorder studies. This assessment includes co-morbidity with depression, severity of disease, agoraphobic avoidance behavior, illness duration, and illness-related social disability. Whether these variables affect the outcome of patients with panic disorder was determined.

Methods and Findings.—Fifty patients seeking care for anxiety disorders at an outpatient clinic were followed prospectively for 5 years. These patients were originally enrolled in a controlled study of imipramine or doxepin in addition to supportive psychotherapy. The strongest predictors of outcomes in a multiple stepwise regression analyses were co-morbidity with current depression, disease severity, and agoraphobic avoidance. Disease-related social impairment at baseline apparently did not affect outcome.

Conclusion.—These findings are consistent with those of earlier studies that co-morbidity with current depression, illness severity, illness duration, and agoraphobic avoidance behavior at baseline are the best predictors of outcome in patients with panic disorder. The degree of illness-related social impairment at baseline was not a relevant predictor of outcome.

► This study documents very clearly the predictors of illness severity in panic disorder. The authors find, as other have, that current depression and severity and duration of the illness, as well as agoraphobic avoidance behaviors, are the best predictors of how well patients with panic disorder will respond to treatment. It is now clear that some patients respond very well and others do not. This paper allows prediction of patients who will need more or different treatment.

J.C. Ballenger, M.D.

Advances in the Psychosocial Treatment of Anxiety Disorders: Implications for National Health Care

Barlow DH, Lehman CL (Boston Univ)

Arch Gen Psychiatry 53:727–735, 1996 8–16

Background.—Controlled studies demonstrate the efficacy of new psychosocial treatments of anxiety disorders, but questions remain regarding whether the improvement is lasting and whether drug treatment is helpful.

The current status of psychosocial treatment and the direction of current research were described for each anxiety disorder.

Discussion.—Panic disorder, with or without agoraphobia, can be successfully treated with panic control therapy or cognitive therapy, both of which target the disorder's cognitive, physiologic, and behavioral components. The addition of drug therapy, with either imipramine or a high-potency benzodiazepine, is producing encouraging results. For generalized anxiety disorder, a combination of relaxation or meditation with cognitive therapy is effective, with as many as 58% of patients still greatly improved after 12 months. Exposure and habituation to the worry itself is under investigation. Patients with obsessive-compulsive disorder appear to respond to exposure and response prevention, plus relapse prevention, as are used in addictive disorders. One multicenter study appears to have found better results from exposure and response prevention than from drug therapy with clomipramine.

For social phobia, cognitive behavioral group treatment, combining group therapy with cognitive therapy, is successful. Current research suggests that treatment with phenelzine or alprazolam is equally effective. Specific phobias are best treated with exposure-based therapy. Research is currently directed at the use of a prolonged single session of exposure to feared stimuli. Posttraumatic stress disorder is generally treated with direct exposure, through therapeutic reliving of the event, or with stress management. There are preliminary indications that preventive therapy is possible soon after the traumatic event.

Conclusion.—Psychosocial treatment using exposure, cognitive therapy, and coping strategies successfully treats anxiety disorders. Many techniques have not proven to be transportable to other institutions. The addition of pharmacotherapy appears promising.

► David Barlow has been one of the principal workers in the field of psychosocial treatments of anxiety disorders. In this article, he reviews and compares psychosocial and pharmacologic treatments of the various anxiety disorders. This is an excellent review.

J.C. Ballenger, M.D.

Hypothalamic-Pituitary-Adrenal Axis Activity in Panic Disorder: Effects of Alprazolam on 24 h Secretion of Adrenocorticotropin and Cortisol

Abelson JL, Curtis GC, Cameron OG (Univ of Michigan, Ann Arbor)

J Psychiatr Res 30:79–93, 1996 8–17

Background.—Both panic disorder and depression have been linked to excessive activity in the hypothalamic-pituitary-adrenal (HPA) axis, driven by corticotropin-releasing hormone (CRH) neurons. Because alprazolam is effective against panic disorder, a demonstration that this agent blocks panic by inhibiting the CRH system would offer strong support for an etiologic role for CRH in panic disorder. Clinical evidence of such a role,

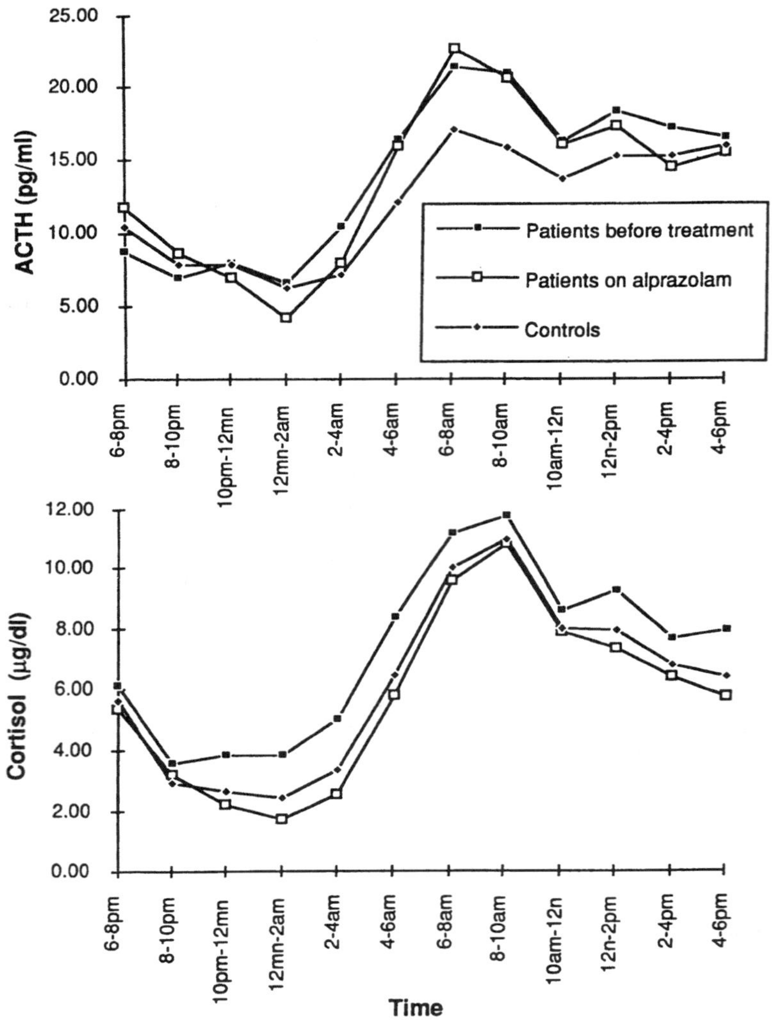

FIGURE 1.—The adrenocorticotropin (*ACTH*) (**upper panel**) and cortisol (**lower panel**) levels measured every 15 minutes and averaged over 2 hour-epochs for 24 hours in panic patients before treatment and after an average of 12 weeks of alprazolam, and in normal control subjects. Graphic presentation is meant to provide a visual depiction of the results but to avoid figures than are too complex to visually process comfortably. Error bars are not included. (Reprinted from the *Journal of Psychiatric Research* 30:79–93, by Abelson JL, Curtis GC, Cameron OG: Hypothalamic-pituitary-adrenal axis activity in panic disorder: Effects of alprazolam on 24 h secretion of adrenocorticotropin and cortisol, copyright 1996 with kind persmission from Elsevier Science Ltd, The Boulevard, Langford Lane, Kidlington OX5 1GB, UK)

however, and of a role for inhibition of HPA axis activity in alprazolam's anti-panic efficacy, is inconsistent. These questions were examined in a study of 20 patients with panic disorder and 12 normal controls.

Methods.—Participants ranged in age from 18 to 42 years; all were medically healthy and none had been exposed to psychoactive medication for a least 2 weeks before the study. Patients met *Diagnostic and Statistical Manual of Mental Disorders*, third edition, revised, criteria for panic disorder, with or without agoraphobia. All participants were evaluated by a Structured Clinical Interview. Patients underwent an initial, detailed evaluation of HPA axis functioning, a 12-week treatment protocol with alprazolam, and a repeat evaluation of the HPA axis.

Results.—Patients and controls were comparable in mean age and sex distribution. At the end of the alprazolam treatment period, patients were taking an average of 4.1 mg/day, most on a 3-times-per-day schedule. All severity-of-illness variables were significantly improved in the patient group. Panic attacks were averaging 0.8 per week, reduced from an average of 3.5 per week at study entry. Patients had elevated overnight cortisol secretion relative to controls at entry; this difference disappeared after the alprazolam treatment period. No significant correlations were found between changes in symptom severity and changes in cortisol measures. The impact of alprazolam treatment on adrenocorticotropin (ACTH) secretion was less clear. The total patient group did not differ from controls in mean ACTH levels before or after treatment, but an apparent elevation of ACTH during the initial 4 hours of monitoring was significant (Fig 1). Levels of ACTH tended to be relatively elevated in patients with low panic attack frequency.

Conclusion.—Twelve weeks of treatment with alprazolam substantially reduced symptoms in patients with panic disorder. The agent also significantly reduced cortisol levels but had little overall effect on ACTH levels. Interpretation of ACTH data was complicated by the effects of panic attack frequency. The mechanism involved in alprazolam's inhibition of activity within the HPA axis must be compatible with an overall reduction in cortisol levels, little change in ACTH, and differential effects on ACTH levels depending on initial panic attack frequency.

► This study examines the issue of whether alprazolam in the treatment of panic disorder has significant effects on the HPA axis, cortisol, and ACTH as has been hypothesized. The authors demonstrate some effects on cortisol but less on ACTH contributing to the importance of the debate around these issues. Part of the importance has to do with the deleterious effect of anxiety and related symptoms on cardiovascular status. Some of these issues are reviewed in this year's Annual Review. Alprazolam has been reported to block the cortisol response, which has been thought to perhaps mediate the deleterious effect of anxiety and depression on cardiovascular measures.

J.C. Ballenger, M.D.

Clinical Features of Cocaine-induced Panic

Louie AK, Lannon RA, Rutzick EA, et al (Univ of California, San Francisco)
Biol Psychiatry 40:938–940, 1996 8–18

Introduction.—A number of studies have noted an association between the use of cocaine and panic disorder. In some cases, an autonomous panic disorder persists after cocaine use is discontinued. A telephone survey of 96 cocaine users was conducted to provide additional evidence for a relationship between the drug and panic disorder.

Methods.—Research subjects were sought through a newspaper article published in 1990. Ninety-five of approximately 400 respondents described experiencing panic attacks after significant cocaine use. During a 45-minute telephone interview with a psychiatrist or a psychiatric social worker, participants were assessed using *Diagnostic and Statistical Manual of Mental Disorders*, edition III, revised criteria for the presence of panic disorder with or without agoraphobia. Information was obtained on cocaine use history, its relationship to panic attacks, use of other recreational drugs, and medical and family history.

Results.—The study group had a mean age of 34.3 years; 52% were women and 81% were white. Panic symptoms had been present for an average of 4.1 years, with an average of 1.4 episodes per day. The attacks were unchanged over time in 42% of respondents, had improved in 26%, were variable in 19%, and had worsened in 13%. Most respondents (72%) reported psychosensory changes in association with the attacks and more than two thirds had agoraphobia. Cocaine use started at an average of 10.9 years and stopped at an average of 3.7 years before the interview; 60% gave up the drug because they thought it caused their panic symptoms. A variety of medications had been prescribed for the panic disorder. Tricyclic antidepressants were not well tolerated and tended to worsen anxiety symptoms; benzodiazepines were better tolerated and relatively efficacious. Both caffeine and marijuana were said to worsen panic symptoms.

Discussion.—Cocaine-induced panic disorder differs from primary panic disorder in several ways. Psychosensory disturbances are more common, agoraphobia less frequent, and responses to medication atypical. A family history of panic disorder was present in only 7% of this sample vs. the 15% to 25% prevalence found in primary panic disorder. Findings are consistent with a model of cocaine-induced panic based on the phenomenon of kindling.

► For some time we have known that in some patients, the use of cocaine actually produces panic attacks and even panic disorder, which is difficult to treat. These patients responded less well to typical treatments with tricyclics, although they did respond reasonably well to benzodiazepines.

J.C. Ballenger, M.D.

A Double-blind Comparative Study of Brofaromine and Fluvoxamine in Outpatients With Panic Disorder

van Vliet IM, den Boer JA, Westenberg HGM, et al (Academic Hosp Utrecht, The Netherlands)

J Clin Psychopharmacol 16:299–306, 1996 8–19

Background.—Panic disorder (PD) has many adverse consequences for social functioning. Selective serotonin reuptake inhibitors and monoamine oxidase inhibitors have been shown to be effective in the treatment of PD. The efficacy of the selective serotonin reuptake inhibitor fluvoxamine was compared with that of the reversible monoamine oxidase inhibitor brofaromine.

Methods and Findings.—Thirty patients with PD with or without agoraphobia were given 150 mg of fluvoxamine or brofaromine in a double-blind fashion. After 12 weeks of therapy, 93% of those receiving brofaromine and 87% receiving fluvoxamine felt much or very much better. Forty-seven percent and 33%, respectively, had a 50% reduction in the Hamilton Rating Scale for Anxiety score. The main adverse effects were middle-sleep disturbance in the brofaromine group, fatigue in the fluvoxamine group, and nausea after taking medication in both groups. During a further 12 weeks of follow-up, both treatment groups had further improvements, with no significant between-group differences.

Conclusions.—Brofaromine and fluvoxamine are equally effective in the treatment of PD. Both agents decrease the number of panic attacks and subsequently reduce agoraphobic avoidance.

▶ Because the monoamine oxidase inhibitors have been an excellent treatment of PD but their use is significantly limited by side effects, the development of the reversible monoamine oxidase inhibitors are of considerable interest. Unfortunately, brofaromine and moclobemide have had serious difficulties getting to market. This study compares fluvoxamine to brofaromine. In this study brofaromine was equally as effective as fluvoxamine and a very effective treatment of panic disorder.

J.C. Ballenger, M.D.

Alcoholism/Substance Abuse

Alcohol and Drugs in Suicides

Ohberg A, Vuori E, Ojanperä I, et al (Univ of Helsinki; Natl Public Health Inst, Helsinki)

Br J Psychiatry 169:75–80, 1996 8–20

Introduction.—Undertreatment for depression is a major problem, and depression is an important risk for suicide. In some cases individuals use their own antidepressants to commit suicide. A nationwide study conducted in Finland sought to determine the role of alcohol and drugs in suicides.

Methods.—Data were collected for the period from April 1997 through March 1988. All officially classified suicides were included in the study. Information was gathered from medical records, records of social and other agencies, and from interviews with relatives and attending health care personnel. Toxicological data were obtained from police investigations, drug screening, and autopsies. When ingested drugs included neuroleptics, antidepressants, barbiturates, and dextropropoxyphene, an attempt was made to determine if these agents had been prescribed for the victim. Suicides were analyzed by age, gender, method of suicide, and toxicological findings.

Results.—During the 1-year study period, 1,397 suicides were reported in Finland. Samples for toxicological screening were available for 1,348 victims: 1,032 men and 316 women. The suicide rate in all age groups was significantly higher in men than in women. Men died most often by hanging and shooting; overdosing and hanging were the most common methods among women. Overall, 41.6% of victims had taken some drug and 35.9% were under the influence of alcohol. The presence of alcohol was significantly higher among men, whereas the use of any drug was observed significantly more often in women. Benzodiazepines were the most frequently detected drugs, although a benzodiazepine was seldom the principal drug used for suicide. In cases of overdosing, the substance detected was the victim's own prescribed drug in 77.4% of suicides where antidepressants were used and in 74.3% of those where neuroleptics were used.

Discussion.—Alcohol, which has a mind-impairing and triggering effect, was detected in 36% of suicides and twice as often in men as in women. One fifth of suicide victims had taken antidepressants and/or neuroleptics. Overall, drugs were present in two thirds of women and one third of men, and prescribed drugs were often involved. Because of the association between depression and suicide risk, prescription drugs should be selected carefully for depressed patients.

► This is one of many studies which suggest that the judgment-impairing effects of alcohol and other drugs are involved in the choice to kill oneself. Should we be more scrupulous in telling depressed people to avoid alcohol (and drugs), especially if they have any suicidal ideation? I have seen that many people who attempt suicide while intoxicated regret it later when sober. However, I have never seen avoidance of alcohol/drugs as a clear part of the treatment regimen of depression and shouldn't it be?

J.C. Ballenger, M.D.

Five-Year Course of Major Depression: Effects of Comorbid Alcoholism
Hasin DS, Tsai W-Y, Endicott J, et al (Columbia Univ, New York; New York State Psychiatric Inst; Brown Univ, Providence, RI; et al)
J Affect Disord 41:63–70, 1996 8–21

Background.—Since the mid-1980s, the effect of alcoholism on major affective disorders has been studied. There is little or no information on the effect of changes in the status of alcoholism on outcome of depression in individuals with alcoholism and an affective disorder. Differences in the effects of unipolar, bipolar, or schizoaffective disorder and of coexisting alcoholism have not been addressed. The effects of changes in status of alcoholism on sustained changes in status of the affective disorder have also not been addressed.

Methods.—The effect of remissions in alcoholism on sustained remissions and relapses in patients with unipolar, bipolar, or schizoaffective disorder was studied in 127 patients. All patients were white, 40% were female, and about two thirds were younger than 40 years.

Results.—Of the 127 patients, 97 were followed up for 5 years. Remission in alcoholism significantly increased the chance of remission in depression. Remission in alcoholism was also associated with a lower chance of depression relapse.

Discussion.—Clinicians who ignore alcoholism in patients with depression may not be able to adequately treat either condition. It appears that many providers of mental health services are uncomfortable addressing issues related to alcoholism and may not be familiar with techniques for treating substance abuse. Perhaps this and similar reports will help the effort to develop more effective treatment for patients with problems from dual diagnoses.

► These doctors document that you cannot ignore alcoholism and expect depressed people to recover. Other articles this year, not in the YEAR BOOK, have demonstrated that the converse is also true.

J.C. Ballenger, M.D.

Schizophrenia

The Course of Schizophrenia Over 13 Years: A Report From the International Study on Schizophrenia (ISoS) Coordinated by the World Health Organization
Mason P, Harrison G, Glazebrook C, et al (Univ Hosp, Nottingham, England)
Br J Psychiatry 169:580–586, 1996 8–22

Background.—The different concepts of schizophrenia and of outcome used in outcome studies of schizophrenia make comparisons of such studies difficult. The 13-year course of schizophrenia in an epidemiologically defined and representative cohort of patients selected during their first episode was reported.

Methods.—Sixty-seven patients with ICD-9 schizophrenia diagnosed between 1978 and 1980 in Nottingham, England, were included. Symptoms, disability, and hospitalization were assessed using standardized instruments administered at disease onset and 1, 2, and 13 years later. Time to first relapse and first readmission were plotted as survival curves.

Findings.—The curves indicated that first relapses and readmissions occurred in the first 5 years. The length of time spent in psychotic episodes and in the hospital was greatest in the first year of follow-up but stable thereafter. Social adjustment improved from study entry to the first-year follow-up assessment. Between 2 and 13 years, a small deterioration in social adjustment was noted.

Conclusion.—After the initial episode of schizophrenia, the course of this illness appears to be relatively stable. Neither the concept of progressive deterioration or progressive amelioration was supported by these findings. Also, no evidence of a "late recovery" was found.

▶ This is a long-term study of patients with schizophrenia in the modern era who were followed for up to 13 years. In this particular sample, there was very little, if any, deterioration after the initial episode. Most of the difficulty occurred early, and this contributes to the modern view of schizophrenia as, in many ways, having a more favorable course.

J.C. Ballenger, M.D.

Relapse and Rehospitalization During Maintenance Treatment of Schizophrenia

Schooler NR, Keith SJ, Severe JB, et al (Univ of Pittsburgh, Pa; National Institute of Mental Health, Rockville, Md; Med College of Pennsylvania, Philadelphia, et al)

Arch Gen Psychiatry 54:453–463, 1997 8–23

Objective.—A range of treatments is needed for successful community tenure of patients with schizophrenia. Dose-reduction strategies can reduce the amount of medication taken by patients with schizophrenia, as long as the dose is not reduced too low, and the patient is not in an active phase of illness. One approach to dose reduction is targeted therapy, in which patients in stable condition take medication only when they experience prodromal signs or psychotic symptoms. Psychoeducational family treatment of schizophrenia has been studied as well; however, the interaction between these treatments has never been determined. Dose reduction of antipsychotic medication and family treatment were studied for their effects on relapse and rehospitalization rates among patients receiving maintenance therapy for schizophrenia.

Methods.—The study included 313 outpatients from 5 centers with a *DSM-III-R* diagnosis of schizophrenia or schizoaffective disorder. The patients were randomly assigned to 1 of 3 drug approaches using fluphenazine decanoate. One group received standard therapy, a continuous, moderate dose of 12.5–50 mg every 2 weeks. Another group received continuous low-dose fluphenazine, consisting of 2.5–10 mg every 2 weeks. The third group, assigned to targeted, early intervention, took fluphenazine only when they were symptomatic.

The patients were further randomized to 1 of 2 family treatment strategies. One group received supportive family management, which relied on monthly group meetings. The other group received a more intensive family management approach, with monthly group meetings supplemented by home visits, and with an emphasis on communication and problem-solving skills. After 2 years, the effects of the treatments on relapse and rehospitalization rates were assessed.

Results.—The relapse rate was increased for patients in both the continuous low-dose and the targeted treatment groups. Use of rescue medication was increased in these groups as well. Targeted treatment was associated with an increased hospitalization rate, although low-dose therapy was not. The outcomes of the various drug groups were similar, regardless of family treatment. Family treatment had no apparent influence on relapse or rehospitalization rate. However, the rehospitalization rate in both dose-reduction groups was lower than that reported with usual care in previous studies of family treatment.

Conclusions.—In outpatients with schizophrenia, continuous low-dose medication and targeted, early intervention are both associated with an increased relapse rate, while targeted intervention also increases the rehospitalization rate. Most patients with schizophrenia probably should receive a moderate dose of medication. Intensive applied family management does not appear to reduce relapse or rehospitalization rate. Both family management conditions used in this study engaged the family members, which may explain the absence of any effect of the intensive intervention.

► The Pittsburgh group in a large NIMH trial clearly documents the failure of two of the treatment strategies proposed for schizophrenia, i.e., the continuous low-dose and the targeted treatment strategies. Neither group did as well as the moderate-dose treatment group.

J.C. Ballenger, M.D.

Clinical Risk Following Abrupt and Gradual Withdrawal of Maintenance Neuroleptic Treatment

Viguera AC, Baldessarini RJ, Hegarty JD, et al (Harvard Med School, Boston; Highland Drive Veterans Affairs Med Ctr, Pittsburgh, Pa)
Arch Gen Psychiatry 54:49–55, 1997 8–24

Background.—Individuals can experience early relapse after abruptly discontinuing their psychotropic medication. It is hypothesized that the risk of psychotic morbidity is highest in the first few months after discontinuing oral neuroleptic medication. This hypothesis is supported by preliminary evidence of a 13-fold increase in risk of relapse in the first 3 months after discontinuing neuroleptic treatment, and a 2-fold increase or less during the second year.

Methods.—Data were collected on studies of the timing of relapses in patients with schizophrenia after they discontinued neuroleptic medication, combined with new data, and reanalyzed. The data were obtained on 1,210 patients; 1,006 discontinued their neuroleptic medication abruptly and 204 discontinued their medication gradually.

Results.—The risk of relapse was 50% within 30 weeks in patients who discontinued drug therapy abruptly. There was little additional risk between 30 weeks and 3.7 years. Relapse was more rapid among inpatients than among outpatients. Studies of patients who stopped taking their oral medication abruptly vs. gradually showed that relapse was earlier after abrupt withdrawal and that a difference in relapse rates was seen for at least 6 months.

Discussion.—Pharmacodynamic stress factors affecting the risk of relapse after abrupt withdrawal of neuroleptic treatment may include supersensitivity of central dopamine receptors. Additional research is needed to determine whether the high risk of relapse is greater than in untreated psychotic illness and whether gradual removal of medication can reduce, rather than postpone, relapse.

► I have said for some time that we ought to gradually taper all of our medications. This study documents that this is true with the gradual withdrawal of maintenance neuroleptic treatment in schizophrenia. This has also been demonstrated with lithium in bipolar illness and antidepressants in depression. It does seem to be a general truth.

J.C. Ballenger, M.D.

Obsessive-Compulsive Disorder in Patients With Schizophrenia or Schizoaffective Disorder

Eisen JL, Beer DA, Pato MT, et al (Brown Univ, Providence, RI)
Am J Psychiatry 154:271–273, 1997 8–25

Background.—Previous studies of the incidence of obsessive-compulsive disorder in individuals with schizophrenia or schizoaffective disorder have reported rates of 3.5% to 25%. This variation partly results from different methodologic approaches in assessing obsessive-compulsive disorder and symptoms.

Methods.—The incidence of obsessive-compulsive disorder in 52 patients with schizophrenia and 25 patients with schizoaffective disorder was analyzed. Structured interviews and standardized criteria for defining obsessions and compulsions were used. Women made up 40% of the sample.

Results.—Of the 77 patients, 6 met the *Diagnostic and Statistical Manual of Mental Disorders*, edition III, revised criteria for both obsessive-compulsive disorder and schizophrenia or schizoaffective disorder. Five patients with schizoaffective disorder and 1 patient with schizophrenia had obsessive-compulsive disorder. The mean age of the patients was 38.4 years and the mean age at onset of obsessive-compulsive symptoms was 15.2 years.

Discussion.—Obsessive-compulsive disorder occurred in 7.8% of these patients with schizophrenia or schizoaffective disorder. The safety and efficacy of combining medications for both these disorders should be investigated.

► It is a surprising but consistent observation that panic disorder, and in this case obsessive-compulsive disorder, does occur in individuals with schizophrenia. This seems to represent an important hint about etiology for us and certainly a challenge for treatment.

J.C. Ballenger, M.D.

Miscellaneous Disorders

Studies of Serotonin Function in Anorexia Nervosa

Brewerton TD, Jimerson DC (Med Univ of South Carolina, Charleston; Harvard Med School, Boston)

Psychiatry Res 62:31–42, 1996 8–26

Background.—Serotonin dysregulation may be related to the eating disorders, including anorexia nervosa (AN). Serotonin modulates several hormones reported to be dysfunctional in AN patients, and it has been linked with alterations in eating behavior, mood, anxiety, and body image. Serotonin function in patients with AN was investigated.

Methods.—Participating in the study were 12 patients with AN and 16 healthy individuals. Participants were challenged with (1) the postsynaptic serotonin receptor agonist *m*-cholorophenylpiperazine (*m*-CPP), (2) the serotonin precursor L-tryptophan (L-TRP), and (3) placebo. Eight patients with AN were rechallenged 3 to 4 weeks after attaining a goal weight.

Results.—Low weights differed from goal weights by an average of 13 kg. Compared with controls, patients with AN had blunted prolactin responses to both *m*-CPP and L-TRP at low weight and goal weight. A tendency toward normalization occurred after weight gain. Only in low-weight patients with AN was there a trend for blunted growth hormone responses after L-TRP and *m*-CPP. Cortisol responses did not differ significantly among groups. Although *m*-CPP decreased meal size in controls, measures of temperature and test meals were generally unaffected by serotonergic agents. Pyschometric responses varied.

Conclusion.—These data indicate that responses in the postsynaptic hypothalamic pituitary serotonergic pathways of patients with AN are altered. Attainment of goal weight resulted in some trends toward normalization, but many differences persisted. Changes in serotonergic function may occur at CNS levels above the hypothalamus.

► This study comes from 2 of the principal workers trying to understand the serotonin abnormalities in eating disorders. They report abnormalities in the postsynaptic hypothalamic pituitary serotonin pathways of anorexic patients which normalized somewhat with attainment of goal weight.

J.C. Ballenger, M.D.

Computerised Psychoeducation for Patients With Eating Disorders

Andrewes DG, O'Connor P, Mulder C, et al (Univ of Melbourne, Parkville, Australia; Swinburne Univ of Technology, Hawthorn, Australia)
Aust N Z J Psychiatry 30:492–497, 1996 8–27

Background.—Psychoeducation is the process of disseminating information to a patient about the disorder as a way of changing attitude and behavior. It is frequently used in eating disorders. These authors have developed DIET, a psychoeducational computer program aimed at communicating health care information and changing attitudes about dieting. The effect of this program on the eating disorder-related knowledge base and attitudes of patients with a diagnosis of bulimia nervosa or anorexia nervosa was evaluated.

Methods.—The study group consisted of 54 patients with eating disorders diagnosed by *Diagnostic and Statistical Manual of Mental Disorders*, edition III, revised. The patients were randomized to receive either DIET or a placebo computer-based program. Each of these 2 groups contained 14 patients with anorexia nervosa, 4 with anorexia and bulimia, and 9 with bulimia. The 2 groups did not differ significantly in severity of eating disorder or premorbid intelligence. Both groups were examined before and after the intervention by questionnaire to assess knowledge of and attitude toward eating disorders.

Results.—The patients who used the DIET psychoeducation program had significantly greater improvement in both knowledge of and attitude toward their eating disorder, compared with the placebo group. The patients rated the DIET program as being helpful and easy to use.

Conclusion.—The DIET psychoeducational computer program appears to be an effective and resource-efficient method of health education for patients with eating disorders. Further research should focus on whether the program has additional therapeutic effects.

► Psychoeducation and therapeutic computerized treatment programs are proving to be surprisingly effective and efficient. This paper reviewed a computerized educational program for patients with eating disorders and found it to be quite helpful.

J.C. Ballenger, M.D.

Adult Attention-Deficit Hyperactivity Disorder: Assessment Guidelines Based on Clinical Presentation to a Specialty Clinic

Roy-Byrne P, Scheele L, Brinkley J, et al (Univ of Washington, Seattle)

Compr Psychiatry 38:133–140, 1997 8–28

Background.—Attention-deficit hyperactivity disorder (ADHD) is estimated to have a 3% to 9% prevalence among school children. Several prospective studies have suggested that 1% to 3% of these children will continue to have disabling symptoms in adulthood. These patients will probably seek care from adult-oriented clinicians, so adult-oriented assessment guidelines are required. A cohort of 143 adults with self-described suspected ADHD who sought fee-for-service examination at a university-based adult ADHD assessment and brief treatment program was evaluated.

Study Design.—The study group consisted of 98 men and 45 women aged 18–64 years, who had complaints of poor concentration, disorganization, distractibility, or procrastination. Some also had complaints of hyperactivity-impulsivity. The evaluation included the Brief Symptom Inventory/Symptom Checklist 53, Drug Abuse Screening Test, Alcohol Use Disorders Inventory Test, Social Adjustment Scale-Self-Report Version, Wender-Utah Rating Scale (WURS), Wide-Range Achievement Test, and Connor's Continuous Performance Test (CPT). Testing was followed by a diagnostic interview.

Findings.—Of the 143 adults who sought assessment for ADHD, 32% clearly met the diagnostic criteria, 32% clearly did not, and 36% did not meet criteria because of a lack of childhood history or a complicating severe psychiatric or substance abuse comorbidity. These 3 groups did not differ significantly in demographics, psychiatric diagnosis, symptom severity, or functional impairment. Patients with a diagnosis of ADHD had more childhood learning disability, poorer reading scores on the Wide-Range Achievement Test, poorer scores on the CPT, and higher scores on the WURS and ADHD. Patients in the ambiguous category had higher rates of substance abuse than either of the other 2 groups. Although this group resembled the ADHD group in their WURS and CPT scores, they resembled the non-ADHD group in their low incidence of learning disability and normal reading scores.

Conclusions.—Of a group of 143 adults who referred themselves for ADHD assessment, approximately one third did not meet criteria for this diagnosis, one third did meet these criteria, and one third had significant confounding variables that made diagnosis difficult. The WURS was the most discriminating psychometric measure for adult ADHD in this population.

► Some have recently joked that the most rapidly growing industry in psychiatry is the "adult ADD" patient. This careful study documents that one third of patients who refer themselves for evaluation of this disorder do, in fact, appear to have this disorder, while the other two thirds do not.

J.C. Ballenger, M.D.

Two-year Follow-up of Inpatients With Dissociative Identity Disorder

Ellason JW, Ross CA (Univ of Texas, Arlington; Colin A. Ross Inst for Psychological Trauma, Richardson, Tex)

Am J Psychiatry 154:832–839, 1997 8–29

Background.—Dissociative identity disorder presents with auditory hallucinations, depression, suicidal tendencies, phobic anxiety, somatization, substance abuse, and borderline features. The ultimate goal of therapy is integration, defined as 3 stable months of continuity of contemporary memory, self-perception of internal unity, and no evidence of behaviorally separate identities. The long-term progress of a large group of inpatients with dissociative identity disorder was monitored to determine prognosis.

Study Design.—The study group consisted of 135 inpatients at Charter Behavioral Health System of Dallas with a clinical diagnosis of dissociative identity disorder. After 2 years of primarily outpatient psychotherapy and medication, the study participants were re-contacted and re-examined using the same assessments as in the initial interviews: the Dissociative Experiences Scale, Dissociative Disorders Interview Schedule, the PTSD section of the National Institute of Mental Health Diagnostic Interview Schedule, the Structured Clinical Interview for DSM-III-R-I and -II, the Beck Depression Inventory, and the Hamilton Depression Rating. Of the original 135 study participants, 62 were located after 2 years and 54 were reinterviewed.

Findings.—Overall, these patients demonstrated significant improvement in Schneiderian first-rank symptoms, mood and anxiety disorders, dissociative symptoms, and somatization, as well as a significant decrease in prescribed psychiatric medicine when compared to their initial evaluation and treatment. Patients who achieved integration were significantly more improved in these parameters than patients who had not achieved integration.

Conclusions.—Dissociative identity disorder is a severe psychiatric illness requiring long-term treatment, but these findings suggest that patients can respond to outpatient treatment within a time-frame of 2 years.

► One of the most controversial and peripheral syndromes in psychiatry is the dissociative identity disorder. This study follows a large sample (n = 135) of patients with this syndrome and documents clear improvement over a two-year follow-up. Studies like this provide empirical support for this condition.

J.C. Ballenger, M.D.

Body Dysmorphic Disorder: A Survey of Fifty Cases

Veale D, Boocock A, Gournay K, et al (Royal Free Hosp, London; Inst of Psychiatry, London; Univ of London; et al)

Br J Psychiatry 169:196–201, 1996 8–30

Background.—Little research has been conducted on body dysmorphic disorder (BDD), a preoccupation with a perceived defect in one's appearance. A survey of patients with BDD was performed and scores obtained from 2 different structured BDD interviews were compared.

Methods.—Referrals of patients with BDD were solicited from psychiatrists, dermatologists, plastic surgeons, and from patients themselves who had read recent articles about the disorder. Patients underwent structured interviews for BDD and axis II personality disorders, based on *Diagnostic and Statistical Manual of Mental Disorders,* edition III, revised; the Body Dysmorphic Disorder Examination (BDDE); and the modified Yale-Brown Obsessive-Compulsive Scale (YBOCS); plus a depression rating scale and questionnaires and interviewer/patient ratings of the perceived defects.

Results.—Fifty (82%) of the 61 referred patients who were assessed were found to have BDD as a primary diagnosis. Thirty-six of the 50 were self-referred. Past suicide attempts were common (24%), as were past depressive episodes (36%). There was a 72% incidence of 1 or more personality disorders. There was moderate correlation between scores on the BDDE and the YBOCS. Most patients (68%) perceived that they had multiple defects. For 86%, the face was involved. Clinically depressed patients were significantly more likely to believe that they would still be unattractive without their defect than were nondepressed patients. Whereas examiners rated the patients' defects as normal (77%) or minor and within normal limits (23%), 71% of patients scored their perceived defects as severe. Of the 62% who had told their general physician of their concern, 83% (25/30) were dissatisfied with the doctor's response.

Conclusion.—Body dysmorphic disorder is associated with a high comorbidity rate of personality disorder and depression. Patients are reluctant to voice their concerns to physicians, who may not respond helpfully. Symptoms of BDD should be sought in patients with depression, OCD, and social phobia.

► Recognition of BDD has grown in recent years but is still inadequately recognized by general physicians, dermatologists, and even plastic surgeons. This article reviews this area and reports that 83% of patients were dissatisfied with their physician's response.

J.C. Ballenger, M.D.

Premenstrual Dysphoric Disorder: An Update

Steiner M (McMaster Univ, Hamilton, Ont, Canada)

Gen Hosp Psychiatry 18:244–250, 1996 8–31

Background.—Premenstrual dysphoric disorder (PMDD) is distinct from premenstrual syndrome, which refers to relatively mild physical symptoms and minor mood changes. Premenstrual dysphoric disorder is less common and more severe, affecting 3% to 8% of menstruating women, primarily those in their late 20s through mid-30s. Symptoms interfering with patient lifestyle—such as irritability, tension, dysphoria, and lability of mood—may occur and do not respond to conventional therapies. Recent advances in the study and classification of PMDD were reviewed.

Findings.—Research criteria for PMDD are now included in the appendix of the fourth edition of the *Diagnostic and Statistical Manual of Mental Disorders*, edition IV (DSM-IV). Confirmation of the diagnosis may be accomplished by use of DSM-IV criteria in conjunction with prospective daily charting for at least 2 cycles. Standardized interviews for past or present axis I or II diagnoses are also essential. Conservative therapy involves lifestyle and stress management techniques; more aggressive therapy may include pyschotropic medications. In extreme cases, hormonal or surgical intervention to eliminate ovulation may be performed. Selective serotonin reuptake inhibitors and oophorectomy (medical or surgical) have been shown to be effective for PMDD by randomized, placebo-controlled trials.

Conclusion.—The published data indicate that either elimination of the hormonal trigger or reversal of the sensitivity of the serotonergic system may be effective, although no single intervention has been proven uniformly or consistently effective. Any therapeutic interventions should include lifestyle and stress management as necessary adjuncts.

▶ This article reviews the severe menstrual syndrome currently called premenstrual dysphoric disorder. It is now clear that conservative therapy involving lifestyle and stress management techniques are effective in some, but the condition many require more aggressive therapy. There are now studies that the selective serotonin reuptake inhibitors are effective, as are medical or surgical oophorectomy. This would seem to be an area needing research, with such radical treatments as oophorectomy being used.

J.C. Ballenger, M.D.

Geriatrics

Mental Disorder in an Elderly Home Care Population: Associations With Health and Social Service Use

Banerjee S, MacDonald A (Inst of Psychiatry, London; Hither Green Hosp, London)

Br J Psychiatry 168:750–756, 1996 8–32

Background.—The social services departments of local authorities in Great Britain have a statutory duty to provide home care services to those in need of practical help within their own homes. This service is primarily used by the elderly population. The prevalence and recognition of mental disorder within the elderly home care population was investigated.

Methods.—A cross-sectional study with random cluster sampling was done involving people over 65 years of age who were receiving home care in Lewisham. An interview was conducted and mental disorder was rated using the Geriatric Mental State Examination (GMS).

Results.—Of the 177 eligible individuals within this area, 169 were interviewed, for a response rate of 96%. In this population, 46% were rated as having a mental disorder by GMS criteria. Of these, 15% of disorders were organic and 26% were depressive in nature. Most of those who were rated as depressive did not appear to be receiving appropriate treatment. None of the home care group were receiving counseling or therapy. Home care provision to those with depression could not be completely explained by their activity limitation.

Conclusion.—There appears to be a high rate of mental disorder, especially depression, among the elderly home care population in Great Britain. Most of this population does not appear to be receiving appropriate treatment for depression. Because home care provision to those with depression could not be completely explained by the activity limitation, it is possible that depression itself may be associated with a need for home care services. This suggests that the delivery of appropriate treatment for depression might reduce the need for home care services and free these resources for those with activity limitations.

► This English study of the elderly receiving home care presents the striking finding that a large percentage of these patients were being treated for depression and were being poorly treated. As such, it is a helpful finding, but it is discouraging to continue to find such poor treatment of psychiatric conditions in nonpsychiatric settings.

J.C. Ballenger, M.D.

Managing Geriatric Syndromes: What Geriatric Assessment Teams Recommend, What Primary Care Physicians Implement, What Patients Adhere To

Shah PN, Maly RC, Frank JC, et al (East Carolina Univ, Greenville, NC; Univ of California, Los Angeles)

J Am Geriatr Soc 45:413–419, 1997 8–33

Background.—Geriatric syndromes, such as urinary incontinence, falls, depression, and functional impairment, are responsible for some of the frailty and morbidity of aging. The comprehensive geriatric assessment (CGA) is an interdisciplinary approach specifically developed to manage geriatric syndromes. Comprehensive geriatric assessment can only be effective if recommendations are followed by both physicians and patients. The response of patients and physicians to CGA recommendations for the management of falls, depression, urinary incontinence, and functional impairment was examined in a case series study.

Study Design.—The study group consisted of 150 older community-dwelling participants who had at least one of the target geriatric syndromes. After a comprehensive geriatric assessment and evaluation, Project Safety Net made recommendations. To increase compliance, the primary care physician was contacted by a geriatrician to convey recommendations and background materials. Patients received a copy of the recommendations, a copy of the CGA consultation, a "how to talk to your doctor" book, and a follow-up call 2 weeks later to encourage compliance. A structured interview was conducted after 3 months to determine compliance rate.

Findings.—Of the 212 CGA recommendations related to the target geriatric syndromes, 59% required a physician's order for implementation and the remainder were patient self-care recommendations. The overall physician implementation rate was 70%. Physician implementation rates were highest for falls and lowest for functional impairment. The overall patient compliance rate was 85% for physician-implemented recommendations and 46% for self-care recommendations. Patient compliance to recommendations for counseling, support groups, or exercise programs was especially low.

Conclusions.—A process of care study of a community-based consultative comprehensive geriatric assessment program revealed that although the older patients in this series were compliant with primary care physician-initiated recommendations, there was less compliance for self-care recommendations. This result emphasizes the importance of understanding and increasing patient compliance to bring about the desired outcome of a consultative CGA program.

► This study usefully explores what geriatric patients do and do not do with out recommendations. It presents an interestingly "realistic" view.

J.C. Ballenger, M.D.

Old Theories Revisited

On the Nature and Consequences of Early Loss
Hofer MA (Columbia Univ, New York)
Psychosom Med 58:570–581, 1996 8–34

Background.—Acute losses—such as that of a spouse, child, or job—increase vulnerability to a wide variety of diseases. However, the process of how loss becomes translated into disease is not understood. Furthermore, even an understanding of why or how loss is so disruptive to mental functioning is not precise. The use of an animal model system to explore basic questions about the nature of loss and the effects of early loss on later vulnerability to disease was described.

Methods and Findings.—The physiologic and behavioral responses of infant rats to separation from their mothers was analyzed. An extensive layer of processes underlying the psychological constructs generally used to understand response to loss was revealed. A number of discrete sensorimotor, thermal, and nutrient-based events with unexpected long-term regulatory effects on specific components of infant physiology and behavior were documented. Release from these inhibitory and excitatory regulators during maternal separation constitutes a novel mechanism by which the experience of loss is translated into a complex patterned response (Fig 1).

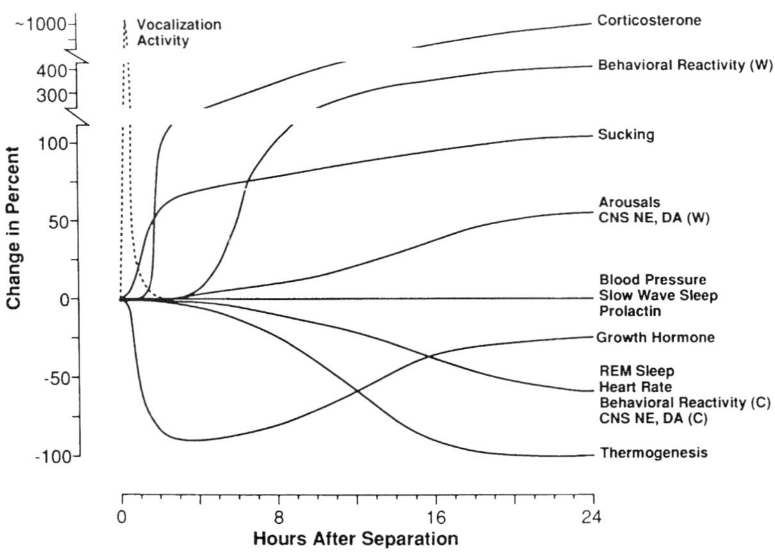

FIGURE 1.—Schematic representation of the time course of changes in physiology and behavior during 24 hours after separation of infant rats from their mothers. Percentage change from baseline in levels of the measures are plotted over time. The *dotted lines* at the extreme left show the immediate response to isolation of a single pup in a novel environment; the *solid lines*, the slower developing responses to removal of the dam from pups left together in a litter group in the home cage. *W* and *C* refer to whether pups are kept warm at nest temperature or allowed to cool in a room temperature environment during separation. *NE* represents norepinephrine and *DA*, dopamine. (Courtesy of Hofer MA: On the nature and consequences of early loss. *Psychosom Med* 58:570–581, 1996.)

Conclusion.—Previous research has documented the long-term effects of loss and selective replacement of regulators on behavioral development and later vulnerability to disease. The data in this study provide a new understanding of early attachment as a developmental force and of human grief as a health risk. Early regulatory processes, also observed in human mother-infant interactions, may constitute the building blocks from which attachment and object representations develop.

► Elsewhere in this volume we review several papers demonstrating the important psychological and physical outcomes of loss in humans. This article reviews a fascinating animal model potentially explaining these observations. This is fascinating intellectually, but it also provides models that might help us convince our generalist friends and colleagues of the importance of these psychological issues and how they might produce physical problems.

J.C. Ballenger, M.D.

Clinical Characteristics of Women With a History of Childhood Abuse: Unhealed Wounds

McCauley J, Kern DE, Kolodner K, et al (The Johns Hopkins Univ, Baltimore, Md; Montgomery County Health Department, Montgomery, Ala; Hahnemann Univ, Philadelphia)

JAMA 277:1362–1368, 1997 8–35

Background.—A variety of psychosocial problems are associated with previous childhood abuse, such as poor self-esteem, depression, and anxiety disorders. Prevalence estimates of childhood sexual and physical abuse vary among settings. The prevalence of such abuse in primary care practices was determined, and the physical and psychologic effects in victims of different types of abuse were compared.

Methods.—The cross-sectional study included 1931 women seen at 4 community-based, primary care internal medicine practices. The women, of various ages and marital, educational, and economic status, completed a self-administered, anonymous survey.

Findings.—Twenty-two percent reported childhood or adolescent physical or sexual abuse. Compared with the 1,257 women who reported no abuse, the 204 women who reported abuse in childhood but not in adulthood had more physical symptoms and higher scores for depression, anxiety, somatization, and interpersonal sensitivity. These women were also more likely to be abusing drugs or to have a history of alcohol abuse, to have attempted suicide, and to have had a psychiatric admission. The number of physical symptoms, emotional distress, substance abuse, and suicide attempts did not differ significantly between women abused only as children and those abused only as adults. Women experiencing both childhood and adult abuse had greater levels of psychological problems and physical symptoms than those with childhood or adulthood abuse alone.

Conclusions.—In this large, socioeconomically diverse, community-based population of primary care patients, 1 in 5 women was the victim of sexual or physical abuse. Physical and psychological problems are associated with such abuse, even in women abused in childhood only. Recognizing this may alter healthcare providers' diagnostic and treatment plans for such patients.

▶ This article reminds us of the secrets of childhood sexual abuse that were so horrible Freud chose not to believe them. Perhaps they were not true in Victorian Vienna, but 20% of women in the modern United States have been assaulted as children or adults with very real psychiatric and medical sequelae.

J.C. Ballenger, M.D.

Enhanced Response to Repeated d-Amphetamine Challenge: Evidence for Behavioral Sensitization in Humans

Strakowski SM, Sax KW, Setters MJ, et al (Univ of Cincinnati, Ohio)
Biol Psychiatry 40:872–880, 1996 8–36

Introduction.—Intermittent stimulant exposure that produces a time-dependent, enduring, and progressively greater or more rapid behavioral response is known as behavioral sensitization. Previous studies with animals have shown that stimuli given too closely together in time produce tolerance, whereas stimuli given further apart produce sensitization. The study of behavioral sensitization enhances knowledge of neural plasticity and a variety of psychiatric syndromes. A double-blind, placebo-controlled, randomized clinical trial with 11 volunteers was designed to examine behavioral sensitization to repeated d-amphetamine challenges.

Methods.—Eleven volunteers with an average age of 24.2 years participated in this 4-day protocol. Each received a daily dose of either d-amphetamine (0.25 mg/kg) or placebo so that each had received 2 doses of placebo and 2 doses of drug by the end of the trial. Measurements were taken of eye-blink rate, mood, rate of speech, and activity level hourly for 5 hours after the drug was administered. The ratings were based on a 0–4 point scale of severity, although there was never a rating of greater than 2 as this would indicate mania and psychosis.

Results.—All 4 measures were significantly enhanced after the second amphetamine dose compared with the first amphetamine dose and both placebo doses. There was a significant treatment effect in increased activity/energy 2 hours post administration in which the response to the second amphetamine dose was significantly greater than to the first dose and both placebo doses (Fig 1). The second dose of amphetamine reached a rating of close to 1.25 compared with a first dose of about 0.50 at 2 hours. For elevated mood, the second dose of amphetamine reached a rating near 0.75, whereas the first dose reached less than 0.25 at 4 hours. In speech ratings, the second dose of amphetamine reached a rating of about 1.0 at 4 hours, whereas the first dose reached a rating of less than 0.50.

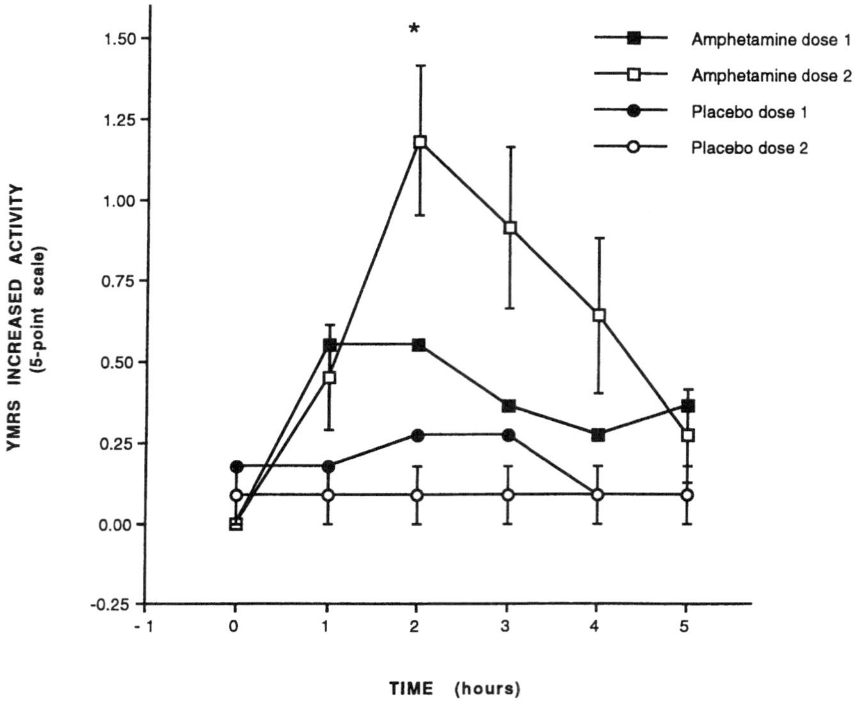

FIGURE 1.—Changes in ratings of the Increased Activity/Energy item from the Young Mania Rating Scale in 11 normal volunteers receiving 2 daily doses of amphetamine (0.25 mg/kg), separated by 48 hours, alternating with 2 daily doses of matched placebo. Two hours post administration, the response after the second amphetamine dose was significantly greater than that after the first amphetamine and both placebo doses ($P < 0.05$, protected t test) (*asterisk*). Error bars for the dose 1 conditions were omitted for clarity. (Reprinted by permission of Elsevier Science Inc., from Enhanced response to repeated d-amphetamine challenge: Evidence for behavioral sensitization in humans, by Strakowski SM, Sax KW, Setters MJ, et al, BIOLOGICAL PSYCHIATRY 40:872–880, copyright 1996 by the Society of Biological Psychiatry.)

Conclusion.—In humans, behavioral sensitization is measurable. Even though a low dose of amphetamine was administered on only 2 occasions separated by 48 hours, an increase in response occurred. In future research, this paradigm may be further developed as a model of human psychopathology.

▶ This study actually provides data on normal humans, supporting the occurrence of behavioral sensitization in a phenomenon akin to kindling. This has long been an area of considerable interest to me as a model for human psychopathology. The study shows evidence of increasing response to repeated doses of amphetamines, providing support for what has, in many ways, been an interesting but theoretical issue. But the issue is one of considerable interest to me and a few of my friends, at least.

J.C. Ballenger, M.D.

New Techniques and Their Contributions to Clinical Psychiatry

Gender Differences in Regional Cerebral Blood Flow During Transient Self-induced Sadness or Happiness

George MS, Ketter TA, Parekh PI, et al (NIH, Bethesda, Md)
Biol Psychiatry 40:859–871, 1996 8–37

Introduction.—The lifetime rates of clinical depression are reported to be at least twice as high for women as for men, but few studies have investigated the neurobiology of gender differences in depression susceptibility. A study of 20 healthy volunteers sought to determine whether women are better able than men to self-induce transient emotional states and whether there are gender differences in regional cerebral blood flow (rCBF) during various emotions.

Methods.—Study participants were 10 women with a mean age of 34.5 years and 10 men with a mean age of 35 years. All were evaluated to confirm their physical and mental health. The 2 groups were similar in mean educational level. Regional cerebral blood flow was mapped while participants performed 4 different tasks: a "resting" period followed by happy, sad, and neutral activation tasks. The happy, sad, and neutral states were evoked by recalling specific life events and by looking at happy, sad, and neutral human faces. Scanning was performed with $H_2{}^{15}O$ positron emission tomography.

Results.—Healthy men and women were both found to have significant changes in regional brain activity during transient emotional states. During the resting period, women had decreased temporal and prefrontal cortex rCBF and increased brain-stem rCBF. Visual analogue ratings yielded no significant differences between groups according to gender on the degree of sadness or happiness induced. Men found the neutral state easiest to induce, followed by happiness and then sadness; the order for women was happiness, then neutral, and lastly sadness. Despite similar self-reported changes in mood, women activated a significantly wider portion of their limbic system than did men during transient sadness. Men had greater variability in self-induced mood states than women, but the difference was not statistically significant.

Conclusion.—Men and women are known to differ significantly in the performance of various cognitive functions. Differences have also been noted in brain volume, both global and regional. This study did not confirm that women are better able than men to self-induce transient emotional states, but there were some gender differences in rCBF during emotional states.

► In this remarkable study, healthy men and women simulated happiness and sadness. Remarkably, changes in rCBF between these states were detected on positron emission tomography scanning. Women activated a significantly larger portion of the limbic system in transient sadness than did men. This study has attracted much national media attention for obvious reasons; however, it also contributes importantly to evolving studies of the brain anatomy of depression.

J.C. Ballenger, M.D.

Advances in Neuroimaging: How Might They Influence Our Diagnostic Classification Scheme?

Rauch SL (Massachusetts Gen Hosp, Charlestown)

Harvard Rev Psychiatry 4:159–162, 1996 8–38

Introduction.—Advances in neuroimaging make the prospect of someday using brain imaging tests in the differential diagnosis of psychiatric disorders less far-fetched than it once was.

Syndrome-based Classification.—The current diagnostic classification scheme of the DSM-IV and ICD-10 reflects the current state of psychiatry. Psychiatric disorders are defined according to signs and symptoms, not pathophysiology. Syndromes, not diseases per se, are diagnosed. These diagnostic criteria, the signs and symptoms, are easily accessible to the clinician and are relatively inexpensive to evaluate. A classification scheme based on pathophysiology could result in more precise treatment with the most effective antidepressants for a particular disorder, or prediction of which patients may develop mania on a particular antidepressant.

Restructuring of Current Diagnostic Criteria.—Findings on brain imaging tests may one day be incorporated into or even replace the current diagnostic criteria for psychiatric disorders. Neuroimaging criteria could be incorporated into diagnostic criteria of specific psychiatric subtypes. Neuroimaging may also result in restructuring of the current classification scheme. For example, the obsessive-compulsive spectrum disorders are currently listed under different categories, but neuroimaging data have revealed that some of them are disorders of corticostriatal dysfunction and may be pathophysiologically related. These disorders may someday be recombined or subdivided.

Discussion.—Neuroimaging is not the only field that is adding information about the neurobiology of psychiatric disease. The techniques of molecular biology and other subspecialties are also providing new information. Neuroimaging is the most powerful means of evaluating brain structure and function. The boundaries of psychiatry and neurology are likely to become blurred as distinctions among specific psychiatric diseases become more clearly defined based on pathophysiology.

► Scott Rauch from the Massachusetts General Hospital group reviews an area of intense interest in the field for a long time, i.e., whether brain neuroimaging or other tests can allow us to make our diagnostic systems more accurate. This has been a "holy grail" for many for a long time, and we do appear to be getting closer to making it a reality.

J.C. Ballenger, M.D.

Increased Prefrontal Sulcal Prominence in Relatively Young Patients With Unipolar Major Depression

Elkis H, Friedman L, Buckley PF, et al (Univ of São Paulo, Brazil; Case Western Reserve Univ, Cleveland, Ohio; Yonsei Univ, Seoul, South Korea)

Psychiatry Res 67:123–134, 1996 8–39

Background.—Several brain imaging studies have demonstrated ventricular enlargement and sulcal prominence in mixed samples of patients with affective disorders. It is not known whether these findings also apply to a homogeneous sample of relatively young patients with unipolar major depression ventricular-to-brain ratio (VBR) and prefrontal sulcal prominence (PSP).

Methods and Findings.—Ventricle/brain ratio and PSP were compared in 24 patients with affective disorders, 40 medical control subjects, and 101 patients with schizophrenia. The mean age of the patients with affective disorders was 39 years. The 3 groups did not differ in VBRs. However, the 2 patient groups were found to have significantly greater PSP than the medical control group. They did not differ significantly from each other on PSP.

Conclusion.—These findings extend previous reports of PSP, but not ventricular enlargement, to relatively young patients with unipolar depression. Patients with schizophrenia and those with affective disorders apparently differ only slightly or not at all in brain morphology at the level of MR resolution used.

► This international group reports increased PSP, but not an increased VBR, in depressed patients as well as schizophrenic patients. Coupled with recent findings of hypometabolism in the frontal lobes in depression, this finding contributes to the growing evidence that depression is associated with pathology in the frontal lobe.

J.C. Ballenger, M.D.

MRI Brain Abnormalities in Chronic Schizophrenia: One Process or More?

Woods BT, Yurgelun-Todd D, Goldstein JM, et al (Texas A & M Med School, Temple, Tex; Harvard Med School, Boston; Harvard Inst of Psychiatric Epidemiology and Genetics, Boston)

Biol Psychiatry 40:585–596, 1996 8–40

Background.—Research has suggested that schizophrenia is mainly a prefrontal-temporal-limbic circuitry disorder. It has been argued that primary neurologic vulnerability to the disease may be established only in the early stages of brain development and is not progressive. Whether brain volume losses in prefrontal and temporal-limbic regions have occurred before or after brain growth is thought to be complete was determined.

Methods and Findings.—Magnetic resonance imaging was performed in 19 patients with chronic schizophrenia and 19 healthy persons matched for age and sex. The scans were segmented into gray and white matter and CSF compartments for the frontal and temporal lobes as well as the posterior cerebral hemispheres. Absolute intracranial cerebrum and subregion volumes, absolute tissue volumes, and tissue-to-intracranial volume (TCV) ratios were analyzed by multivariate analysis of variance. Significant intracranial volume reductions in the frontal lobes and very significantly lower TCV ratios in all 3 major regions were observed in the patients.

Conclusion.—The decreases found in frontal intracranial volumes in schizophrenic patients appeared to reflect a pathologic process that affected the frontal regions before brain growth was complete. The generalized lower TCV ratios in the patients may be attributable to a process that affected the whole cerebrum over a period after the brain volume had reached its maximum levels.

▶ This sophisticated study and review provides evidence that the brain damage in patients with schizophrenia occurred, at least in part, before brain growth was complete. This is consistent with conclusions of many other recent studies and techniques.

J.C. Ballenger, M.D.

Schizophrenia and Cognitive Dysmetria: A Positron-emission Tomography Study of Dysfunctional Prefrontal-Thalamic-Cerebellar Circuitry

Andreasen NC, O'Leary DS, Cizadlo T, et al (Univ of Iowa, Iowa City)

Proc Natl Acad Sci U S A 93:9985–9990, 1996 8–41

Background.—Schizophrenia is marked by cognitive abnormalities, which may be related to dysfunction in the circuitry that coordinates interaction of perception, retention, retrieval, and response. A key role in such interaction may be played by a network between the prefrontal cortex and the cerebellum, linked through the thalamus. Positron emission tomography (PET) scans were performed on patients with schizophrenia while the patients performed cognitive tasks to explore the possibility that such patients manifest a cognitive dysmetria with abnormalities in the above-mentioned circuitry. Differences in activation patterns between patients with and without schizophrenia, in brain regions known to have anatomical connectivity, are suggestive of dysfunctional circuitry in schizophrenia.

Methods.—Participating in the study were 13 healthy volunteers and 14 patients with schizophrenia. Patients underwent PET scanning during performance of 2 tasks (practiced and novel free recall of complex narrative material) that required monitoring of the retrieval and expression of remembered information (prefrontal regions and the cerebellum are activated during retrieval). The 2 tasks were likely to recruit similar neural components, but patients with schizophrenia would be expected to perform equally with the controls during "practiced" recall but poorer than the controls during novel recall.

Results.—Controls had activation of similar brain regions during the 2 tasks. Patients with schizophrenia had decreased blood flow in fronto-thalamic-cerebellar regions during both tasks, suggesting a fundamental deficit in this circuitry in schizophrenia.

Conclusion.—These data suggest that patients with schizophrenia may have dysfunctional prefrontal-thalamic-cerebellar circuitry that results in cognitive dysmetria. Specific variations in circuit abnormalities occurred in schizophrenic patients during the novel vs. practiced tasks; these variations are believed to result from a disruption in functional or anatomical connectivity rather than a generalized decrease in cerebral blood flow. The consistency of the basic pattern of flow across 2 different tasks suggests that connectivity of multiple nodes is associated with schizophrenia.

► This fascinating study from the Iowa group provides support for their hypothesis that there is decreased blood flow in the fronto-thalamic-cerebellar circuit in schizophrenia.

J.C. Ballenger, M.D.

Striatal Dopamine D_2 Receptor Quantification and Superior Temporal Gyrus: Volume Determination in 14 Chronic Schizophrenic Subjects

Tune L, Barta P, Wong D, et al (Emory Univ, Atlanta, Ga; Johns Hopkins School of Medicine, Baltimore, Md; Univ of Alabama-Birmingham)

Psychiatry Res 67:155–158, 1996 8–42

Background.—Multiple brain regions, including the temporal lobe and basal ganglia, have been implicated in the pathophysiology of schizophrenia. The structural and functional interrelationships between these areas (which are connected via the basal ganglia–thalamocortical circuit) in schizophrenic and normal individuals are, therefore, of interest. The authors hypothesized that schizophrenia is associated with elevated striatal D_2 receptor density (B_{max}) and decreased superior temporal volumes.

Methods.—Participating in the study were 14 patients with schizophrenia and 15 healthy individuals. Caudate dopamine D_2 receptor densities were estimated by 2 positron emission tomography scans. The volume of the superior temporal gyrus was measured by MRI.

Results.—Patients with schizophrenia had significantly higher average values for B_{max} and significantly smaller average volumes for the left superior temporal gyrus than did controls. There was also a tendency for patients with schizophrenia to have smaller average volumes for the right superior temporal gyrus.

Conclusion.—The relationships between structure and function in selected brain regions in schizophrenia can be explored through a combination of structural and functional neuroimaging techniques. An inverse relationship was found between elevated B_{max} values and reduced superior temporal gyral volume. These findings should be considered preliminary and should be confirmed with studies including a larger patient base.

► This report from several of the most active neuroimaging groups provides further evidence of increased dopamine receptors in certain regions, in patients with schizophrenia as well as smaller average volume of the superior temporal gyri. The report contributes to the slowly coalescing evidence in this area.

J.C. Ballenger, M.D.

Magnetic Resonance Image-guided Stereotactic Cingulotomy for Intractable Psychiatric Disease

Spangler WJ, Cosgrove GR, Ballantine HT Jr, et al (Massachusetts Gen Hosp, Boston; McLean Hosp, Boston; Harvard Med School, Boston)

Neurosurgery 38:1071–1078, 1996 8–43

Introduction.—Cingulotomy was once widely used in the treatment of intractable psychiatric disease, but it was largely replaced by other techniques. However, there are still some patients who do not respond to treatment and remain severely disabled. If cingulotomy would improve the treatment and functional results in this group, it might be considered. An experience with MRI-guided stereotactic cingulotomy in 34 patients with intractable psychiatric disease is reported.

Patients.—The patients were 18 men and 16 women, whose mean age was 37 years. Of these, 31 were monitored for longer than 6 months. The primary diagnosis was intractable major affective disorder in 15 patients and obsessive-compulsive disorder (OCD) in 15, 12 of whom had coexistent major depression. The other patient had an unclassifiable diagnosis. All operations were done using an MRI-compatible stereotactic frame and radiofrequency thermocoagulation. Fourteen patients had repeat cingulotomy, for a total of 50 procedures.

Results.—Of the patients, 38% were considered complete responders, 23% were positive responders, and 38% were nonresponders. Of the patients undergoing repeat cingulotomy, 36% were responders, 36% were possible responders, and 28% were nonresponders. The response rate was 53% for patients with major affective disorder, vs. 27% for those with OCD. Two patients committed suicide. The results were similar to historical results of cingulotomy using earlier methods, and they compared favorably with other neurosurgical procedures performed for intractable psychiatric disease. Side effects were uncommon.

Conclusions.—In patients with intractable psychiatric disease, MRI-guided cingulotomy is a safe procedure with a response rate of 33.3% or better. Longer follow-up is needed to establish the treatment role of this procedure. The response appears to be better in patients with major affective disorder than in patients with OCD.

► This article employs new MRI capabilities to "modernize" stereotactic cingulotomy for intractable OCD and depressed patients. The authors report good results in more than a third with the first surgery, and a similar percentage on a second try. Surprisingly, the results were better in the depressed patients. These are essentially the same findings seen in multiple studies of psychosurgery. It would appear that the available scientific evidence would make psychosurgery a treatment option for more patients who have not been helped by our treatments. Unfortunately, it is even more shrouded in stigma and bias than electroconvulsive therapy.

J.C. Ballenger, M.D.

Applicability of Telemedicine for Assessing Patients With Schizophrenia: Acceptance and Reliability

Zarate CA Jr, Weinstock L, Cukor P, et al (Harvard Med School, Boston; McLean Hosp, Belmont, Mass; Massachusetts Gen Hosp, Boston)

J Clin Psychiatry 58:22–25, 1997 8–44

Background.—Telemedicine, the use of communications technology to deliver health care, is not frequently used in the psychiatric setting. Interest has recently increased because of economic pressures. If telemedicine is to be applied to increase the availability of health care to underserved populations, its acceptance and reliability with patients with major psychiatric disorders must be documented. A study of patients with well-characterized DSM-IV schizophrenia was conducted to determine the acceptability and reliability to telemedicine for this patient group.

Methods.—The study group consisted of 45 patients who met DMS-IV criteria for schizophrenia from the Bipolar and Psychotic Disorders Program at McLean Hospital. The reliability of the Brief Psychiatric Rating Scale, the Scale for the Assessment of Positive Symptoms, and the Scale for Assessment of Negative Symptoms was assessed when administered in person, by videoconferencing at low bandwidth, and by videoconferencing at high bandwidth. All patients and interviewers rated the study interviews by comparing them to previous experience with live interviews.

Results.—The total scores on the Brief Psychiatric Rating Scale and the Scale for the Assessment of Positive Symptoms were equally reliable by all 3 interview methods. The total score on the Scale for the Assessment of Negative Symptoms was less reliable at the low bandwidth, especially those symptoms that rely on nonverbal cues. Video interviews were accepted by patients in both groups, although the patients who had high bandwidth interviews were more likely to prefer the videoconferences to live interviews.

Conclusions.—The reliability of video evaluations was compared to that of live interviews of schizophrenic patients in a systematic, controlled study. Live interviews, video at low bandwidth, and video at high bandwidth were all equally reliable in determining global schizophrenia severity and a summary score of positive symptoms. Assessment of negative symptoms was less reliable at lower bandwidth. This technology was accepted by all patients in this study. Telemedicine appears to provide a reliable method of evaluating schizophrenic patients in remote locations who would otherwise have limited access to psychiatric services.

► Getting psychiatric expertise to remote regions has been almost impossible until the recent advent of telemedicine links. This is one of several articles describing how reliable and well-accepted the technique is.

J.C. Ballenger, M.D.

Managed Care and Psychiatry

Differences in 4-year Health Outcomes for Elderly and Poor, Chronically Ill Patients Treated in HMO and Fee-for-Service Systems: Results From the Medical Outcomes Study

Ware JE Jr, Bayliss MS, Rogers WH, et al (New England Med Ctr, Boston)
JAMA 276:1039–1047, 1996 8–45

Background.—Enrollment in HMOs has increased 10–fold since 1976, and government policies now seek to shift publicly insured patients to HMOs. The Medical Outcomes Study compared 4-year health outcomes for chronically ill patients treated in well-established HMOs with fee-for-service (FFS) plans serving the same medical marketplaces in Boston, Chicago and Los Angeles. Only those with hypertension, non–insulin-dependent diabetes mellitus, recent acute myocardial infarction, congestive heart failure, and depressive disorder were followed. This study focused on patients aged at least 65 years covered by Medicare and those near or below the poverty line.

Methods.—The study group consisted of 2,235 adult patients with one of the 5 index conditions who were sampled in 1986 and followed through 1990. Medicare and low income patients were analyzed separately. The Short-Form Health Survey (SF-36) was used to determine differences in physical and mental health over the 4-year study period.

Results.—Overall, physical health declined and mental health remained stable over the 4-year follow-up period of this study. These physical declines were significantly larger for the elderly than for the nonelderly in the study group. For the average patient, physical and mental health outcomes were not different between the HMO and FFS systems. For elderly Medicare patients, physical health declines were significantly more common in HMOs than in FFS plans. For patients near or below the poverty line, outcomes were more favorable in the FFS system than in HMOs.

Conclusion.—Although for the average patient there was no difference in medical outcome between the HMO and FFS systems, for poor and elderly patients, health outcomes were worse in HMOs than in FFS systems. These results indicate that vulnerable subgroups need to be separately monitored by health care plans to ensure that their needs are being adequately met.

▶ This study followed more than 2,000 patients, comparing their outcomes in HMO vs. FFS systems. Most patients did equally well in the 2 payment systems; however, the elderly and the poor did less well in the HMOs than in the FFS system. It is not surprising that certain groups would fare less well in 1 system than in another because the systems are quite different. It will be incumbent on all of us to pay special attention to vulnerable subgroups, 2 of which are identified in this study.

J.C. Ballenger, M.D.

Does Managed Care Permit Appropriate Use of Psychotherapy?
Borenstein DB (Univ of California, Los Angeles)
Psychiatric Serv 47:971–974, 1996 8–46

Introduction.—The coverage of psychiatric care has been reduced by managed care plans since the late 1980s, and there have been restrictions placed on access to treatment. Nervous and behavioral health benefits began to be managed separately from other medical benefits. Outpatient treatment became very restricted, forcing inpatient hospital psychiatric treatment to be extended. One study has shown that psychoanalysis and psychotherapy could be provided for less than 7.5% of the total medical expense when the risk is spread across a significant proportion of the population. Trends in managed care and their restrictions on psychotherapy were examined.

Considerations.—There is a high correlation between the use of psychotherapy and nervousness, depression, general health problems, and functional impairments. In cancer patients, survival time is increased when treatment includes psychotherapy. Patients with depression require psychotherapy. Patients with anorexia nervosa have mortality rates 5 times less when receiving long-term psychotherapy compared with those of patients receiving brief, general medical care. Significant economic loss results among the depressed because of work impairment. Only 4.3% of the population used outpatient psychotherapy when care was free.

Quality Concerns.—A problem has been that psychiatrists, who prescribe the medication, have had little contact with the patient's psychotherapist. A recent study showed that it was more cost effective for the psychiatrist to provide the medication and the psychotherapy than to split the treatment. Whereas managed care has brought the cost of mental health care down to some 4% from about 10% of medical expenses, access and quality have also been reduced. Adverse health outcomes are likely to result from programs that restrict long-term treatment. Nevertheless, some managed care plans hope to further reduce mental care costs to 2% of medical expenses.

Conclusion.—There appears to be no way to further reduce the cost of treating mental illness without jeopardizing quality of care. The cost-based constraints on care are not acceptable until carefully constructed outcome studies demonstrate that they produce no adverse effects on established psychiatric treatments.

► This study examines the explosive question in our field as to whether there will be a place for psychotherapy in managed care. It points out that some studies show that it is more effective for a psychiatrist to provide both medication and psychotherapy than to split the treatment between psychiatrist and psychotherapist, as has become a frequent strategy in managed care. The paper also presents multiple nuggets of data, including the fact that only 4.3% of the population uses psychotherapy even when it is free and that multiple groups, such as depressed anorectic patients, can be treated cost effectively.

J.C. Ballenger, M.D.

Is Psychotherapy Ever Medically Necessary?

Bennett MJ (Harvard Med School, Boston)

Psychiatric Serv 47:966–970, 1996 8–47

Background.—Mental health care has become controversial, as the needs of patients and the allocation of resources are rethought by managed care providers. The usefulness of psychotherapy is no longer taken for granted. This paper presented a framework for providing mental health care to populations rather than individuals and suggested a role for psychotherapy.

Psychotherapy Before Managed Care.—Studies of the mental health care system that existed before the advent of managed health care have revealed that mental disorder was common, whereas treatment was not common. Among those who did receive mental health treatment, most did not have a diagnosable mental disorder at the time of treatment. Mental health care specialists frequently practiced long-term psychotherapy, which accounted for most mental health expenditures. There does not appear to have been a strong relationship between need for treatment and receipt of treatment under the system that existed before managed care. At least some mental health care appeared to be discretionary.

Medically Necessary Psychotherapy.—Most managed care organizations consider treatments to be medically necessary if they establish or re-establish normality or limit disability associated with a diagnosable disorder. Because mental health treatment is heterogeneous and large, long-term, controlled clinical trials are often unavailable, it is difficult for exact treatment paradigms to be created. Managed care systems determine a need for mental health services based on the presence of a mental disorder and either a state of clinical instability or impaired function resulting from the specific disorder. Within this context, psychotherapy will be viewed as medically necessary if it is effective in treating defined mental disorders by itself, as short-term adjunctive therapy or as the best therapy when effective therapy has not been defined. Treatment is most controversial for patients who have complex disorders that are refractory to treatment. These patients function poorly on a chronic basis and require long-term treatment. For these complex patients, brief periods of psychotherapy to achieve stabilization or remediation could be interspersed with longer periods of case management and support for rehabilitation.

Conclusion.—Despite its limitations, the *Diagnostic and Statistical Manual of Mental Disorders* system has value in setting thresholds beyond which need for treatment can be defined. These thresholds are important in rational resource application by managed care entities. Psychotherapy is a treatment tool and will continue to be considered useful as long as it can be shown to be effective in treating mental disorder.

► This is a thoughtful article by Michael Bennett who practiced psychotherapy in the Harvard Community Health Plan for a long time and now is employed by an HMO company. Because of that background, the article is both a little more readable and a little more understandable to the rest us.

J.C. Ballenger, M.D.

Psychiatry, Primary Care, and General Medicine

Somatic Symptoms of Distress: An International Primary Care Study

Simon G, Gater R, Kisely S, et al (Group Health Cooperative, Seattle; Univ of Manchester, England; Universita di Verona, Italy)

Psychosom Med 58:481–488, 1996 8–48

Introduction.—Psychological distress–related somatic symptoms are linked to significant disability and health utilization. A large, cross-national cohort was evaluated to determine cross-national differences in somatic symptoms associated with psychological distress.

Methods.—The Psychological Problems in General Health Care investigation evaluated the prevalence, management, and outcomes of common psychological disorders among patients in primary care from 15 centers in 14 countries. Consecutive or randomized samples of patients from each center completed a 28-item General Health Questionnaire, Composite International Diagnostic Interview, and questions regarding medical history, use of health care services, and functional disability.

Results.—A total of 5,438 patients completed all evaluations. The number of somatic symptoms was associated with psychological distress at all sites. Anxiety and depressive symptoms were correlated with somatic symptom counts; specific somatic symptoms or symptom clusters did not indicate differential correlation with anxiety or depression. Somatic symptoms clustered into significant groups but did not reveal differential association with anxiety or depression (Table 2). Evaluation of individual somatic symptoms and symptom clusters did not show clear patterns of association by geography or level of economic development.

TABLE 2.—Point-Biserial Correlation of Specific Somatic Symptoms With Current Distress Scores for All Sites Combined

	Anxiety	Depression	Distress
Weakness	.21	.21	.24
Headache	.21	.18	.23
Palpitations	.22	.17	.22
Shortness of breath	.20	.16	.20
Dizziness	.20	.15	.20
Heavy/light feelings	.19	.16	.19
Chest pain	.17	.15	.18
Lump in throat	.18	.14	.18
Nausea	.18	.14	.18
Excessive gas	.19	.10	.18
Trouble walking	.14	.16	.17
Abdominal pain	.17	.13	.17
Ears ringing/buzzing	.15	.14	.17
Arm/leg pain	.16	.13	.17
Joint pain	.16	.11	.16
Back pain	.15	.12	.15
Numbness/tingling	.14	.12	.15
Bad taste	.12	.10	.13
Vomiting	.12	.09	.12
Skin crawling/creeping	.11	.09	.12
Blurred vision	.10	.09	.11
Diarrhea	.10	.06	.10
Shaking spells	.06	.09	.08

(Courtesy of Simon G, Gater R, Kisely S, et al: Somatic symptoms of distress: An international primary care study. *Psychosom Med* 58:481–488, 1996.)

Conclusion.—Findings indicate several similarities in symptoms patterns and strong correlations between somatic symptoms and psychological distress across a diverse range of primary care sites.

▶ This study is one that helps us as we struggle to approach the patients with somatic symptoms related to psychiatric problems. In a sample of more than 5,400 patients, these authors clearly correlate psychological distress with somatic symptoms. It is no surprise that they found that depression and anxiety were the most frequent psychiatric causes of somatic symptoms.

J.C. Ballenger, M.D.

Multisomatoform Disorder: An Alternative to Undifferentiated Somatoform Disorder for the Somatizing Patient in Primary Care

Kroenke K, Spitzer RL, deGruy FV III, et al (Uniformed Services Univ of the Health Sciences, Bethesda, Md; New York State Psychiatric Inst, New York; Columbia Univ, New York, et al)

Arch Gen Psychiatry 54:352–358, 1997 8–49

Background.—At least one quarter of all physical symptoms that are seen in outpatient visits are never adequately physically explained and may be considered somatoform. Somatization Disorder, which was introduced in the *Diagnostic and Statistical Manual of Mental Disorders*, ed III, revised, is a well-validated construct useful in classifying patients with extreme somatization symptoms, but the majority of patients seen in an outpatient setting do not meet that high symptom threshold. During the Primary Care Evaluation of Mental Disorders (PRIME-MD) 1000 Study, criteria were developed for a new somatoform disorder, multisomatoform disorder, defined as at least 3 current somatoform symptoms from a 15-symptom checklist and at least a 2-year history of somatoform symptoms. The 15 symptoms were chosen to account for greater than 90% of outpatient visits for physical complaints. The data from the PRIME-MD Study of 1,000 patients were used to evaluate the validity of this new somatoform diagnosis.

Study Design.—The PRIME-MD study population consisted of 1,000 patients seen for medical care at 4 primary clinics. The average age of these patients was 55 years. Of the study group, 60% were women, 58% were white, and 28% were college graduates. All participants were examined with PRIME-MD, a validated diagnostic interview, and the 20-item Short Form General Health Survey (SF-20). Outcomes included 6 areas of health-related quality of life, self-reported disability and health care use, and physician-rated interview difficulty.

Findings.—Of the 1,000 patients included in this study, 139 had a PRIME-MD somatoform diagnosis, including 82 with a multisomatoform diagnosis. Compared to patients without somatoform disorder, patients with somatoform disorder were more likely to be younger, women, and less educated. Psychiatric co-morbidity was common, as 61% had a co-existing mood disorder and 50% had anxiety disorder. Multisomatoform disorder was associated with similar impairment in health-related quality of life, more self-reported disability days and health care use, and greater clinician-determined patient difficulty than mood and anxiety disorder.

Conclusions.—Multisomatoform disorder, defined as at least 3 current medically unexplained physical symptoms and a history of somatization, appears to be a valid diagnosis of relevance to the outpatient population. The impairment in people with a diagnosis of this disorder is at least as great as that of many Axis I disorders. This diagnosis should not be precluded because of co-morbid psychiatric symptoms, as multisomatoform disorder has a large and independent effect on impairment.

► This work is from Kroenke, Spitzer, and deGruy studying patients who have multiple puzzling physical symptoms in primary care. These patients make up one out of every seven visits to primary care physicians and one quarter of visits to internists. This group has been an important contributor to this area. This is an interesting, affirmative article.

J.C. Ballenger, M.D.

Consultation-Liaison Psychiatry in General Practice

Carr VJ, Lewin TJ, Walton JM, et al (Univ of Newcastle, Callaghan, Australia)
Aust N Z J Psychiatry 31:85–94, 1997 8–50

Background.—In Australia, an estimated 74% of patients with a mental disorder are treated in general practice; more than 40% of these patients may have serious or chronic mental disorders. In the last 25 years, there have been many studies of the incidence of psychiatric illness in patients treated by general practitioners. This incidence has been estimated at 25% or more, although about half are undetected by the general practitioner. In response to these findings, educational programs in the detection and management of psychiatric problems in the primary care setting have been developed, as well as the provision of consultation-liaison psychiatric services to general practitioners. The characteristics of patients referred to such services were described.

Methods.—During a 12-month period, 303 patients were referred to consultation-liaison psychiatric services provided to 8 group general prac-

TABLE 3.—Diagnostic and Statistical Manual of Mental Disorders, Edition III, Revised Axis I Diagnoses for Patients Referred to the Consultation-Liaison Service

DSM-III-R Clinical Audit Diagnosis (n=303)	n	%
Organic mental disorder	11	3.6
Any substance abuse/dependence	37	12.2
Alcohol	21	6.9
Other drugs	22	7.3
Schizophrenia/other psychoses	3	1.0
Any mood disorder	87	28.7
Bipolar disorder	2	0.7
Major depressive disorder	53	17.5
Dysthymia	36	11.9
Other	9	3.0
Any anxiety disorder	43	14.2
Panic disorder with agoraphobia	13	4.3
Panic disorder without agoraphobia	5	1.7
Agoraphobia without panic attacks	1	0.3
Generalised anxiety disorder	7	2.3
Simple phobia	1	0.3
Social phobia	0	0.0
Obsessive-compulsive disorder	2	0.7
Posttraumatic stress disorder	10	3.3
Other	7	2.3
Somatoform disorder	4	1.3
Eating disorder	5	1.7
Other specific Axis I disorder	8	2.6
Mental disorder not otherwise specified	21	6.9
Adjustment disorder	46	15.2
V Codes	42	13.9
No Axis I disorder/condition	16	5.3

(Courtesy of Carr VJ, Lewin TJ, Walton JM, et al: Consultation-liaison psychiatry in general practice. *Aust N Z J Psychiatry* 31:85–94, 1997.)

tices. Information was collected regarding patient demographic characteristics, reasons for referral, psychiatric diagnoses, use of psychotropic medication, clinical management, and prognosis. Patients were also invited to participate in a separate, prospective study to evaluate outcome using interviews and questionnaires.

Results.—Of 303 eligible patients, 86 agreed to participate; 79 of these were assessed by the Composite International Diagnostic Interview and by questionnaire; 7 patients completed the questionnaire only. A sample of 535 nonreferred patients also completed the questionnaire. The most common reasons for referral were depression, anxiety, diagnostic assessment, and impaired relationships. The most common psychiatric diagnoses were mood disorders; mild, transient conditions; anxiety; and substance abuse disorders (Table 3). The general practitioners were actively involved in treatment in 53% of cases after the psychiatric consultation. The rate of referral to another mental heath agency was 44%.

Discussion.—The diagnoses of these patients differ from the diagnoses of patients treated in general hospitals, primarily in the lower rates of organic brain syndromes, suicide risk evaluations, and differential diagnosis of somatic symptoms. In both settings, trained general practitioners rather than specialist mental health clinicians may be able to treat patients with mild, transient problems. The ability of general practitioners to detect anxiety disorders and somatoform disorders needs improvement. A description of the consultation-liaison psychiatric services is provided in the paper.

► In Australia, 75% of the care rendered to people with psychiatric conditions is in primary care, even higher than in the United States. After instituting a consult/liaison service, the authors found that 44% of these patients actually needed a referral to a mental health agency, cetainly more than occurs in the U.S. Have they had the courage or foresight to discover something we are reluctant to discover?

J.C. Ballenger, M.D.

Gender, Quality of Life, and Mental Disorders in Primary Care: Results From the PRIME-MD 1000 Study

Linzer M, Spitzer R, Kroenke K, et al (Division of Gen Medicine, Madison, Wis; Columbia Univ, New York; Uniformed Services Univ, Bethesda, Md; et al)

Am J Med 101:526–533, 1996 8–51

Introduction.—Many studies indicate that women in primary care have an excess of certain mental disorders, particularly mood disorders, and that physicians often fail to diagnose these disorders. Data from a large primary care study (PRIME-MD 1000) were analyzed for gender differences in the frequency of mental disorders in the primary care setting and the potential impact of these differences on health-related quality of life (HRQL).

TABLE 3.—Health-related Quality of Life in Women and Men

HRQL*: Mean (SD)	Women	Men	P
Physical function	67 (28)	76 (26)	.0001
Pain	56 (27)	63 (28)	.0005
Social	79 (30)	85 (26)	.001
General health	53 (26)	59 (28)	.001
Role function	70 (42)	76 (40)	.02
Mental health	69 (20)	76 (18)	.0001
Disability days (mean, past 3 months)	6.1	3.7	.02
MD office visits (mean, past 3 months)	1.5	1.8	.14
ER visits (mean, past 3 months)	.34	.19	.01

*All health-related quality of life scales scored from 1–100, 100 indicating best health.
Abbreviations: HRQL, health-related quality of life; *ER*, emergency room.
(Reprinted by permission of the publisher from Linzer M, Spitzer R, Kroenke K, et al: Gender, quality of life, and mental disorders in primary care: Results from the PRIME-MD 1000 Study. AMERICAN JOURNAL OF MEDICINE, 101:526–533, copyright 1996 by Excerpta Medica, Inc.)

Methods.—One thousand patients were evaluated during the PRIME-MD Study at 4 primary care sites to diagnose mood, anxiety, somatoform, alcohol, and binge-eating disorders. The instrument used contained 2 parts: a 1–page patient questionnaire (PQ) and a clinician's evaluation guide (CEG). The CEG is a structured clinical interview designed to follow

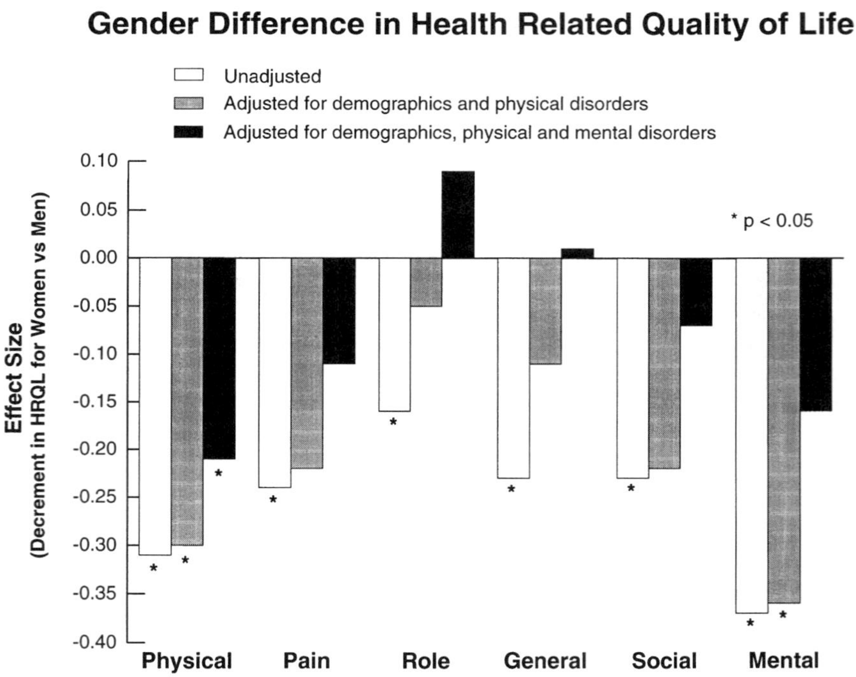

FIGURE.—Gender difference in health-related quality of life. (Reprinted by permission of the publisher from Linzer M, Spitzer R, Kroenke K, et al: Gender, quality of life, and mental disorders in primary care: Results from the PRIME-MD 1000 Study. *American Journal of Medicine*, vol. 101, pp. 526–533. Copyright 1996 by Excerpta Medica, Inc.)

up on positive responses to the PQ. Health-related quality of life was assessed with the Medical Outcomes Study SF-20 General Health Survey. Patients in the study had a mean age of 55 years; 56% were women and 58% were white. Sixty-one percent of physicians were men. The most common physical disorders in the group were hypertension (48%) and arthritis (23%); 39% had 1 or more mental disorders.

Results.—Men and women differed significantly in certain baseline demographic characteristics. Women were less likely to have a college degree or to be married and more likely to be nonwhite. Half of the women were obese, but only one third of the men were. Women were significantly more likely than men to have any mental disorder (43% vs. 33%) and to have psychiatric co-morbidity (26% vs. 15%). Particularly prominent among the women patients were mood disorders, anxiety disorders, somatoform disorders, and binge eating. Women had significantly worse HRQL than men, scoring lower in all 6 domains of the SF-20 (Table 3). After controlling for number of mental disorders, however, differences in HRQL were eliminated in 5 of 6 domains (Figure). Female physicians were more sensitive than male physicians to PRIME–MD–diagnosed psychiatric caseness, but women patients were not less satisfied with care from male physicians.

Discussion.—Women in this sample of primary care patients were significantly more likely than men to have mood, anxiety, and somatoform disorders and psychiatric co-morbidity. Largely as a result of these mental disorders, women scored significantly lower on HRQL. It is important for primary care physicians to screen for and treat common mental disorders in their female patients.

► This study is similar to Abstract 8–52, a brief survey for detection of psychiatric problems in primary care. PRIME-MD questionnaire reviewed in this study also proves to be reliable, sensitive, and predictive. The authors found a much higher rate of psychiatric problems in women than in men in primary care, and they make a plea for closer attention to this issue. If you followed this section this year and in previous years, you know that I think this is an extremely important issue for both female and male patients in primary care. If we are going to use primary care physicians as gatekeepers for most patients, we need to help our primary care colleagues to identify and effectively treat psychiatric patients to a much greater degree than we are currently able to do.

J.C. Ballenger, M.D.

Brief Screens for Mental Disorders in Primary Care

Leon AC, Olfson M, Weissman MM, et al (Cornell Univ, New York; Columbia Univ, New York; Kaiser Permentante, Oakland, Calif; et al)

J Gen Intern Med 11:426–430, 1996 8–52

Introduction.—For individual and multiple psychiatric disorders, there have been efforts to develop screens for internists in outpatient practice who serve as gatekeepers to more specialized services. To facilitate diagnosis of mental disorders, there is the Symptom Driven Diagnostic System for Primary Care, which consists of diagnostic screens, diagnostic modules, and a longitudinal tracking form. Included are self-administered screens for alcohol dependence, drug dependence, generalized anxiety disorder, major depressive disorder, obsessive-compulsive disorder, panic disorder, and suicidal ideation. This system was updated for the *Diagnostic and Statistical Manual of Mental Disorders,* fourth edition. The results of the validation of the diagnostic screens were reported.

Methods.—There were 1,001 patients, two thirds of whom were women, who completed the self-administered screening questionnaire, which contained 26 items on multiple mental disorders. A research nurse administered brief diagnostic modules, structured for psychiatric diagnoses.

Results.—Nearly 90% of those with 1 of the 6 disorders were detected by this screen, and more than half who screened positively met the criteria for the disorder. Alcohol dependence had a sensitivity of 0.75 and a predictive value of 0.58. Drug dependence had a sensitivity of 0.74 and a predictive value of 0.44. Major depressive disorder had a sensitivity of 0.71 and a predictive value of 0.52. Obsessive compulsive disorder had a sensitivity of 0.71 and a predictive value of 0.15. Panic disorder had a sensitivity of 0.71 and a predictive value of 0.43. Patients with symptoms who met established diagnostic criteria and those who did not were distinguished with this screen.

Conclusion.—This screen proved valuable in distinguishing between patients with and without psychiatric disorders. Previously unrecognized patients with disorders were detected with this screen; the screening would prove to be valuable for primary care physicians in psychiatric diagnosis. The brief screens would serve as the first in a 2-stage assessment procedure. However, this screen cannot alter patient outcomes if mental health support personnel are not accessible.

► An important issue for our field, and one I have followed in the YEAR BOOK for the last few years, is the presentation of psychiatric disorders in primary care or general medical care. This article reviews a short screening instrument which has been recently studied. It identified patients with a high level of sensitivity and predictive value. It can be of considerable value if primary care physicians use it and—as the authors themselves pointed out—if mental health personnel are available to help manage these patients. Our availability to help our primary care physicians is a central issue and one that we must approach aggressively, in my opinion, in the very near future. I, personally, favor more extensive use of psychiatrists actually co-practicing with primary care physicians because the idea is so popular with patients and with our colleagues. It also avoids the difficulty in getting patients to accept a psychiatric referral to another facility and physician. We will continue to follow this issue.

J.C. Ballenger, M.D.

Psychological Symptoms, Somatic Symptoms, and Psychiatric Disorder in Chronic Fatigue and Chronic Fatigue Syndrome: A Prospective Study in the Primary Care Setting

Wessely S, Chalder T, Hirsch S, et al (King's College School of Medicine and Dentistry, London; Charing Cross and Westminster Med School, London; Royal Free Hosp School of Medicine, London)

Am J Psychiatry 153:1050–1059, 1996 8–53

Background.—Controversy persists over possible connections between chronic fatigue syndrome and psychiatric disease. The relationship of chronic fatigue and chronic fatigue syndrome to somatic and psychological symptoms and to psychiatric diagnoses was studied.

Methods.—Patients seen at 6 general practice clinics with viral symptoms were matched with same-age control patients. Six months later, patients from each group were screened for persistent fatigue by means of a fatigue questionnaire and a general health questionnaire. Those from both groups who had experienced significant fatigue returned for blood testing, a psychiatric interview, and administration of a number of questionnaires covering fatigue, somatic symptoms, psychiatric health, and the outcome of the index illness. Chronic fatigue and chronic fatigue syndrome were diagnosed based on the 1994 revised criteria of the Centers for Disease Control (CDC).

Results.—Patients with chronic fatigue and chronic fatigue syndrome were significantly more likely than nonfatigued respondents to have a previous or current psychiatric diagnosis and to have taken psychotropic drugs. Of the 185 patients with chronic fatigue completing the evaluation, 64 (34.6%) were probably depressed and 31 (16.8%) were definitely depressed. Also, 113 (61.1%) had probable anxiety disorder and 81 (43.8%) had definite anxiety disorder. Sixteen (44.4%) of the 36 patients with chronic fatigue syndrome were probably depressed, 10 (27.8%) were definitely depressed, 24 (66.7%) had probable anxiety and 19 (52.8%) had definite anxiety.

The probable presence of psychiatric disorder at first evaluation was significantly greater for patients with chronic fatigue syndrome than for those without fatigue. The mean number of reported somatic symptoms was linearly related to the number of reported symptoms from the 1994 CDC definition of chronic fatigue syndrome, with no specific symptom profile being seen.

Conclusion.—Primary care patients with chronic fatigue and chronic fatigue syndrome are more likely to exhibit a diagnosis of depression or anxiety disorder than nonfatigued patients.

► This careful study contributes to the continuing evolution of our understanding of the chronic fatigue syndrome. The authors found a high rate of anxiety and depression in these patients, a rate similar to those of most previous studies.

J.C. Ballenger, M.D.

Treatment Outcomes for Primary Care Patients With Major Depression and Lifetime Anxiety Disorders

Brown C, Schulberg HC, Madonia MJ, et al (Univ of Pittsburgh, Pa)

Am J Psychiatry 153:1293–1300, 1996 8–54

Background.—Among psychiatric patients, major depression is seen as often as 60% of the time with co-morbid panic or generalized anxiety disorder. The clinical outcome for primary care patients with major depression was compared with that of depressed patients with co-morbid lifetime anxiety disorders, when they received either psychotherapy or pharmacotherapy.

Methods.—Adults who were found on screening to meet criteria for major depression were randomzied to receive usual care by the primary care physician, interpersonal psychotherapy, or nortriptyline. Patients were also evaluated for other psychiatric (axis I) disorders or personality (axis II) disorders and any lifetime history of generalized anxiety or panic disorders. Patient depressive symptoms, anxiety levels, and mental and physical health-related functioning were evaluated at intervals.

Results.—Depressed patients with lifetime co-morbid anxiety were significantly older than those with depression alone, and they reported significantly more depression, anxiety symptoms, and suicidal thoughts. Personality disorder was significantly more likely to be diagnosed in those with co-morbid anxiety, and those patients exhibited significantly poorer function in psychosocial and health realms. Patients with co-morbid anxiety were initially more depressed, improved more slowly than those with only depression, and showed less symptom improvement with either psychotherapy or pharmacotherapy. The difference was most pronounced for those with panic disorder. With psychotherapy, patients with depression with or without anxiety disorder improved significantly more than those with co-morbid panic. Pharmacotherapy was not related to any difference in improvement between groups.

Conclusion.—Pharmacotherapy and psychotherapy are equally effective for treating depressed patients, with or without co-morbid anxiety disorder, but not those with co-morbid panic disorder. It is crucial for primary care physicians to seek symptoms of panic disorder in their depressed patients.

▶ This important study from the Pittsburgh group shows that although depressed patients in primary care do equally well with pharmacotherapy or psychotherapy, this is clearly not true if the patient has co-morbid panic disorder. Those patients appear to require pharmacotherapy to improve. One important issue that we will need to help our primary care colleagues to understand is the critical importance of the presence of panic disorder in their patients.

J.C. Ballenger, M.D.

A Preliminary Study to Examine the Adequacy of Long-term Treatment of Depression and the Extent of Recovery in General Practice

Hawley CJ, Quick SJ, Harding MJ, et al (Queen Elizabeth II Hosp, Hertfordshire, England; Woodbridge Hill Surgery, Guildford, England; Hertfordshire, England)

Br J Gen Pract 47:233–234, 1997 8–55

Background.—In general outpatient practice, once depression has been diagnosed and treatment initiated, many patients receive prescriptions for long-term therapy to avoid unnecessary office visits. It is not known whether these patients are receiving adequate medication to remain symptom-free.

Study Design.—The study site was a training practice of 9 partners in a relatively affluent area. All 193 patients with mood disorder who received repeat prescriptions of amitriptyline, dothiepin, fluoxetine, or paroxetine for at least a 6-month period were identified and 100 were randomly selected to participate in this study. Current dosage was obtained from computer records. The participants were mailed the Beck Depression Inventory (BDI) and a short drug history questionnaire. A BDI score of no more than 11 was defined as remission, 11–24 as subsyndromal illness, and greater than 24 as syndromal major depression.

Results.—The response rate was 78%, including 24 men and 45 women aged 20–91 years. There were 55 patients receiving tricyclics and 23 receiving selective serotonin reuptake inhibitors (SSRIs). Patients receiving tricyclics were less likely to be receiving adequate medication doses than patients receiving SSRIs (Table 1). The average dose of tricyclic antidepressants was 70 mg, although 75 mg/day is the smallest dose that has been shown to be better than placebo in a controlled clinical trial. Of the 78 patients in the study group, only 35% had a BDI score less than 11, 44% had scores between 11 and 24, and 21% had a BDI score greater than 24. The average BDI score was 17.5 in patients receiving tricyclic antidepressants and 15.8 in patients receiving SSRIs.

Conclusions.—In a group of 78 outpatients receiving long-term therapy for depression, only 35% were in full remission and 21% appeared to have persistent syndromal major depression. Most patients appeared to be receiving suboptimal dosages of tricyclic antidepressant medications. The results of this study suggest that more effort is required to ensure that

TABLE 1.—Distribution of Doses and Beck Depression Inventory Scores

	Daily dose (mg)			BDI score		
AMI/DOT	≥ 125	<125, ≥75	<75	≤11	>11, <24	≥24
n=55	13%	43%	44%	31%	45.5%	23.5%
PAR/FLU	≥20	<20		≤11	>11, <24	≥24
n=23	100%	0%		43.5%	39%	17.5%

Abbreviations: AMI, amitriptyline; *DOT,* dothiepin; *PAR,* paroxetine; *FLU,* fluoxetine; *BDI,* Beck Depression Inventory.
(Courtesy of Hawley CJ, Quick SJ, Harding MJ, et al: A preliminary study to examine the adequacy of long-term treatment of depression and the extent of recovery in general practice. *Br J Gen Pract* 47:233–234, 1997.)

patients are receiving adequate, effective therapy and are monitored regularly to ensure remission is achieved and maintained.

► There is a common practice in primary care to give prescription renewals for antidepressants to depressed patients rather than see them multiple times on return visits. This study supports what has been previously found, i.e., that patients on tricyclics are generally not receiving adequate doses but do receive higher doses if SSRIs are prescribed. They also document that only one third of patients were in full remission and again document that this routine strategy is definitely not a wise one.

J.C. Ballenger, M.D.

Sustained Change in Parents Receiving Preventative Interventions for Families With Depression

Beardslee WR, Salt P, Versage EM, et al (Judge Baker Children's Ctr, Boston; Children's Hosp, Boston)

Am J Psychiatry 154:510–515, 1997 8–56

Background.—Depression is a major public health concern. Depression in an individual can affect an entire family, and it is estimated that up to 50% of children of parents with serious affective disorders will themselves experience depression by the end of adolescence. There have been promising results of studies on preventing affective disorders in adults but little information on evaluation of other family members. Sustained effects in parents receiving 1 of 2 psychoeducational preventive interventions were evaluated.

Methods.—There were 37 families with at least 1 child between 8 and 15 years of age and at least 1 parent with affective disorder. One intervention was clinician-facilitated (6 to 10 sessions) and the other was in lecture/discussion format (2 lectures attended by parent only). The 2 interventions differed in the degree of involvement of the children and the linking of information to the family's life experience.

Results.—Sustained effects from the psychoeducational preventive interventions were reported 1.5 years after enrollment. More positive changes reported by both the patient and clinician were associated with the clinician-facilitated intervention. There were no harmful effects from either intervention reported or observed.

Discussion.—Relatively short clinical interventions can have sustained effects on individuals with affective disorders. Although both interventions communicated the same information, the clinician-facilitated approach was better able to translate the information into changes in attitude and behavior within the family.

► This article reports a set of activities we should be doing more of. Beardslee and his group have intervened with depressed adults and their children in the home and have demonstrated how this helps the children.

J.C. Ballenger, M.D.

Effect of Primary Care Treatment of Depression on Service Use by Patients With High Medical Expenditures

Katzelnick DJ, Kobak KA, Greist JH, et al (Dean Found for Health, Research, and Education, Middletown, Wis)

Psychiatric Serv 48:59–64, 1997 8–57

Background.—A previous study of patterns of utilization by members in a prepaid HMO found that 13% accounted for approximately one third of services. Greater utilization of services was not related to patient marital status, income, or occupation, but was related to higher degrees of psychological distress, especially depression. Other reports have confirmed a relationship between high use of nonpsychiatric medical services and depressive symptomatology. Data on 50,000 patients of an HMO were reviewed for high users, and their rates of depression were compared with those of patients identified as average users. The effects of treatment of depression on use of health care services, disability, and quality of life were assessed.

Methods.—Eligible patients were 18 years of age or older and were continuously enrolled for the 2 most recent 12-month periods before the study. The Medical Outcomes Study (MOS) depression screen was administered to 786 high users of services and an equal number of randomly selected patients who were not high users. Those in the high-use group who screened positive were subsequently seen by their primary care physician and offered treatment if given a diagnosis of depression. Twenty of 150 patients who screened positive on the MOS were confirmed as having depression, were not already receiving psychiatric treatment, and agreed to a 6-month course of open-label antidepressant treatment.

Results.—The 786 high users made up 8.7% of the HMO population and accounted for 37% of total HMO utilization. High users were significantly older than those who were not high users (mean, 52 vs. 47.7 years) and significantly more likely to be women. The 20 high users with depression all completed the 6-month study. Antidepressant therapy led to significant reductions in depression and significant improvement in measures of quality of life. The percentage of patients who reported that they were not impaired by their depression at work increased from 10% to 40%. The mean total cost for HMO in-plan use of services decreased in treated patients from $13.28 a day for the 6-month period before screening to $6.75 a day during the 6-month study period. Treatment study costs, however, increased the daily service use cost to $12.55.

Conclusion.—With identification and treatment, patients with depression and a history of high medical expenditures experienced significant improvement in general health, mental health, occupational functioning, and overall quality of life. Their service use decreased as well, suggesting that medical expenditures might be reduced if depression were more widely recognized and treated.

► This study examined an important group of patients in primary care (i.e., those who have been called high utilizers). This small group, often described as 10% to 15% of patients, has been reported to use 33% to 50% of health care services. In this study, the group proved to be 8.7% of an HMO population, and they utilized 37% of the resources. The study showed that treatment of depressed high utilizers cut their general medical expenditures in half. When psychiatric costs were added in, total costs were still less than they were before identification and treatment, and the patients experienced significantly greater symptom relief and improved quality of family and occupational life. This study and those like it are important to our argument that these patients should be identified and treated. In my opinion, there is no valid argument why they should not be treated.

J.C. Ballenger, M.D.

Borderline Personality Disorder and Health Care Utilization in a Primary Care Setting

Sansone RA, Sansone LA, Wiederman MW (Univ of Oklahoma, Tulsa; Medical Care Associates of Tulsa, Okla; Ball State Univ, Muncie, Ind)
South Med J 89:1162–1165, 1996 8–58

Background.—Studies have indicated that those with psychiatric disorders use more primary care services than those without such disorders. Borderline personality disorder is characterized by a superficial veneer of normalcy in transient social encounters coupled with significant underlying psychological dysfunction. The impact of borderline personality disorder on health care utilization in the primary care setting of an HMO was examined.

Study Design.—The study group consisted of 194 consecutive female patients between the ages of 17 and 52 years who were seen for nonemergency medical care by a single HMO physician. Each participant completed the borderline personality scale of the Personality Diagnostic Questionnaire-Revised (PDQ-R), the Self-Harm Inventory (SHI), and a demographic inquiry. The preceding year of health care utilization was investigated for each participant in a blinded fashion.

Findings.—Study participants with scores on either test suggestive of borderline personality disorder made significantly more contacts with the HMO and received more prescriptions. Use of health care resources increased with increasing severity as measured by the PDQ-R.

Conclusions.—Study participants with borderline personality symptoms, as assessed by the PDQ-R, used significantly more primary health care resources than those without these symptoms. Increasing symptom severity was associated with increased utilization of these resources.

► I've always wondered how a primary care physician could possibly understand and/or deal with borderline patients. This article documents some of the problems individuals with this disorder create in primary care, and they wouldn't surprise any psychiatrist. However, this is an area where we might be particularly helpful (and appreciated) by our primary care colleagues.

J.C. Ballenger, M.D.

Are Symptoms of Anxiety and Depression Risk Factors for Hypertension? Longitudinal Evidence From the National Health and Nutrition Examination Survey I Epidemiologic Follow-up Study

Jonas BS, Franks P, Ingram DD (Ctrs for Disease Control and Prevention, Hyattsville, Md; Univ of Rochester, NY)

Arch Fam Med 6:43–49, 1997 8–59

Background.—Some studies have suggested that anxiety and depression may have a pressor effect on the cardiovascular system that could lead to hypertension. To examine the role of anxiety and depression in the subsequent development of hypertension, data from the National Health and Nutrition Examination I (NHANES I) Epidemiologic Follow-Up Study were used.

Study Design.—The NHANES I study was conducted from 1971 to 1975 with a nationwide probability sample of the civilian noninstitutionalized population of the United States. The Epidemiologic Follow-Up Study is a longitudinal study of 14,407 of the original NHANES I participants. The participants for this study included 2,992 white and black participants from NHANES I who were 25 to 64 years old at baseline and normotensive at the beginning of the study period. These participants were observed for 7–16 years. The association between anxiety and depression at baseline and hypertension at follow-up was analyzed.

Results.—Multivariate analysis indicated that for whites and blacks aged 45–64 years, high anxiety and depression at baseline assessment were independent predictors of subsequent hypertension and treatment for hypertension. For whites aged 25–44 years, intermediate anxiety and depression were independent predictors of treated hypertension.

Conclusions.—This prospective study suggests that among both whites and blacks aged 25–64 years there was an association between self-perceived anxiety and depression and subsequent hypertension. Further studies are required to understand the mechanism by which anxiety and depression exert their effects on blood pressure to increase the incidence of subsequent hypertension.

► We are finding in study after study that anxiety and depression appear to have long-term adverse implications for the cardiovascular stystem. This study suggests this risk may be mediated by hypertension.

J.C. Ballenger, M.D.

Effects of Mental Stress on Myocardial Ischemia During Daily Life
Gullette ECD, Blumenthal JA, Babyak M, et al (Duke Univ, Durham, NC; Ohio State Univ, Columbus; Uniformed Services Univ, Bethesda, Md)
JAMA 277:1521–1526, 1997 8–60

Objective.—Myocardial ischemia, an important indicator of future cardiac events in patients with coronary artery disease (CAD), can be triggered by stress. A prospective case–crossover investigation was conducted to determine the effect of generalized versus specific emotional stress on initiation of ischemia.

Methods.—Ambulatory ECG monitoring was performed over a 48-hour period on 132 patients with CAD and recent evidence of exercise-induced ischemia. Patients received no anti-ischemic medication and kept a diary of major activities during the monitoring period. Information about emotional arousal, time of day, and physical activity were correlated with ST segment episodes.

Results.—Of the 58 patients experiencing myocardial ischemia during the monitoring period, 2 were excluded from the study. No physical activity was recorded for 2,311 of the 2,760 hours during the monitoring period. Although most patients did not report high levels of negative emotion, the percentage of ischemic hours was highest during high levels of negative emotion which included 101 hours of tension levels greater than 2 (on a 5-point scale), 98 hours of high frustration, and 28 hours of sadness. The percentage of ischemic hours was lower during high levels of positive emotions. Unadjusted relative risk for high levels of negative emotion was 3.0 for tension, 2.9 for sadness, and 2.6 for frustration. When adjusted for time and day and level of activity, the relative risk diminished to 2.2 for all 3 emotions.

Conclusion.—These findings indicate that everyday mental stress can trigger myocardial ischemia. Stress management techniques are recommended and should be evaluated for use with CAD patients.

▶ This study documents again that negative emotions lead to ischemia of the coronary arteries, at least after they are diseased. For me, this article and the next two provide convincing evidence that psychiatry can be of significant help in the treatment of coronary patients.

J.C. Ballenger, M.D.

A Prospective Study of Anger and Coronary Heart Disease: The Normative Aging Study
Kawachi I, Sparrow D, Spiro A III, et al (Harvard Med School, Boston)
Circulation 94:2090–2095, 1996 8–61

Introduction.—Earlier findings indicate that anger and hostility are related to the incidence of coronary heart disease (CHD). The relationship between anger and overall CHD risk was prospectively evaluated in the

Veterans Administration Normative Aging Study, on ongoing cohort of older, community-dwelling men.

Methods.—The mean participant age was 61 years. The revised Minnesota Multiphasic Personality Inventory (MMPI-2) was administered to 1,305 men with no diagnosis of CHD. Research subjects were categorized according to their responses to the MMPI-2 anger content scale. All participants underwent physical examination, medical history update, measurement of a variety of biochemical values, and assessment for morbidity and mortality. The average follow-up was 7 years.

Results.—Research subjects who scored high on anger were younger, heavier, more likely to be current smokers, and somewhat more likely to drink at least 2 alcoholic beverages daily. During follow-up, 110 new coronary events occurred in 1,305 men. They included 30 nonfatal myocardial infarction (MIs), 20 cases of fatal CHD, and 60 cases of angina pectoris. Men with higher levels of anger experienced increased risks of CHD. Men who scored in the highest category of anger had about a 60% excess risk of nonfatal MI and an increased risk of incident angina pectoris. Men with higher levels of anger had shorter periods of CHD-free survival. A dose-response association was observed between level of anger and overall CHD risk.

Conclusion.—Anger was associated with a twofold to threefold increased risk of total CHD and angina pectoris in older men. These findings need to be explored in other populations before anger management programs can be suggested as a means of helping reduce the risk of CHD events.

► This article contributes the very interesting finding that men with higher levels of anger had a significant increase in risk of CHD and MI. This is another finding that should help us reorient our activities to becoming more involved with primary care generalists and physicians in internal medicine and cardiology.

J.C. Ballenger, M.D.

Is Worrying Bad for Your Heart? A Prospective Study of Worry and Coronary Heart Disease in the Normative Aging Study

Kubzansky LD, Kawachi I, Spiro A III, et al (Harvard School of Public Health, Boston; Channing Lab, Boston; Harvard Med School, Boston)

Circulation 95:818–824, 1997 8–62

Background.—Anxiety has been linked to an increased incidence of coronary heart disease (CHD), although the psychological and biological mechanisms of this relationship are unclear. Worry plays an important role in the cognitive component of anxiety. Although worrying can be constructive, it also can have negative effects. Previous studies have linked chronic worry to reduced heart rate variability. The possible association between high levels of worry and CHD risk was prospectively examined.

Methods.—The study used data collected for the Normative Aging Study, an ongoing longitudinal study of aging. On entry into the study in 1975, 1,759 men with no diagnosis of CHD completed a Worries scale, in which they graded their level of worry in the following domains: social, health, financial, self-definition, and aging. Other cardiovascular risk factors were assessed as well. The men were then followed up for CHD for an average of 14 years. Age-adjusted odds ratios of CHD were analyzed according to worry levels.

Results.—During follow-up, 323 patients developed CHD—nonfatal myocardial infarction (MI) in 113, fatal CHD in 86, and angina pectoris in 124. The social domain of worry was the one most strongly related to CHD. Men with the highest levels of worry in the social domain had an adjusted relative risk of 2.41 for nonfatal MI and 1.48 for total CHD, compared with men with the lowest levels of social worries. As the level of worry increased, so did the risk of nonfatal MI and total CHD. Social worry was unrelated to risk of angina pectoris or fatal CHD. Health and financial worries bore some relationship to health. Self-definition and aging worry did not affect CHD risk. Worry about social conditions was moderately correlated with worry over aging and finances and strongly correlated with health worry.

Conclusions.—High levels of worry—particularly about social conditions—are linked to an increased risk of CHD. Confirmatory research is needed. Behavioral consequences of worry may play a role in this relationship.

► Like two of the previous articles, this documents that an emotion, in this case worry, is involved in the etiology or pathophysiology of coronary heart disease.

J.C. Ballenger, M.D.

Psychological Rehabilitation After Myocardial Infarction: Multicentre Randomised Controlled Trial

Jones DA, West RR (Univ of Wales, Cardiff)

BMJ 313:1517–1521, 1996 8–63

Background.—Although studies of psychological rehabilitation after acute myocardial infarction have suggested possible benefits regarding morbidity and cardiac mortality, the reduction in mortality failed to achieve significance, even after all the data from all the trials were pooled. In addition, most such studies included only men under the age of 65 years. Thus, the effects of psychological rehabilitation after myocardial infarction were further investigated.

Methods.—The subjects were 2,328 patients with confirmed myocardial infarction admitted to 6 hospitals during a 2-year period. All were discharged home within 28 days. The patients were randomly assigned to intervention or no intervention after discharge. Rehabilitation consisted of psychological therapy, counseling, relaxation training, and stress management training during 7 weekly group outpatient sessions for patients and spouses.

Findings.—The prevalences of anxiety and depression (33% and 19%, respectively) did not differ significantly between the patients receiving rehabilitation and those who did not. The patients in rehabilitation had a lower frequency of angina, medication, and physical activity. Clinical complications, clinical sequelae, and mortality did not differ between groups at 12 months.

Conclusion.—Patients who have had myocardial infarction apparently do not benefit from rehabilitation programs based on psychological therapy, counseling, relaxation training, and stress management. The objective benefits documented in this study were less than those reported previously.

► Perhaps one of the areas in which psychiatry can and should expand in the future is in helping our general medical colleagues in multiple areas, not only with psychiatric problems but with medical problems as well. This study followed over 2,000 patients with confirmed myocardial infarction and studied the rehabilitation issues afterward. In this particular study, the psychosocial interventions studied actually had no benefit. It is this kind of objectivity that will be necessary to define what does and does not work for our efforts to be accepted more fully in general medicine.

J.C. Ballenger, M.D.

The Relationship of Current Psychiatric Disorder to Functional Disability and Distress in Patients With Inflammatory Bowel Disease

Walker EA, Gelfand MD, Gelfand AN, et al (Univ of Washington, Seattle; Virginia Mason Med Ctr, Seattle; Univ of Manchester, England)

Gen Hosp Psychiatry 18:220–229, 1996 8–64

Background.—Patients with chronic medical illnesses who experience anxiety and depression may exhibit a worsening of their medical condition, poor compliance with treatment, changes in immune system activity, and increased mortality. To examine the hypothesized relationship between psychiatric disorders and worsening of chronic medical illness, researchers studied the effects of anxiety and depression on gastrointestinal symptoms in patients with inflammatory bowel disease (IBD).

Methods.—Forty patients with IBD were evaluated with selected portions of the National Institutes of Mental Health Diagnostic Interview Schedule. The patients were also interviewed for functional gastrointestinal symptoms and previous episodes of emotional, physical, or sexual abuse and completed a battery of self-report measures of personality and disability. Eight patients who met criteria for major depression were administered the Hamilton Depression Inventory (HAM-D), then treated in an open label design with paroxetine. These patients were reinterviewed after 8 weeks and completed a second HAM-D and an SF-36. A logistic regression analysis was used to compare patients with IBD with and without a current psychiatric disorder, while controlling for disease severity.

Results.—The 40 patients with IBD appeared to have numerous medically unexplained gastrointestinal symptoms and disorders unrelated to their IBD. Fourteen were found to have a current psychiatric disorder and 26 were not. These 2 groups were comparable in age, percentage who were female, percentage who were married, social class, and severity of IBD. Patients with a current psychiatric diagnosis had a significantly higher mean number of medically unexplained physical symptoms, mean number of lifetime psychiatric diagnoses, and mean number of current anxiety symptoms. The prevalence rates of prior sexual and physical victimization were also significantly higher in patients with a current psychiatric disorder. A logistic regression equation, using mean number of lifetime psychiatric diagnoses, dissociation score, and mean number of functional gastrointestinal symptoms, correctly classified 87% of cases. Functional disability was improved in those receiving antidepressant treatment, despite a lack of objective changes in gastrointestinal disease severity.

Discussion.—The presence of a current psychiatric disorder in patients with IBD appears to alter their perception of disease severity. Unnecessary and aggressive interventions may be offered such patients if their psychiatric illness is not recognized. Patients with IBD and unexplained gastrointestinal symptoms may, thus, benefit from psychiatric evaluation and treatment.

▶ Our field is increasingly recognizing the relationship between gastrointestinal symptoms and psychiatric difficulties, especially depression and anxiety. Although these studies are often performed with irritable bowel syndrome, this study examines patients with frank inflammatory bowel disease. The authors found that psychiatric problems significantly complicate the care of these patients. Again, it was also found that the rates of prior sexual and physical victimization are very high in these patients, especially in the patients with a concurrent psychiatric disorder.

J.C. Ballenger, M.D.

Impact of Irritable Bowel Syndrome on Quality of Life

Whitehead WE, Burnett CK, Cook EW III, et al (Univ of North Carolina at Chapel Hill; Univ of Alabama, Birmingham)

Dig Dis Sci 41:2248–2253, 1996 8–65

Background.—Determining the impact of irritable bowel syndrome (IBS) on quality of life would be useful for judging the efficacy of treatment and comparing IBS severity among patients. A well-standardized measure, the Medical Outcome Study Short Form (SF-36), was used to determine the impact of IBS on quality of life and whether such impairments are caused by neuroticism.

Methods.—The study subjects were 83 undergraduate students with IBS who had consulted a physician, 165 students with IBS who had not consulted a physician, and 122 asymptomatic controls. The subjects completed questionnaires on quality of life, neuroticism, and psychological distress.

Findings.—Quality of life was more impaired in subjects consulting physicians than in those with IBS who did not consult physicians. The latter group had greater quality-of-life impairment than the control subjects. All quality-of-life measures were correlated with neuroticism and psychological distress. However, IBS still significantly, negatively affected quality of life after the partialling out of neuroticism and psychological distress.

Conclusion.—Irritable bowel syndrome has a negative impact on quality of life, independent of neuroticism. The SF-36 may be a useful outcome measure in IBS treatment studies, although its scales are highly correlated with neuroticism.

► Psychiatrists should be more involved with patients with IBS because they have so many psychiatric difficulties. This study shows clearly how profound the impact is on quality of life in patients with IBS.

J.C. Ballenger, M.D.

Psychiatric Interview and Psychometric Predictors of Cardiac Transplant Survival

Chacko RC, Harper RG, Gotto J, et al (Baylor College of Medicine, Houston; Methodist Hosp, Houston)

Am J Psychiatry 153:1607–1612, 1996 8–66

Background.—Because of the extraordinary stresses associated with organ failure, terminal illness, and the selection of candidates for the transplantation of scarce organs, psychiatric consultation has become increasingly commonplace in this setting. The relationship between pretransplant assessment of psychiatric diagnosis, coping skills, and social support and the outcome measures of survival and health utilization was prospectively investigated in 1 group of cardiac transplant recipients.

Methods.—Ninety-four patients were interviewed and completed a battery of self-report psychometric tests of coping style, health status, and psychosocial supports. Follow-up ranged from 9 to 56 months.

Findings.—The 63 survivors and 31 nonsurvivors were comparable in pretransplant cardiac status and illness severity. Survival was best predicted by dimensional psychometric measures of coping and social support based on patient self-assessment. Considered separately, other potential predictors were interview-determined ratings of social support and pretransplant compliance with treatment regimens. Formal DSM-III-R diagnoses were specifically associated with posttransplant hospital utilization and posttransplant health behavior.

Conclusions.—Psychiatric diagnosis, coping style, and psychosocial support may all contribute differently to mortality and health care utilization among cardiac transplant recipients. Thus, multifaceted assessment is useful.

► In my own institution, the number of times we are involved with transplant candidates has literally exploded over the past few years. The field is still full of controversies of what in the psychiatric consultation can validly help the transplant team. This article provides evidence that diagnoses and pretransplant compliance do matter in these heart transplant patients, contradicting findings from another study in this issue with liver transplant patients.[1] Coping skills and social support also appear to be important in this study.

J.C. Ballenger, M.D.

Reference

1. Tringali RA, Trzepacy PT, DiMartini A, et al: Assessment and follow up of alcohol dependent liver transplant patients: A clinical cohort. *Gen Hosp Psych* 18:70–77, 1996.

Assessment and Follow-up of Alcohol-dependent Liver Transplantation Patients: A Clinical Cohort

Tringali RA, Trzepacz PT, DiMartini A, et al (Univ of Pittsburgh, Pa)

Gen Hosp Psychiatry 18:70S-77S, 1996 8–67

Introduction.—The most common types of fatal liver disease are alcohol-related cirrhosis and alcoholic hepatitis. Many liver transplant recipients are alcoholic cirrhotics, and treatment for this group is controversial. Some view alcoholism as a contraindication to transplantation, whereas others require specified periods of sobriety before consideration for transplantation. Previous studies have shown that liver transplantation outcomes for alcoholic and nonalcoholic cirrhotics appear to be similar. Pretransplantation characteristics of liver transplant patients with a history of heavy alcohol abuse and dependence were reported. The predictive value of pretransplantation variables for posttransplantation outcomes was assessed.

Methods.—During a 28-month period, 103 alcoholic cirrhotics had orthotopic liver transplantation. Of 82 survivors, 52 were followed for their characteristics, including pretransplantation psychiatric and demographic variables, whether they were sober for more than 6 months, and whether those who died after transplantation had longer hospital stays. Statistical analysis was conducted on all of these variables.

Results.—Statistical trends toward predicting shorter posttransplant survival duration were found with age older than 50 years and index hospital stays greater than 1 month. Posttransplant survival duration was not predicted by pretransplant sobriety, gender, or duration of pretransplant heavy drinking. The relapse rate was doubled for females and for pretransplant unemployment; however, all other variables—including preoperative sobriety or participation in alcohol rehabilitation programs during the transplantation period—did not predict relapse. The relapse rate of 21% in this study is similar to that found in other centers and for the general alcoholic population.

Conclusion.—Presumed predictive variables in selecting the best candidates for liver transplantation have been challenged by these results. Posttransplant survival rates did not differ among alcoholic and nonalcoholic cirrhotics. Decreased patient or graft survival did not necessarily result from a return to drinking post transplant.

► It has been a source of controversy almost from the beginning in liver transplants as to whether alcoholism predicts a poor outcome. This debate has often taken on ethical overtones, and, at some centers, treatment of alcoholism and cirrhosis or poor adherence to alcoholism treatment have been taken into consideration, formally or informally, regarding transplant. This study definitively shows that the issues of pretransplant alcoholism and adherence to alcoholism treatment are not predictive of success post transplant.

J.C. Ballenger, M.D.

Quality of Life in Peritoneal Dialysis Patients

Steele TE, Baltimore D, Finkelstein SH, et al (Med Univ of South Carolina, Charleston; New Haven CAPD, Conn)

J Nerv Ment Dis 184:368–374, 1996 8–68

Background.—Issues of efficient and effective resource allocation in medicine will cause increased attention to be paid to patients' quality of life. The relationship between a patient's perceived quality of life and that patient's medical, psychological, and symptomatic status was examined for persons undergoing continuous ambulatory peritoneal dialysis (CAPD).

Methods.—A series of 49 CAPD patients was selected to undergo evaluation, which included an assessment of the adequacy of dialysis, the Beck Depression Inventory, and the Patient-Rated Anxiety Scale. The Kupfer-Detre-System-2 was used to assess somatic symptoms. The Patient-Assessed Quality of Life Index and the Staff-Assessed Quality of Life Index were obtained for each patient.

Results.—The clinicians' quality-of-life scores for patients correlated significantly with the overall quality-of-life scores of the patients themselves. Taken singly, measures of depression, anxiety, dialysis adequacy, somatic symptoms, and life circumstances correlated significantly with the patients' overall quality of life index. However, only the patients' depressive symptoms remained significantly correlated with the Patient-Assessed Quality of Life Index, after adjustment for dialysis adequacy, anxiety, and somatic symptoms.

Conclusion.—Depressive symptoms were more closely correlated with patients' rating of their quality of life than with the other factors examined, suggesting the need for heightened awareness of depressive symptoms in CAPD patients.

► With procedures such as dialysis, we can extend people's lives, making the issues of quality of life of great importance. This study showed that it is the depressive symptoms that are most important in the patients' ratings of their own quality of life, suggesting that we should all pay greater attention to depression in this setting.

J.C. Ballenger, M.D.

Severe Life Stress as a Predictor of Early Disease Progression in HIV Infection

Evans DL, Leserman J, Perkins DO, et al (Univ of Florida, Gainesville; Univ of North Carolina, Chapel Hill)

Am J Psychiatry 154:630–634, 1997 8–69

Background.—There is a popular belief that stress affects the immune system, as well as the onset and course of immune-based physical diseases such as cancer and AIDS. Numerous studies have shown changes in immunity associated with stress and depression, but there is little information on the ability of stress to change the progression of immune-based diseases. The multifactorial nature of HIV disease is now appreciated, and there are more attempts to identify factors that account for the variance in the progression of this disease. Such factors could affect the management of individuals with HIV infection or AIDS. Whether stress can accelerate the progression of HIV disease was investigated.

Methods.—There were 93 male, homosexual subjects who did not have clinical symptoms at the start of the study. Every 6 months up to 42 months, the subjects had comprehensive medical, neurologic, neuropsychological, and psychiatric evaluations. Assessments included evaluation of stressful life events.

Results.—A proportional hazard survival method was used to analyze the time of the first disease progression. This showed that the risk of early HIV disease progression was higher with greater severe life stress (Fig 1). The risk of early disease progression doubled for each 1 severe stress episode per 6-month period. A subset of 66 subjects was also analyzed by logistic regression after a minimum of 24 months in the study. In this subset, the odds of HIV disease progression increased almost fourfold with greater severe life stress. Analysis by a proportional odds logistic regression model showed that the degree of disease progression was predicted by severe life stress.

Discussion.—These prospective findings indicate that severe life stress can predict the degree of HIV disease progression in men. Greater severe stress is associated with a greater risk of disease progression, as well as

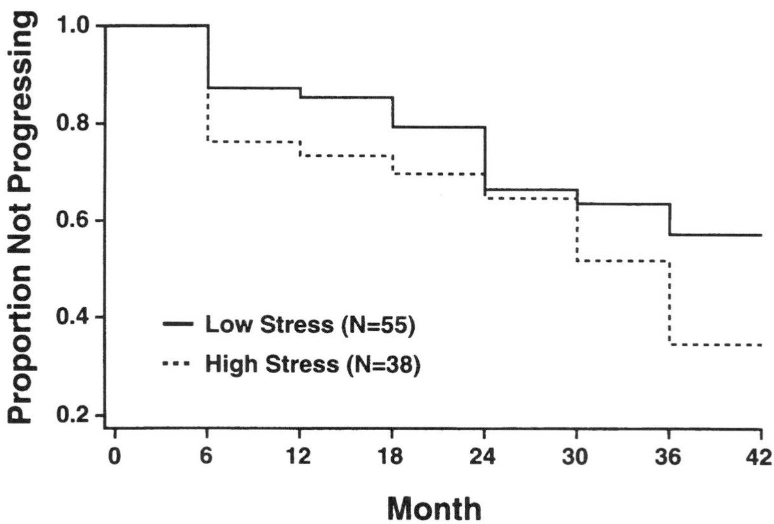

FIGURE 1.—Effect of high and low stress on HIV disease progression in 93 men without control for other variables. (Reprinted by permission from Evans DL, Leserman J, Perkins DO, et al: Severe life stress as a predictor of early disease progression in HIV infection. *Am J Psychiatry* 154:630–634, 1997. Copyright 1997, the American Psychiatric Association. Reprinted by permission.)

greater severity of disease progression. In these subjects, only severe stress affected disease progression, not levels of stress experienced in everyday living. Further research is needed to clarify the underlying immune or biological factors of this relationship, and to replicate these findings in women with HIV infection.

▶ Dwight Evans and his colleagues provide us with the first evidence that life stress hastens the progress of HIV infection. Like the previous articles in this section, this underscores again, and forcefully, the importance of our perspective in the care of medically ill patients.

J.C. Ballenger, M.D.

9 Biological Psychology

Introduction

A diverse group of excellent studies in the biology of schizophrenia and mood disorders awaits the interested reader. Similarly, some very exciting and excellent preclinical papers have been selected from a very large group of neuroscience reports with potential relevance to neuropsychiatric disorders. There is relatively little about obsessive-compulsive disorder or anxiety disorder to be found, a perennial problem. The evidence for schizophrenia as a neurodevelopmental disorder (Abstract 9–5) with both structural and functional disturbances continues to mount from studies that are methodologically sound. The hippocampus and dorsolateral prefrontal cortex remain the area of greatest interest (Abstracts 9–7, 9–8, and 9–9). While no characteristic lesion has yet been found, it is apparent that there are cellular abnormalities in the prefrontal cortex and hippocampus. There is evidence for both increased dopamine (DA) release in the striatum (Abstract 9–2) and down regulation of D1 receptors in the frontal cortex (Abstract 9–1) which conceivably might be related to increased DA release in the cortex. While the importance of DA in the pathophysiology of schizophrenia remains unchallenged, the role of serotonin and glutamate in the pathophysiology of schizophrenia, possibly through the modulation of dopaminergic activity, is gaining more and more credence (Abstracts 9–3, 9–14, and 9–15).

This year's most interesting papers on mood disorders include a group on the genetics of depression (Abstracts 9–16 through 9–20 and 9–24) and identification of polymorphisms that may point toward the role of serotonin (Abstracts 9–20 and 9–24) in particular to the etiology of major depression or bipolar disorder. The finding of Berrentini et al. (Abstract 9–19) that a bipolar susceptibility gene exists near the centromere of chromosome 18 has been well replicated and may become useful as a genetic marker for this disorder. However, the full range of genes involved must be further elucidated. The evidence that increased glucocorticoids may be involved in the pathophysiology of major depression is further strengthened by both structural brain imaging studies (Abstract 9–21) and evidence that clarifies the pattern of increased secretion of ACTH and cortisol in major depression (Abstract 9–28). The finding of markedly increased serotonin synthesis in males compared to females using a novel new PET method may be relevant to the higher rate of depression in females (Abstract 9–25). Identification of a possible gene for obsessive-compulsive disorder (COMT, Abstract 9–33) could be of great significance if it holds up with further research.

Basic research papers report some exceptionally interesting findings. The first antipsychotic drug which does not directly block a DA receptor may be MDL 100907 (Abstract 9–35). It is a highly selective 5–HT2a receptor antagonist. A number of studies show the power of molecular genetics via knockout mice, or antisense oligonucleotides to reveal the role of genes in particular behaviors of interest to neuropsychiatric disorders (Abstracts 9–36, and 9–38 through 9–40). The ability of an enriched environment during the postnatal period to improve survival of hippocampal neurons (Abstract 9–41) is encouraging to those who believe in the nature-nurture view of man. It certainly reemphasizes the importance of psychosocial research and treatment modalities in interaction with biological psychiatry.

Herbert Meltzer, M.D.

Schizophrenia

Decreased Prefrontal Dopamine D1 Receptors in Schizophrenia Revealed by PET

Okubo Y, Suhara T, Suzuki K, et al (Tokyo Med and Dental Univ)
Nature 385:634–636, 1997 — 9–1

Background.—Altered activation of dopamine receptors is believed to be involved in schizophrenia. One of the classic signs of schizophrenia is dysfunctional working memory, and the brain area associated with working memory, the prefrontal cortex, is dense with D1 receptors. Thus, these authors used positron emission tomography (PET) to investigate whether the prefrontal cortex D1 receptor density changes in patients with schizophrenia, as well as to determine any clinical or pathologic correlations.

Methods.—Two PET scans were performed in 17 patients with schizophrenia and 18 normal controls. Patients had been free of neuroleptic drugs for more than 2 weeks (n = 7) or had never taken neuroleptics (n = 10). Two labels were used in the PET studies, one that binds to D1 receptors ([^{11}C]SCH23390) and one that binds to D2 receptors ([^{11}C]NMSP). The D1 binding potential was determined as the association rate constant (k_3) divided by the dissociation rate constant (k_4). Investigators rated the symptoms of schizophrenia. Also, patients performed the Wisconsin Card Sorting Test.

Findings.—In the striatum, D1 and D2 receptor densities did not differ between patients and controls. In the prefrontal cortex, however, the D1 binding potential was significantly lower in the patients with schizophrenia, compared with controls. Furthermore, patients with a reduced D1 receptor density in the prefrontal cortex had significantly worse symptoms of schizophrenia and performed more poorly on the card sorting test.

Conclusions.—Patients with schizophrenia have a decreased D1 receptor density in the prefrontal cortex. This pathologic finding correlates strongly with poor working memory and negative symptoms. Further research should target D1 receptor agonists in the treatment of this disorder.

► Numerous studies have suggested a relationship between cognitive dysfunction and negative symptoms in schizophrenia. The ability of clozapine to increase dopamine antagonist release in the prefrontal cortex has been suggested to be the basis for its ability to improve negative symptoms and cognitive function. Decreased D1 receptor density in the prefrontal cortex was found to be correlated with deficient working memory and executive function, as measured by the Wisconsin Card Sorting test, and negative symptoms, thus linking the 2 major features of schizophrenia to the same pathophysiologic process. Postmortem studies that assess D1 receptor density or mRNA in various brain regions in schizophrenia are needed to corroborate these findings. Previous failures of D1 antagonists to ameliorate schizophrenia are consistent with these data. Clinical trials with D1 agonists would be of interest.

H. Meltzer, M.D.

Schizophrenia Is Associated With Elevated Amphetamine-induced Synaptic Dopamine Concentrations: Evidence From a Novel Positron Emission Tomography Method

Breier A, Su T-P, Saunders R, et al (Natl Inst of Mental Health, NIH, Bethesda, Md)

Proc Natl Acad Sci U S A 94:2569–2574, 1997 9–2

Background.—Dopamine overactivity is the most widely accepted hypothesis for the pathophysiology of schizophrenia. Supporting this concept is the psychomimetic potential of amphetamine and other agents that stimulate dopamine outflow. A new technique of positron emission tomography (PET) can provide an indirect indicator of in vivo synaptic dopamine concentration. Studies were performed in animals and humans to determine the association between schizophrenia and amphetamine-induced elevations of synaptic dopamine.

Methods.—In the first study, the dopamine D_2/D_3 PET radioligand ^{11}C-raclopride was used to assess the relationship between amphetamine-induced changes in striatal extracellular dopamine levels and in vivo microdialysis and striatal binding levels in monkeys. In the human study, ^{11}C-raclopride PET was used to determine whether patients with schizophrenia had greater amphetamine-induced striatal synaptic dopamine concentrations than controls.

Results.—In monkeys, doubling the dose of amphetamine resulted in a doubling of ^{11}C-raclopride-specific binding reductions. Small changes in binding led to large changes in dopamine outflow—the ratio of percent mean dopamine increase to percent mean binding reduction for amphetamine was 44:1. In the human study, the mean amphetamine-related decrease in ^{11}C-raclopride-specific binding was 22.3% for schizophrenic patients vs. 15.5% in controls. This finding, combined with the data from the animal study, suggested that the patients with schizophrenia had a significantly greater increase in synaptic dopamine concentrations than the controls did.

Conclusions.—Studies with ^{11}C-raclopride PET support the hypothesis that patients with schizophrenia have elevated amphetamine-induced synaptic dopamine concentrations. The increase in amphetamine-induced dopamine outflow in schizophrenia may be explained by changes in the distribution of intracellular dopamine, perhaps an increased ratio of free-to-bound intracellular dopamine.

▶ This study is of interest because it provides some of the first evidence for an abnormality of the dopamine (DA) system in schizophrenia. The methodology used here needs further documentation. About one third of 12 patients with nonacute schizophrenia had an excessive increase in DA release in the striatum after amphetamine challenge. The clinical significance of this finding is unclear because it involves the striatum rather than the mesolimbic system. The latter is more relevant to psychosis. In addition, there were no apparent clinical correlates of the potential to respond to amphetamine with increased extracellular DA levels. It is remarkable how little direct evidence there is for a dopaminergic abnormality in schizophrenia.

H. Meltzer, M.D.

Serotonergic Modulation of Dopamine Measured With [^{11}C]-Raclopride and PET in Normal Human Subjects

Smith GS, Dewey SL, Brodie JD, et al (New York Univ; Brookhaven Natl Lab, Upton, NY; State Univ of New York, Stonybrook; et al)

Am J Psychiatry 154:490–496, 1997 9–3

Introduction.—The much-debated dopamine hypothesis of schizophrenia holds that this disorder is characterized by a hyperdopaminergic state. Positron emission tomography (PET) techniques are now available to test the hypothesis that neuropsychiatric symptoms result from the inability of one neurotransmitter system to modulate the activity of a functionally linked system. Serotonergic modulation of dopamine was studied in normal human beings.

Methods.—The study used ^{11}C-raclopride, a radiotracer for the striatal dopamine D_2 receptor. Eleven normal men underwent 2 ^{11}C-raclopride PET studies, before and 3 hours after pharmacologic challenge with the serotonin-releasing agent and reuptake inhibitor fenfluramine (6 mg orally). The distribution volume of D_2 receptors was assessed by graphic analysis of the ^{11}C-raclopride PET data. The subjects also underwent measurement of plasma fenfluramine, norfenfluramine, homovanillic acid (HVA), cortisol, and prolactin.

Results.—During the postchallenge PET scan, the subjects had elevated levels of fenfluramine and prolactin. No such elevations were noted for HVA or cortisol. This scan showed significant reductions in specific (striatal) and nonspecific (striatal minus cerebellar) binding of ^{11}C-raclopride. Fenfluramine had no significant effect on the metabolic rate or nonspecific binding of ^{11}C-raclopride.

Conclusions.—Carbon-11–raclopride binding is decreased in normal subjects receiving a fenfluramine challenge of the serotonin system. The findings seem to reflect an increase in dopamine concentration and the stimulation of dopamine activity by serotonin. Carbon-11–raclopride PET offers a way of measuring serotonergic modulation of dopamine in vivo, which may be useful in studying the causes and treatment of such disorders as schizophrenia, major depressive disorder, obsessive-compulsive disorder, and substance abuse.

► The use of PET to study drug action in man has often focused on receptor changes. This study provides data on presynaptic neuronal activity by analyzing the impact of a 5-hydroxytryptamine (HT) drug, fenfluramine, on the binding of ^{11}C-raclopride to postsynaptic D_2 receptors. The observed decrease in binding may well be the result of increased release of dopamine (DA). How fenfluramine is achieving this is unclear. It might be indirectly via effects on 5-HT in the dorsal raphe or on projections to the striatum. However, fenfluramine may also have a direct effect to release DA in the striatum. There is considerable evidence that serotonin can inhibit nigrostriatal dopaminergic activity via 5-HT2a receptor mechanisms.

H. Meltzer, M.D.

Measuring Age-related Changes in Dopamine D_2 Receptors With ^{11}C-Raclopride and ^{18}F-*N*-Methylspiroperidol

Volkow ND, Wang G-J, Fowler JS, et al (Brookhaven Natl Lab, Upton, NY; State Univ of New York, Stony Brook)

Psychiatry Res 67:11–16, 1996 9–4

Introduction.—With advancing age, brain dopamine activity usually decreases along with a decline in the concentration of D2 receptors. Most studies looking at D2 receptors used postmortem brains, which showed many discrepancies. The problems associated with postmortem studies have been overcome with positron emission tomography (PET) and single photon emission CT, which permit quantitation of D2 receptors. Studies with living individuals have shown a decrease in striatal D2 receptor density with aging; however, estimates for loss per decade of life have varied. In 2 series of PET studies, age-related changes in D2 receptors were compared; 1 study used ^{11}C-raclopride, and the other used ^{18}F- or ^{11}C-labeled *N*-methylspiroperidol (NMS).

Methods.—For the NMS study, 20 male healthy volunteers ranging in age from 20 to 49 years were selected, and for the ^{11}C-raclopride study, 24

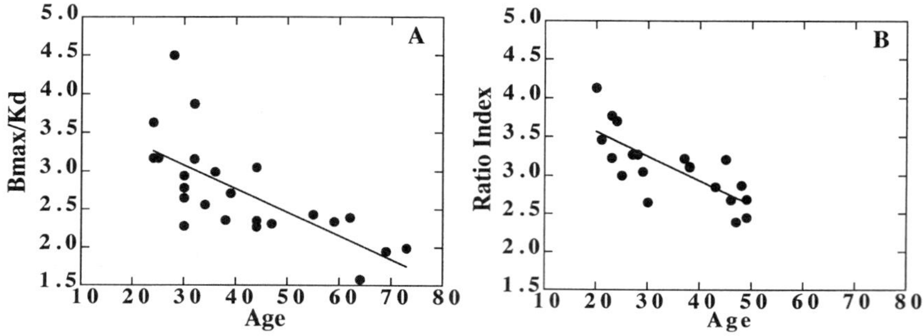

FIGURE 1.—**A**, correlation between age and B_{max}/K_d (DV_{STR}/DV_{CBL}^{-1}) for the ^{11}C-raclopride study ($r = -0.71$, $P < 0.0001$). **B**, correlation between age and the ratio index ($r = -0.62$, $P < 0.005$) for the ^{18}F-*N*-methylspiroperidol study. *Abbreviations: DV*, distribution volume; *STR*, striatum; *CBL*, cerebellum. (Courtesy of Volkow ND, Wang G-J, Fowler JS, et al: Measuring age-related changes in dopamine d_2 receptors with ^{11}C-raclopride and ^{18}F-*N*-methylspiroperidol. *Psychiatry Res* 67:11–16, 1996.)

healthy volunteers, 21 men and 3 women ranging in age from 24 to 73 years, were selected. The participants, were assessed with different tracers and different kinetic models to evaluate the consistency for the estimates of age-induced losses of D2 receptors. The ^{11}C-raclopride group was assessed using the ratio of the distribution volume in striatum to that in cerebellum, and the NMS group was measured using the ratio index of the slope of the striatum-to-cerebellum ratio as a function of time.

Results.—For both ligands, the findings of correlational analysis between age and dopamine D2 receptor availability were significant. The ratio index from NMS corresponded to $r = -0.62$, and the ratio index from ^{11}C-raclopride corresponded to $r = -0.71$ (Fig 1). For the ^{11}C-raclopride study, estimates of dopamine D2 receptor loss per decade corresponded to 7.9%. For the NMS study, estimates of dopamine D2 receptor loss per decade corresponded to 7.8%. Significant age-related decreases in dopamine D2 receptors were found to occur relatively early in life, such as at 40 years of age, according to documentation from both ligands.

Conclusion.—Healthy research subjects showed marked age-related decrements in D2 receptors without evidence of motor impairment, and the magnitude was similar with both tracers. The degeneration of the dopamine pathway may be viewed as a loss of a system that enables the individual to compensate for stressors in the environment, leaving an individual more vulnerable to certain types of cerebral pathologic conditions.

▶ The concordance between the 2 methods of quantitating the decrease in dopamine D2 receptor density in the striatum is interesting. These 2 methods have previously produced discrepant results in quantitating the density of D2 receptors in patients with schizophrenia, which suggests that the differences may be caused more by differences in populations studied than by PET models. The fact that D2 receptor density declines markedly at a relatively early age may be a factor in why psychotic symptoms tend to diminish with age in some patients with schizophrenia.

H. Meltzer, M.D.

Maldistribution of Interstitial Neurons in Prefrontal White Matter of the Brains of Schizophrenic Patients

Akbarian S, Kim JJ, Potkin SG, et al (Univ of California, Irvine)

Arch Gen Psychiatry 53:425–436, 1996 9–5

Background.—In fetal development, the cortical subplate is a temporary zone of early neurons and synaptic neuropil that is believed to play a role in the development of connections in the cerebral cortex. The subcortical white matter (WM) of the normal adult brain contains interstitial neurons that have escaped the programmed cell death that destroys most subplate neurons. One type of interstitial neuron is reportedly maldistributed in the WM of brains of schizophrenic patients, suggesting a possible subplate defect during brain development. The distribution of interstitial neurons in the prefrontal WM of schizophrenic patients was studied.

Methods.—The investigators analyzed WM from beneath the middle frontal gyrus of 20 patients with schizophrenia and 20 matched controls. The distributions of 3 populations of neurons—defined by histochemistry or immunocytochemistry—were studied.

Results.—The distributions of all 3 neuronal populations were altered in the brains of patients with schizophrenia. For microtubule-associated protein 2 and nonphosphorylated neurofilament-immunoreactive neurons, density was decreased in the superficial WM and increased in the deeper WM. For nicotinamide adenine dinucleotide phosphate-diaphorase neurons, density was decreased in the superficial WM and variable in the deeper WM. In 35% of brains from schizophrenic patients, at least 2 of the 3 neuronal populations was maldistributed toward the deeper WM. None of the control brains had this pattern. The neuronal distribution patterns were independent of age, sex, autolysis time, or schizophrenia subtype.

Conclusion.—The frontal lobes of patients with schizophrenia show selective displacement of interstitial WM neurons. The findings suggest that schizophrenia may involve changes in the migration of subplate neurons or in the pattern of programmed cell death. The evidence for altered distribution of WM neurons varies, being most apparent in about one third of patients. The rest have less striking evidence for dysfunction of the subplate, suggesting that other causative factors leading to prefrontal dysfunction are involved.

▶ This follow-up study of the hypothesis of maldistribution of interstitial neurons in schizophrenia produced a variety of confirmatory findings for the theory of abnormal connectivity in schizophrenia. Two of the findings are novel: (1) decreased density of microtubule-associated protein 2 and (2) nonphosphorylated neurofilament-immunoreactive neurons in superficial subcortial WM and an increased density in deeper WM. The increased density in the deeper WM suggests an alteration in the migration of subplate neurons or the pattern of programmed cell death.

These findings complement the previous reported findings of reduced presence of nicotinamide adenine dinucleotide phosphate-diaphorase neurons in superficial WM. Only 35% of the patients had evidence for abnormal distribution of these interstitial neurons. With the limited data available as to the characteristics, it is not surprising that they could not be distinguished from those patients without such abnormalities. The next paper (Akil and Lewis, "Cytoarchitecture of the Entorhinal Cortex in Schizophrenia") used a different method and failed to support the hypothesis of abnormal neuronal migration in schizophrenia.

H. Meltzer, M.D.

Cytoarchitecture of the Entorhinal Cortex in Schizophrenia

Akil M, Lewis DA (Univ of Pittsburgh, Pa)

Am J Psychiatry 154:1010–1012, 1997 9–6

Introduction.—Studies of the entorhinal cortex of patients with schizophrenia have found some evidence of abnormal neuronal migration, which has greatly affected hypotheses of schizophrenia as a neurodevelopmental disorder. However, it is important to establish which subdivisions of the entorhinal cortex are abnormal. Three cytoarchitectonic subdivisions of the entorhinal cortex were compared in the brains of schizophrenic patients vs. normal controls.

Methods.—The study included postmortem brain specimens from 10 patients with schizophrenia and 10 normal controls. The investigators examined Nissl-stained sections through 3 cytoarchitectonic subdivisions, specifically, the olfactory, rostral, and intermediate subdivisions, in which previous studies have reported cytoarchitectural abnormalities.

Results.—The study revealed cytoarchitectonic differences across subdivisions involved in all cortical layers. However, the arrangement of neurons—-especially in layers II and III—differed across entorhinal cortex subdivisions in each subject. Both schizophrenic and control specimens had the typical features of olfactory, rostral, and intermediate regions, with no qualitative differences in cytoarchitecture between groups. None of the schizophrenic patients had obvious displacement of layer II neurons.

Conclusion.—In contrast to previous reports, this study finds no evidence of cytoarchitectural disturbances in the entorhinal cortex of subjects with schizophrenia. The findings do not support the hypothesis that abnormal neuronal migration plays a role in schizophrenia. However, they do not rule out the presence of other disturbances of the neural circuitry of the entorhinal cortex in schizophrenia.

► This study is important because it failed to replicate 1 of the cornerstones of the neurodevelopmental hypothesis of schizophrenia: the report by Jakob and Beckmann[1] that there was displacement to deeper cortical layers of the layer II neurons in some schizophrenic patients. The most logical explanation for the failure is inadequate control for differences between regions of the entorhinal cortex in layer II cellular patterns in both controls and schizophrenics. These negative data do not disprove the neurodevelopmental hypothesis, which has many other bases. They do suggest the need for exquisite care in carrying out neuropathologic studies of schizophrenia in which it is unlikely that any consistent gross abnormalities are to be found.

H. Meltzer, M.D.

Reference

1. Jakob H, Beckmann H: Prenatal development disturbances in the limbic allo cortex in schizophrenia. *J Neural Transmission* 65:303–326, 1986.

The Hippocampus in Schizophrenia: Lateralized Increase in Neuronal Density and Altered Cytoarchitectural Asymmetry

Zaidel DW, Esiri MM, Harrison PJ (Univ of California, Los Angeles; Radcliffe Infirmary, Oxford, England; Warneford Hosp, Oxford, England)

Psychol Med 27:703–713, 1997 9–7

Objective.—On the histologic level, schizophrenia appears to involve changes in the hippocampal and neocortical cytoarchitecture. In the normal brain, some cytoarchitectural variables differ from 1 hemisphere to the other. There is evidence of changes in cerebral asymmetry in schizophrenia, but this issue has not been fully considered in previous cytoarchitectural studies of schizophrenia. A postmortem study was performed to see whether neuronal density or its correlates differ in the left or right hippocampus of subjects with schizophrenia, compared with normal controls.

Methods.—The study included sections of the left and right hippocampus from 22 schizophrenics and 18 normal subjects. Specimens were taken from the dentate gyrus, CA4, CA3, CA1, and subiculum. The neuronal density of the left and right hippocampi were compared. Correlations of neuronal density between paired subfields were assessed as an indicator of their interrelationship. Such correlations had been reported in the left hippocampus of normal subjects, but not in the right side.

Results.—Compared with controls, the schizophrenic subjects had a 25% increase in neuronal density in right CA3 and a 22% increase in right CA1. In schizophrenic patients, neuronal density in the homologous left and right subfields was strongly correlated for CA4, CA3, CA1, and subiculum. In normal subjects, such correlations were observed only for dentate gyrus and CA4. In schizophrenic subjects, the 2 hippocampi had similar intrahippocampal correlations of neuronal density between pairs of subfields, whereas controls had asymmetric distribution.

Conclusion.—This study adds further evidence of cytoarchitectural hippocampal abnormalities in patients with schizophrenia. The findings support the hypothesis that schizophrenia has complex interactions with cerebral asymmetries. The findings must be replicated, and sex differences must be sought. Also, other parameters must be measured to provide a more complete cytoarchitectural profile of the brains of patients with schizophrenia.

▶ This study provides additional morphologic evidence for cytopathologic changes in the hippocampus of patients with schizophrenia. This sample size is considerably larger than those of previous studies and the methodology is much stronger than that of previous studies. The pattern of quantitative and correlative changes in hippocampal structure strongly suggests a neurodevelopmental origin. These types of findings provide a basis for the memory and learning deficits in schizophrenia. They still leave open the question as to why these functional deficits do not emerge until late adolescence.

H. Meltzer, M.D.

Cortical Gray Matter Volume Deficit in Patients With First-Episode Schizophrenia

Lim KO, Tew W, Kushner M, et al (VA Palo Alto Health Care Systems, Calif; Stanford Univ, Calif; State Univ of New York, Stony Brook; et al)
Am J Psychiatry 153:1548–1553, 1996 9–8

Background.—Studies of patients with chronic schizophrenia have shown deficits in cortical gray matter, but not whether the deficits are present early in the disease's course. Ventricular enlargement has also been reported, but that earlier study included all patients entered into the Stony Brook First Episode Study, irrespective of diagnostic outcome.

Methods.—In 22 patients with first-episode schizophrenia within 6 months of onset and 51 control subjects from the Stony Brook First Episode Study, MRI was used. Only patients meeting DSM-III-R criteria for schizophrenia at 2 years were included, after age matching with control subjects, screening for drug and substance abuse, and elimination of technically inappropriate scans.

Results.—Significant cortical gray matter deficits and lateral and third ventricular enlargements were seen in patients with schizophrenia compared with control subjects.

Conclusions.—Cortical gray matter deficit and ventricular enlargement are present early in the course of schizophrenia and may be used as a sign as early as 6 months after onset.

▶ This study provides additional evidence that there are cortical structural abnormalities in schizophrenia at the onset of the illness. The same group has also presented evidence that the cortical volume deficit and ventricular enlargement increase during the course of the first several years of illness. Although this clearly suggests that these deficits are an early feature of the illness, it does not address the issue of specificity and clinical correlates. It could be that these deficits are the results of stress and corticoids rather than a vulnerability factor which preceded the full-blown psychotic episode.

H. Meltzer, M.D.

Hypofrontality in Schizophrenia: Distributed Dysfunctional Circuits in Neuroleptic-Naïve Patients

Andreasen NC, O'Leary DS, Flaum M, et al (Univ of Iowa, Iowa City)
Lancet 349:1730–1734, 1997 9–9

Background.—Patients with schizophrenia have been reported to have decreased prefrontal cortex metabolic activity, but various factors have confounded confirmation. Is abnormal metabolism or blood flow confined to specific prefrontal cortex regions? Are such abnormalities related to symptoms, cognitive state, or treatment? How do toxic medications or illnesses affect the prefrontal cortex?

Methods.—Cerebral blood flow was measured with positron emission tomographic imaging and statistical analysis to detect gyral level abnormalities in 17 patients with early schizophrenia who had never received neuroleptic agents and in matched control subjects.

Results.—In patients, separate prefrontal regions (lateral, orbital, medial) showed decreased perfusion, as did anatomically connected inferior temporal and parietal cortex regions. Increased perfusion was seen in the thalamus, cerebellum, and retrosplenial cingulate, suggestive of imbalance in distributed neural circuits.

Conclusions.—Treatment and chronicity were controlled for by studying neuroleptic-naïve patients during early illness, and other factors were controlled for by closely matching the control group. Flow abnormalities thus were unrelated to neuroleptic medication or chronic psychosis, easing some previous concerns. Use of the term *hypofrontality* to designate these flow deficits should perhaps be discouraged in favor of terms designating specific dysfunctional regions. Although characterized by prefrontal cortex dysfunction, schizophrenia is more complex, involving imbalances in circuits throughout the brain. Psychotic symptoms arise from this imbalance, with impairments in priority setting, information acquisition and processing, meaningful thought, and appropriate behavior.

► Measurement of blood flow in the brain is a surrogate for metabolic activity. The first important brain imaging findings in schizophrenia were the pioneering work of Ingvar and Franzen using the xenon method developed by Seymour Kety. Since their 1974 publication, there have been numerous reports of decreased blood flow and metabolic activity in the frontal cortex of schizophrenic patients. This study advances our knowledge because it utilized never-medicated schizophrenic patients. It may be concluded that medication is not the cause of the decreased activity in these regions. This study also demonstrated 3 specific regions of the frontal cortex in which blood flow was decreased: lateral, orbital, and medial cortex. Previous studies from other groups have shown that these areas are involved in working memory, attention and arousal (lateral cortex), emotional memory (orbital), and willed intention or initiation of behavior (medical cortex).

H. Meltzer, M.D.

Neuropsychological Correlates of Syndromes in Schizophrenia

Norman RMG, Malla AK, Morrison-Stewart SL, et al (Univ of Western Ontario, London, Ont, Canada; North Bay Psychiatric Hosp, Canada)

Br J Psychiatry 170:134–139, 1997 9–10

Background.—Liddle and others advocate a 3-domain model of schizophrenia: psychomotor poverty, from dorsolateral prefrontal cortex dysfunction; reality distortion, from medial temporal lobe dysfunction (in particular, the left medial temporal lobe); and disorganization, from mediobasal prefrontal cortex dysfunction. This model leads to 3 expected correlations: (1) psychomotor poverty symptoms with impaired performance on neuropsychologic tests of dorsolateral prefrontal cortex function, (2) disorganization with impaired mediobasal prefrontal function, and (3) reality distortion with impaired temporal lobe function.

Methods.—The 3 predicted correlations were examined in 87 subjects with confirmed schizophrenia. After scoring of symptoms for all 3 syndromes, patients took 6 neuropsychologic tests specific to the brain areas of interest.

Results.—Two of the 3 expected correlations were not seen, but reality distortion did correlate with neuropsychological performance reflective of temporal lobe function.

Conclusions.—Theories of discrete cortical-subcortical circuits for psychomotor poverty and disorganization were borne out in general, but predicted localizations were not seen. Reality distortion appears to be particularly associated with temporal lobe function.

► There is much interest in the notion that the primary deficit in schizophrenia is in cognition and that various syndromes of psychopathology may be understood as the result of primary abnormalities in cognition. A prediction of this model is that there should be correlations between cognitive measures that reflect specific brain function and measures of psychopathology. This study found little evidence to support this view. Reality distortion, i.e., positive symptoms, was correlated with tests of verbal memory, which are dependent mainly on temporal lobe function, but the correlation was relatively weak. The correlations between psychopathology and the 2 other syndromes that have been identified, psychomotor poverty (negative symptoms) and disorganization, were not consistent with previous findings from Liddle and colleagues. It may be that these results are sensitive to the medication and chronicity of this particularly patient group. The hypothesis is a very compelling one and should receive further testing before it is rejected.

H. Meltzer, M.D.

Neuropsychological Dysfunction in Schizotypal Personality Disorder: A Profile Analysis

Voglmaier MM, Seidman LJ, Salisbury D, et al (Harvard Med School, Boston; Brockton/West Roxbury Veterans Affairs Med Ctr, Mass)

Biol Psychiatry 41:530–540, 1997 9–11

Purpose.—Several lines of evidence suggest a biological relationship between chronic schizophrenia and schizotypal personality disorder (SPD). There are few data on the neuropsychological functioning of patients with SPD, however, though the available information suggests deficits similar to but less severe than those seen in schizophrenia. The neuropsychological profile of 10 subjects with SPD was studied.

Methods.—The study included 10 right-handed men meeting the *Diagnostic and Statistical Manual of Mental Disorders*, ed 3, revised criteria for SPD. Ten matched normal controls were studied as well. The SPD group was of at least normal intelligence, but had problems with social and occupational functioning. The men were tested on a wide range of cognitive functions, including abstraction, verbal and spatial intelligence, memory and learning, language, attention, and motor skills. Test scores were standardized according to the results in the normal controls to construct a neuropsychologic profile for the subjects with SPD.

Results.—The SPD group showed significantly reduced performance on the California Verbal Learning Test, reflecting problems with semantic clustering. They also had problems with concept formation, abstraction, and mental flexibility on the Wisconsin Card Sort Test. After correction for verbal ability and education, the SPD subjects still showed relatively severe deficits of verbal learning and abstraction. There was also evidence of a milder reduction in other cognitive domains.

Conclusions.—This study identifies some areas of specific neuropsychological dysfunction in patients with SPD. The findings support notions of left-temporal and prefrontal brain dysfunction in schizophrenia. The social and occupational difficulties of patients with SPD may arise from both character features and cognitive deficits. More research into the behavioral, functional, and structural correlates of brain function in SPD is needed.

► This study, along with previous research, has demonstrated significant cognitive impairment in patients with SPD. Only 2 of the 10 patients studied had a first-degree relative with schizophrenia, but the cognitive profile was comparable to that of relatives with schizophrenia. In the 2 areas where this group differed from controls, abstraction and executive function and verbal learning, the deficit was appreciable but less severe than that found in schizophrenia. The authors suggest that the cognitive impairment was the basis for the patients' relatively poor social and work function, but the importance of psychopathology in this regard requires further study. Whether the process(es) that lead to cognitive dysfunction in SPD are the same as those in schizophrenia and when they occur in SPD (adolescence or later) could be important in helping to understand the greater cognitive impairment in schizophrenia.

H. Meltzer, M.D.

The Relationship Between Smooth Pursuit Performance, Motion Perception and Sustained Visual Attention in Patients With Schizophrenia and Normal Controls

Stuve TA, Friedman L, Jesberger JA, et al (Case Western Reserve Univ, Cleveland, Ohio)

Psychol Med 27:143–152, 1997 9–12

Background.—Patients with schizophrenia exhibit impaired smooth-pursuit eye movement, perhaps related to impaired motion perception, a potential link between visual perception and ocular motor programming. Area MT, a cortical area in the parieto-occipital region of monkeys selectively involved in motion processing (corresponding to area V5 in humans), is critical in smooth-pursuit performance. It was hypothesized that schizophrenic smooth-pursuit impairment is related to impaired motion perception.

Methods.—Smooth pursuit, motion perception, and sustained attention were assessed in 19 patients with schizophrenia treated with clozapine and 19 control subjects.

Results.—A statistically significant negative correlation was found between smooth-pursuit gain and motion perception threshold ($r = -0.6018$). This correlation remained after controlling for attention deficit determined by 2 measures ($r = -0.5995$ and $r = -0.6013$).

Conclusions.—Smooth-pursuit gain is strongly correlated with motion perception in patients with schizophrenia, a relationship not resulting from sustained visual attention impairment. A dysfunction in area V5 is quite probably responsible for smooth-pursuit impairment in schizophrenia.

► Abnormalities in smooth-pursuit eye movement in schizophrenia are among the most robust of biological correlates of this disease. The finding of a strong negative correlation between smooth-pursuit gain and motion perception threshold, independent of any deficits in attention, is the first evidence to suggest that the deficit in smooth-pursuit gain is related to a possible abnormality in brain area V5, which is located in the parieto-occipital regions and plays an important role in both motion perception and gain. These results were obtained in clozapine-treated patients and must be replicated in neuroleptic-free patients. Abnormalities in smooth pursuit are also present in first-degree relatives of schizophrenic patients and some patients with mood disorders. Further research is needed to determine whether motion perception threshold and smooth-pursuit gain are related in these groups as well.

H. Meltzer, M.D.

Regionally Specific Pattern of Neurochemical Pathology in Schizophrenia as Assessed by Multislice Proton Magnetic Resonance Spectroscopic Imaging

Bertolino A, Nawroz S, Mattay VS, et al (Intramural Research Programs, NIMH Neurosciences Ctr at Saint Elizabeths, Washington, DC)

Am J Psychiatry 153:1554–1563, 1996 9–13

Background.—Proton magnetic resonance spectroscopy (^{1}H-MRS) has provided in vivo evidence of pathologic changes in the brain in schizophrenia. The ^{1}H-MRS method detects strong signals from *N*-acetyl-aspartate (NAA), choline compounds (CHO), creatine and phosphocreatine (CRE), and lactate. Located within neurons but of uncertain intracellular function, NAA has the most prominent ^{1}H-MRS peak (other than water). Brain choline stores are reflected in the CHO signal. The CRE signal reflects compounds of cellular energy metabolism. Lactate is indicative of glycolysis in excess of capacity for oxidative metabolism.

Methods.—Subjects were 10 inpatients (8 men and 2 women, mean age 37.4 years, fulfilling DSM-IV criteria for chronic schizophrenia and receiving neuroleptic drugs) and a control group of 10 healthy sex-, age-, and handedness-matched volunteers. Multislice ^{1}H-MRS was used to determine ratios of metabolite peak areas for multiple cortical and subcortical regions, and findings were examined for correlation with hippocampal region tissue volume.

Results.—Reductions of NAA/CRE and NAA/NAA ratios in the centrum semiovale indicated neurochemical abnormality confined to the hippocampal region and the dorsolateral prefrontal cortex bilaterally and in none of the other surveyed regions. There was no correlation between NAA ratios and volume of the hippocampal region. No surveyed region showed differences in centrum semiovale CHO/CRE, CHO/CHO, or CRE/CRE.

Conclusions.—Neuronal abnormality in patients with schizophrenia is suggested by the NAA reduction; absence of active gliosis is suggested by the stable CHO signal. This absence of gliosis—consistent with neuropathologic studies describing neuronal loss, dysplasia, or hypoplasia but not gliosis—is further evidence that schizophrenia is not a neurodegenerative disorder.

► The major import of this MRI study is that it provides further evidence for the role of the dorsolateral prefrontal cortex and the hippocampus in schizophrenia. The biological significance of *N*-acetyl-aspartate is less clear. There is no evidence to indicate that the decreased concentrations reported here indicate neurodegeneration. Magnetic resonance spectroscopy has considerable promise for further elucidating the neurochemical abnormalities in schizophrenia and other psychiatric disorders.

H. Meltzer, M.D.

Decreased Serotonergic Responsivity in Platelets of Drug-Free Patients With Schizophrenia

Yao JK, van Kammen DP, Moss HB, et al (Dept of Veterans Affairs Med Ctr, Pittsburgh, Pa; Univ of Pittsburgh, Pa)

Psychiatry Res 63:123–132, 1996 9–14

Introduction.—5-Hydroxytryptamine$_2$ receptors in the brain are thought to play a regulatory role in behavioral function because of their affinity for serotonin. In patients with schizophrenia who were either drug free or treated with neuroleptic agents, increased levels of blood or platelet 5-HT have been reported. To study the brain 5-HT transporter in neuropsychiatric disorders, investigators validated the use of human platelets as a peripheral model. The effect of neuroleptic treatment on serotonin-amplified platelet aggregation responses was assessed in unmedicated patients with schizophrenia and in patients with schizophrenia treated with haloperidol.

Methods.—In 27 patients with schizophrenia, the effects of neuroleptics on peripheral serotonergic function were studied by measuring physiologic responsivity of the platelet 5-HT$_2$ receptor complex before and after haloperidol withdrawal. These effects were compared with those in 18 healthy volunteers. To measure platelet secretion using a sensitive luminescent assay for extracellular adenosine triphosphate, investigators used a luminaggregometer. Platelet aggregation was determined by measuring the increase in impedance across collagen-coated electrodes to which platelets and platelet aggregates adhere.

Results.—5-Hydroxytryptamine amplifies the adenosine diphosphate-induced platelet aggregation and dense granule secretion in human platelets. In platelets from normal volunteers and patients stabilized with haloperidol, such an amplification was significantly enhanced in patients not receiving any drugs; however, the magnitude of the 5-HT-amplified dense granule secretion response was no longer significant after haloperidol withdrawal, which demonstrated a decreased serotonergic responsivity in schizophrenia. The net changes of adenosine diphosphate-induced dense granule secretion with and without the presence of 5-HT in the patients who were drug free were correlated significantly and negatively with the Brief Psychiatric Rating Scale and with the Bunney-Hamburg psychosis ratings; however, they were not correlated with the scores on the scale for the Assessment of Negative Symptoms. Between patients with and without relapses, there were no significant differences in 5-HT amplification in the drug-free group.

Conclusion.—A reduced physiologic responsivity mediated through the platelet 5-HT$_2$ receptor complex has been demonstrated in patients with schizophrenia who were not receiving drugs, and this can be modified by haloperidol treatment. Serotonergic mechanisms may account for the pharmacologic action of haloperidol. The magnitude of 5-HT-amplified dense granule secretion may be useful for predicting the therapeutic outcome after haloperidol treatment.

► The finding of a decreased responsivity of the platelet 5-HT_{2A} receptor in patients with schizophrenia who were neither receiving drugs nor treatment with haloperidol is most interesting, especially because the more blunted the response, the higher the scores on the Bunney-Hamburg psychosis ratings. This suggests that the blunted 5-HT_{2A} response may be related to the disease process rather than to a reactive downregulation. Of course, platelet findings, even when replicated, may have little to do with what is happening in the brain. Further studies with patients who have never received medication and studies after treatment with other antipsychotic agents are needed. It would also be of interest to see how well the platelet measures compare with central measures of 5-HT_{2A} function.

H. Meltzer, M.D.

Role of Cortical *N*-Methyl-*D*-Aspartate Receptors in Auditory Sensory Memory and Mismatch Negativity Generation: Implications for Schizophrenia

Javitt DC, Steinschneider M, Schroeder CE, et al (Albert Einstein College of Medicine, Bronx, NY)

Proc Natl Acad Sci U S A 93:11962–11967, 1996 9–15

Introduction.—The capability of the brain to store and manipulate information over brief time periods, ranging from seconds to minutes, is called working memory. Critical substrates for working memory are distributed throughout the cortex, whereas long-term memory is critically dependent on hippocampal long-term potentiation. A model for attention-dependent forms of working memory is auditory sensory memory or echoic memory, which refers to the capability of the brain to store representations of the physical characteristics of simple auditory stimuli for seconds to minutes. In the initiation of long-term memory, *N*-methy-D-aspartate (NMDA) receptors play a crucial role. Mismatch negativity refers to the generation of a specific auditory event-related potential component. Critical substrates for echoic memory and mismatch negativity reside in the region of the primary auditory cortex.

Methods.—Intracortical records through the auditory cortex were combined with focal infusion of NMDA and non–NMDA antagonists into the microregion of the recording electrode to investigate neurochemical mechanisms underlying mismatch negativity generation in awake monkeys. Linear array, multichannel electrodes inserted on a short-term basis into the cortical region of interest were used to obtain recordings

Results.—Without affecting prior obligatory activity in the primary auditory cortex, both competitive and noncompetitive NMDA antagonists block the generation of mismatch negativity. It is suggested that through open, unblocked NMDA channels, mismatch negativity represents selective current flow.

Conclusion.—In the assessment of stimulus familiarity–unfamiliarity, which is a key process underlying working memory performance, a crucial role of cortical NMDA receptors is suggested. Important insights into the pathophysiology of cognitive dysfunction in schizophrenia may be provided by the present findings, which suggest that intracortical mechanisms underlie mismatch negativity generation.

► Deficits in working memory are among the key findings in schizophrenia. Such short-term memory is critical for normal cognitive functioning. This monkey study demonstrates that so-called mismatch negativity, an event-related brain potential that can be readily measured in humans, is linked to working memory. It further demonstrates that stimulation of a specific class of glutamate receptors, the NMDA receptor, which is blocked by the psychotomimetic drug phencyclidine, is necessary for working memory and the accompanying mismatch negativity. Mismatch negativity is diminished in patients with schizophrenia, but there is, as yet, no research relating the deficit in mismatch negativity and deficits in working memory. These data are consistent with the evidence for decreased glutamatergic activity in schizophrenia and reinforce the need for treatment strategies that enhance glutamatergic activity without causing excitotoxicity as a result of excessive stimulation of cortical and subcortical glutamate receptors.

H. Meltzer, M.D.

Clozapine for the Treatment of Psychosis in Parkinson's Disease: A Review

Auzou P, Özsancak C, Hannequin D, et al (Hôpital Charles Nicholle, France; CHU de Rouen, France)

Acta Neurol Scand 94:329–336, 1996 9–16

Introduction.—About 20% of patients with Parkinson's disease have psychiatric symptoms such as depression, hypomania, delirium, delusions, hallucinations, or paranoid psychoses. In up to 60% of patients with terminal-stage Parkinson's disease, acute psychoses exist, indicating a link between increasing neurotransmitter disturbances and antiparkinsonian medication. Mental function improves by reducing the dose of dopaminomimetic therapy or by increasing classic neuroleptics, but extrapyramidal motor symptoms worsen. There is great interest in new antipsychotic agents such as clozapine, which produces few extrapyramidal effects. The efficacy and side effects of clozapine are reviewed. Clozapine has been proposed as a treatment for the psychosis due to L-DOPA or direct acting dopamine agonists such as bromocriptine and pergolide for Parkinson's disease since 1985.

Literature Review.—A literature review was conducted that included 200 patients whose ages ranged from 52 to 80 years. The mean duration of Parkinson's disease was more than 10 years. In these patients, doses to remove psychoses were much lower than doses needed for patients with schizophrenia. Patients with Parkinson's disease had doses ranging from

6.25 mg every other day to 275 mg/day. Generally, it remained at less than 125 mg/day.

Results.—Good results were found in 90% without extrapyramidal symptoms worsening. The improvement occurs within 1–7 days in most patients. There was even improvement noted among some patients when treated by clozapine alone or as dopatherapy was secondarily increased. In patients with dementia or depression, less efficacious results were obtained. One of the most frequently encountered side effects was sedation; however, the withdrawal of clozapine was rarely indicated.

Conclusion.—Regular blood cell counts should be conducted even if the risk of agranulocytosis is slight. When an increase of dopaminergic agonists is necessary, clozapine can prevent psychosis. Treatment should be initiated at 6.25 mg/day and increased to the point at which there is a clinical response and tolerability. The most important advantage of clozapine is the absence of aggravation of motor status.

► This is a good source of information about the clinically and theoretically significant observation that clozapine, at doses between 10% to 20% of those needed to treat schizophrenia in middle-aged adults, is capable of rapidly treating the psychosis caused by L-DOPA or direct-acting dopamine agonists in patients with Parkinson's disease without worsening and sometimes even improving the motor symptoms. The likelihood that this effect is not caused by direct blockade of D dopamine receptors is very high. It may reflect the capability of clozapine to modulate the serotonergic system at very low concentrations and to modulate the indirect effects of serotonin on the dopamine system.

H. Meltzer, M.D.

Mood and Anxiety Disorders

A Complete Genome Screen for Genes Predisposing to Severe Bipolar Disorder in Two Costa Rican Pedigrees

McInnes LA, Escamilla MA, Service SK, et al (Univ of California, San Francisco; Universidad de Costa Rica, San Jose; Hosp Calderon Guardia, San Jose, Costa Rica; et al)

Proc Natl Acad Sci U S A 93:13060–13065, 1996 9–17

Background.—Bipolar (BP) mood disorder has a major genetic component, but no BP mood disorder genes have been definitively localized. Gene mapping used for simple mendelian disorders may be inappropriate for complex psychiatric disorders, in which high single-locus logarithm of odds (lod) scores may be misleading.

Methods.—Two Costa Rican pedigrees were chosen for high densities of BP (only severe, clinically distinctive BP [BP-I] and schizoaffective disorder, manic type [SAD-M], not milder BP or unipolar disorder) and lineages traceable to the area's founding. Linkage simulations selected the most informative cases for genotyping studies under a 90% dominant model.

Results.—Two-point linkage tests were used on 473 microsatellites, and 23 markers exceeded predesignated thresholds for coverage in one or both lineages. Suggestive lod scores in 18q22–q23 were clustered adjacent to but not overlapping a recently reported potential localization to 18q21 of BP-I and BP-II together. Other promising regions, including 11p13–p14 and the telomere of 18p, were not near previously suggested locations for broadly defined BP disorder.

Conclusions.—Suggestive lod scores were found in 18q22–q23, where more extensive studies support a BP-I gene. Positive lod score clustering supports further investigation of 11p13–p14 and the telomere of 18p. Despite possible false positive results with isolated suggestive lod scores, scores in one lineage at markers *D3S1285* and *D7S510* are sufficiently high that these regions should be examined further.

▶ This study is of interest because it produced a number of important leads for the further study of genes that may predispose to BP disorder, especially segments on chromosomes 11 and 18, and because of its methodologic differences between the previous generation of studies, which used linkage analysis to identify genes at a single location. These findings often proved unstable, in part because of broader definitions of the phenotype. This study considered only individuals with BP-I disorder as affected. Surprisingly, they also included schizoaffective disorder, manic type, which does run the risk of including patients whose illness is primarily related to schizophrenia. The stage of the work that has been completed to date is to scan nearly the entire genome by means of 473 microsatellite markers. In the next stages, the most likely candidate regions will be determined and then one of several approaches to identify specific genes will be used. These multi-stage strategies have been used to map complex nonpsychiatric disorders.

H. Meltzer, M.D.

A Follow-up Report of a Genome Search for Affective Disorder Predisposition Loci in the Old Order Amish

LaBuda MC, Maldonado M, Marshall D, et al (Johns Hopkins Med Insts, Baltimore, Md; Washington Univ, St Louis)

Am J Hum Genet 59:1343–1362, 1996 9–18

Introduction.—Disturbances in mood ranging from extreme elation, or mania, to severe depression characterize affective disorders, which can be associated with hyperactivity, weight changes, sleep disturbances, feelings of worthlessness, and suicidal ideation. There has been documentation for a tendency of the mood disorders to cluster within families, suggesting genetic vulnerability to bipolar disorder (mania and depression) and unipolar disorder (depression without mania). In 1984, the first formal linkage analysis of affective disorder in the Old Order Amish was published, and since then, a complete genome screen has been conducted, using data from this family. The logarithm of odds (LOD) score results for an addi-

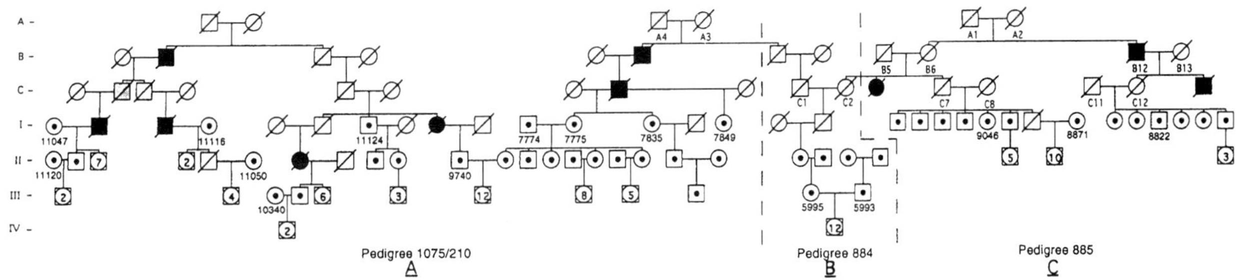

FIGURE 1.—Genotyped members of the Old Order Amish pedigree. The individuals for whom DNA exists are indicated by *dots* or by a *circle within a square* within which is the number of individuals in that sibship. The diagnostic status is unknown to the individuals doing the genotyping and is therefore not shown, except in some members of the earlier generations for whom DNA does not exist. (Courtesy of LaBuda MC, Maldonado M, Marshall D, et al: A follow-up report of a genome search for affective disorder predisposition loci in the Old Order Amish. *Am J Hum Genet* 59:1343–1362, 1996. The University of Chicago Press, publisher.)

tional 367 markers throughout the genome are presented, along with allele- and haplotype-sharing analyses on chromosomes sufficiently saturated with markers.

Methods.—Members of the Old Order Amish were genotyped by extended pedigree (Fig 1). Using a 4-stage process, analyses were conducted: 2-point LOD scores were calculated for all loci under a dominant model with reduced penetrance; for the sharing of alleles in similar affected individuals, a screen was used to highlight areas for further analysis; the affected-pedigree-member method was used to analyze the preceding areas and markers on densely covered chromosomes; in areas showing apparent clustering of significant allele sharing, the sharing of extended haplotypes in affected individuals was examined.

Results.—No statistically significant LOD scores resulted among the 367 markers analyzed. At 74 loci, some degree of allele sharing was found. More stringent significant criteria suggestive of linkage were passed by 3.8% of 14 of all markers analyzed.

Conclusion.—Areas that were clearly involved in the etiology of affective disorder in this population were not identified; however, this analysis provided methods for more informative exploration of potentially suggestive results, such as using 2-gene models and examining extended haplotypes by analyzing for benign recurrent intrahepatic cholestasis.

► Previous studies have identified genetic markers for affective disorder on chromosomes 5, 16, and 18. This large scale, very well-conducted screen of nearly 400 genetic loci across all chromosomes failed to find any significant linkage between any of the loci and affective disorder in this Old Amish population. The failure to replicate previous work may be because of heterogeneity but it could also be because of the previous results reflecting chance occurrences that will not be replicated. It is inevitable that genomic research with sufficient numbers of well-ascertained probands will identify a group of genes that predispose to affective disorder. It is likely that this will occur in the next decade.

H. Meltzer, M.D.

A Linkage Study of Bipolar Illness

Berrettini WH, Ferraro TN, Goldin LR, et al (Thomas Jefferson Univ, Philadelphia; Natl Inst of Mental Health, Bethesda, Md; Indiana Univ, Indianapolis; et al)

Arch Gen Psychiatry 54:27–35, 1997 9–19

Background.—A heritable component of bipolar (BP) disorder is supported by epidemiologic studies, but specific inherited factors remain unknown. Linkage strategies, including genome-wide search, can be used to find BP disorder susceptibility loci.

Methods.—Twenty-two families, in which 173 of almost 400 members had BP-I, schizoaffective disorder, BP-II with major depression, or recurrent unipolar illness, underwent linkage studies. Linkage analyses were performed on 310 DNA markers on chromosomes 1, 5p, 6, 8, 10q, 11q, and 12–18.

Results.—No examined loci compellingly demonstrated linkage by logarithm of odds scores, but model-independent analysis of affected pedigree members did reveal statistically significant evidence ($P < 0.0001$) of a susceptibility gene in pericentromeric chromosome 18. Multilocal analysis by affected sibling pairs concurred in this localization ($P < 0.00008$).

Conclusions.—A BP disorder susceptibility gene may be located near the centromere of chromosome 18. Independent confirmation in other pedigrees suggests that this disease linkage is valid.

▶ This linkage study of BP disorder explored about 5% of the genome using 310 microsatellite markers. There were no promising leads developed by logarithm of odds score analysis. However, using a less stringent model-independent method, the pericentromeric region of chromosome 18 that was not identified in the study of McInnes et al. (see preceding abstract) was found to have a BP susceptibility gene. The differences between the 2 studies may result from the differences in phenotype criteria, which were broader in this study, and the use of more highly inbred, homogeneous families in the study of McInnes et al. There are 3 other studies that replicate the results of Berrettini et al. All 4 studies find the pericentromeric region of chromosome 18 to be related to paternal transmission. There are 2 candidate genes in this region. The genes for the α subunit of a guanosine triphosphate-binding protein and for the ACTH receptor have been localized to this region. Further association studies of these genes with BP disorder are the next step.

H. Meltzer, M.D.

Polymorphism in Serotonin Transporter Gene Associated With Susceptibility to Major Depression

Ogilvie AD, Battersby S, Bubb VJ, et al (Royal Edinburgh Hosp, Univ of Edinburgh, Scotland)

Lancet 347:731–733, 1996 9–20

Background.—The primary target of action for selective antidepressant drugs is the brain's serotonin transporter. Genetic polymorphisms could be related to affective disorder.

Methods.—A polymorphic region of the human serotonin transporter gene was compared between a study group of 83 patients with major affective disorders (39 with unipolar depressive and 44 with bipolar disorder) and a control group of 122 anonymous blood donors and 71 volunteers screened for psychiatric disorders.

Results.—Three novel alleles of variable-number-tandem-repeat element *(STin2.9, STin2.10,* and *STin2.12)* were found to contain 9, 10, and 12 copies, respectively. Frequencies of allelic forms differed significantly between groups, mainly because of excess *STin2.9* allele in unipolar disease ($\chi^2 = 10.05$, $P < 0.004$); *STin2.9* with 9 repeat copies carried a significant risk for unipolar disorder (odds ratio 6.95).

Conclusions.—Susceptibility to affective disorder is probably polygenic, but this strong candidate gene is a starting point for further understanding.

▶ This is the first study to report linkage of a polymorphism in the serotonin transporter gene, which is located on chromosome 17, and major (unipolar) depression. Previous studies have found no evidence of an abnormality in the coding region of the gene in affective disorder. A subsequent study found no association between this polymorphism and bipolar disorder.[1] This particular polymorphism is within a noncoding region (intron) of the gene. It may be a marker for affective disorder (i.e., in linkage disequilibrium) with a mutation elsewhere within the transporter gene not yet discovered or a susceptibility locus nearby. It is also possible that the variable- number-tandem-repeat polymorphism may itself be implicated in the disease process by regulating transcription of the gene. Some of the variance in response to serotonin reuptake inhibitors could be related to these variations in the 5–HT transporter gene. Replication of these findings in an independent sample of patients with unipolar depression is essential.

H. Meltzer, M.D.

Reference

1. Bellivier F, Laplanche JL, Leboyer M, et al: Serotonin transporter gene and manic depressive illness: An association study. *Biol Psychiatry* 41:750–752, 1997.

Hippocampal Atrophy in Recurrent Major Depression

Sheline YI, Wang PW, Gado MH, et al (Washington Univ, St Louis)

Proc Natl Acad Sci U S A 93:3908–3913, 1996 9–21

Introduction.—As a biological characteristic of acute major depression, dysregulation of the hypothalamo–pituitary-adrenal axis resulting in hypercortisolemia has been studied for many years. A recent study using MRI found that right-sided hippocampal volume decreased in combat-related posttraumatic stress syndrome; however, there has been no study to evaluate the association between hippocampal volume loss and depression. In older women with recurrent major depression, hippocampal volume was evaluated by using high-resolution MRI and stereological measurement. It was hypothesized that hippocampal volume loss related to depression, would be duration- and age-dependent.

Methods.—By using volumetric MR images, investigators compared the hippocampal volumes of 10 matched normal controls with the hippocampal volume of 10 women ranging in age from 51 to 86 years with histories of major depressive episodes but who were in remission with no known medical comorbidity. All women were selected to eliminate brain differences. Images were reviewed from the sagittal, axillary, and coronal per-

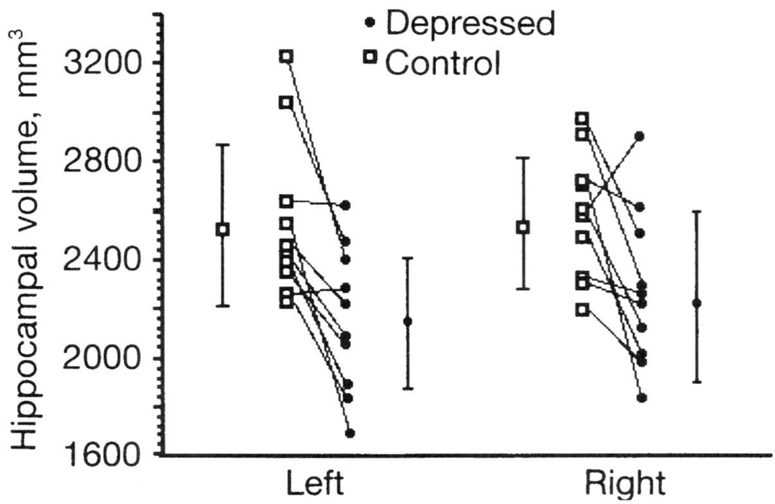

FIGURE 2.—Left and right hippocampal volumes for each pair of research subjects with depression and the age, sex, education, and height-matched case controls; the mean and standard deviation for each group are also shown. (Courtesy of Sheline YI, Wang PW, Gado MH, et al: Hippocampal atrophy in recurrent major depression. *Proc Natl Acad Sci USA* 93:3908–3913, 1996. Copyright 1996 National Academy of Sciences, U.S.A.)

spectives. The women with depression had a mean of 4.5 lifetime episodes of major depression and a lifetime mean of 1,303 days of depression.

Results.—Significantly smaller left and right hippocampal volumes were found in women with histories of major depression (Fig 2), but there was no difference in total cerebral volumes. The total duration of major depression correlated with the degree of hippocampal volume reduction. Within the hippocampus, large hippocampal low-signal foci with diameters of greater than or equal to 4.5 mm were found within the hippocampus. The total number of days of depression correlated with the number of large, low-signal foci.

Conclusion.—Perhaps as a result of a progressive process mediated by glucocorticoid neurotoxicity, depression may be associated with hippocampal atrophy.

► This study provides clear evidence for decreased hippocampal volume in patients with depression. The possible role of glucocorticoid excess causing this decrease in hippocampal volume is very intriguing and provides further reason for treatment strategies designed to reduce glucocorticoid production or responsivity in depression. The correlations between severity of depression and decrease in hippocampal volume are strong evidence for the clinical significance of these observations.

H. Meltzer, M.D.

Adult Major Affective Disorder After Prenatal Exposure to an Influenza Epidemic

Machón RA, Mednick SA, Huttunen MO (Loyola Marymount Univ, Los Angeles; Univ of Southern California, Los Angeles; Univ of Helsinki)
Arch Gen Psychiatry 54:322–328, 1997 9–22

Introduction.—A number of studies published during the past decade report an increase in schizophrenia diagnoses among individuals exposed to an influenza epidemic during the second trimester of gestation. Disruptions in the neural processes during this critical period are hypothesized to increase the probability of adult schizophrenia. Recent MRI findings suggest that affective illness also may have a neurodevelopmental origin. The role of influenza exposure in affective disorders was examined in individuals exposed to the 1957 epidemic in Helsinki, Finland.

Methods.—The period of the epidemic in greater Helsinki was defined as lasting from October 8, 1957 to November 14, 1957. The index cohort consisted of all children born between November 15, 1957 and August 14, 1958 in the county of Uusimaa and admitted as inpatients before the age of 29 years 10 months to a psychiatric hospital in Uusimaa county. Controls were all children fulfilling the same criteria, but who were born 6 years before (from November 15, 1951 to August 14, 1957) the influenza epidemic.

Results.—Index and control groups were compared separately by the 3 trimesters for distribution of major affective disorders. Exposure to the influenza epidemic during trimesters 1 or 3 did not increase the proportion of major affective disorders, compared with controls. Exposure during the second trimester, however, was associated with a significantly elevated proportion of major affective disorders in the index group (13%), relative to the control group (2%). The second-trimester effect appeared to be somewhat stronger in men than it was in women and was unchanged when population-based rates of major affective disorder were estimated. The increase in major affective disorder after second-trimester exposure to influenza was significant for the proportion of unipolar forms of major affective disorder, compared with nonexposed controls (7.1% versus 0.5%, respectively).

Conclusion.—These data support the hypothesis that some forms of major affective disorder, particularly unipolar depressive disorder, may have a neurodevelopmental origin. Specifically, disruptions in the neural processes may result from exposure to maternal influenza during the second trimester.

► This study reports for the first time that there is an increased risk of affective disorder, especially unipolar depression, in the offspring of women who contracted influenza during the second trimester of pregnancy. This parallels the previous findings of these investigators and others that there is an increased risk of schizophrenia associated with second trimester infection with the flu as well. Indeed, the effect on incidence of mood disorders is greater than that for schizophrenia. If these findings are confirmed by subsequent study, it would suggest that both affective disorder and schizophrenia may be considered neurodevelopmental. Thus, these results are consistent with a great deal of other literature, which suggests there are many important biological similarities between these groups of mental disorders.

H. Meltzer, M.D.

Positron Emission Tomography Measurement of Cerebral Metabolic Correlates of Tryptophan Depletion–induced Depressive Relapse

Bremner JD, Innis RB, Salomon RM, et al (Yale Univ, New Haven, Conn; Natl Ctr for Posttraumatic Stress Disorder, West Haven, Conn)

Arch Gen Psychiatry 54:364–374, 1997 9–23

Introduction.—Alterations in central serotonergic function play a role in the pathogenesis of depression, and there is some evidence that reduced serotonin availability in the brain is associated with depressive relapse. In patients with major depression, short-term depletion of plasma tryptophan was shown to result in depressive relapse. This study tested the hypothesis that tryptophan depletion-induced depressive relapse is associated with decreases in metabolism in various brain regions.

Methods.—Study participants were 21 patients age 18 to 65 years. All met criteria for a lifetime history of major depression, and all were clinically improved at the time of the study. Nineteen were treated with fluoxetine hydrochloride and 2 with paroxetine. A tryptophan-depleting drink and placebo were ingested in a double-blind manner. Positron emission tomography (PET) was performed 6 hours after each was administered. Brain metabolism was compared in patients with and without a tryptophan depletion-induced depressive relapse.

Results.—Tryptophan depletion resulted in a marked reduction of plasma tryptophan levels in all patients and led to a depressive relapse in 7 of 21 patients. These 7 patients were found to have a decrease in brain metabolism in the middle frontal gyrus, thalamus, and orbitofrontal cortex. This decrease was not present in the 14 patients without a tryptophan depletion-induced depressive relapse. There was a correlation between decreased brain metabolism in the 3 regions and increased depressive symptoms. Relapse-prone patients had increased baseline metabolism in the prefrontal and limbic regions.

Discussion.—As suggested by findings of previous studies, tryptophan depletion was associated with a decrease in brain metabolism in the thalamus, middle frontal gyrus, and orbitofrontal cortex in patients with a tryptophan depletion-induced depressive relapse. The increased baseline metabolism in the relapse group contributed substantially to the difference between patients who relapsed and those who did not.

▶ This elegant study provides additional evidence to support recent suggestions that the dorsolateral prefrontal cortex, thalamus, and orbitofrontal cortex are key areas of the brain that are involved in major depression. The finding that brain metabolism decreased in these areas only in those serotonin uptake inhibitor–treated patients (7 of 21) who relapsed during a tryptophan–depletion protocol and that the change in metabolism in all 3 regions was correlated with the severity of the depression is impressive support for the importance of these 3 regions. The finding that baseline metabolism in the middle frontal gyrus, orbitofrontal cortex, hippocampus, and pons increased in those patients who relapsed during tryptophan depletion is important evidence for the persistence of metabolic changes in these regions during the recovery period. The nature of their significance requires and is worthy of intensive study. The low relapse rate during this paradigm is abundant evidence that serotonin deficiency, of and by itself, is not the crucial factor in most depressed patients.

H. Meltzer, M.D.

Serotonin$_{2A}$ Receptor Gene Polymorphism in Mood Disorders

Zhang H-Y, Ishigaki T, Tani K, et al (Hamamatsu Univ, Shizuoka, Japan; Univ of Southern California, Los Angeles)
Biol Psychiatry 41:768–773, 1997 9–24

Introduction.—There is growing evidence that the serotonergic (5–HT) system plays a role in the pathogenesis of mood disorders, and the 5–HT$_2$A receptor appears to be of particular importance. A group of patients with mood disorders was screened for possible DNA polymorphisms in the 5–HT$_2$A receptor by means of single-strand conformation polymorphism (SSCP) analysis.

Methods.—The 102 patients were diagnosed according to *DSM-IV* criteria. Seventy-one had depressive disorder and 31 had bipolar disorder. Of those with depressive disorder, 33 had recurrent depressive episodes. Nine in the depressive disorder group and 6 in the bipolar disorder group had attempted suicide. Also studied were 150 healthy controls with no history of psychiatric disorders. Genomic DNA was obtained from whole blood for amplification and sequencing. Patients with mood disorders were studied by means of the nonradioactive SSCP analysis method to screen for DNA polymorphisms in the gene.

Results.—The gene encoding the 5–HT$_1$A receptor had been sequenced in 34 of the mood disorder cases, but no disease-specific polymorphism was identified. The previously reported (Warren et al.) substitution of C for T at position 102 in exon 1 was confirmed. Serine, the corresponding amino acid, did not change. Compared with healthy controls and patients with bipolar disorders, patients with depressive disorders exhibited a significantly higher allele frequency of T at position 102. Patients heterozygous for the T and C alleles had a lower mean age of onset of mood disorder than those homozygous for the C allele. There was a slight association between the genotype and suicide attempts.

Discussion.—Findings provided confirmation of the substitution from T to C at position 102, reportedly a normal DNA polymorphism that does not result in an amino acid change. Patients with depressive disorders had a higher allele frequency of T at position 102 than those with bipolar disorders and healthy controls. Alternatively, it is possible that modulation of the 5–HT_2A receptors is secondary to the disease process rather than the primary cause of mood disorders.

► This is the first study to report an increase in the allele frequency of a polymorphism of the 5–HT_2A receptor in patients with major depression compared to bipolar disorder and normal controls. Findings such as this require extensive replication. If confirmed, the results would be important because postmortem studies have shown increased density of 5–HT_2A receptors in patients with depression who have committed suicide.

Whether these 2 findings are related requires further study. It may be that factors such as a 5–HT_2A or serotonin transporter polymorphism may influence whether major depression is more sensitive to serotonin than other neurotransmitters, and hence whether serotonin reuptake inhibitors or tryptophan depletion are more likely to be therapeutic or induce relapse, respectively.

H. Meltzer, M.D.

Differences Between Males and Females in Rates of Serotonin Synthesis in Human Brain

Nishizawa S, Benkelfat C, Young SN, et al (McGill Univ, Montreal)
Proc Natl Acad Sci U S A 94:5308–5313, 1997 9–25

Introduction.—Reduced levels of serotonin in the brain have been implicated in a number of psychiatric disorders. A recently developed method for measuring serotonin synthesis in the brain uses positron emission tomography (PET) and α-[^{11}C]methyl-L-tryptophan as a tracer. Healthy volunteers were recruited for measurements of serotonin synthesis in the brain.

Methods.—Study participants were 8 men and 7 women, age 18–35 years. All had good mental and physical health, and none had first-degree relatives with an axis I or axis II *DSM-III-R* diagnosis. Participants arrived at the test site at 7 AM for MRI of the head, followed by an evaluation of mood. A venous blood sample was then taken and a PET scan performed. Five hours after ingestion of a tryptophan-deficient amino acid mixture, mood was reevaluated and a second PET scan performed. Participants had ingested a prepared, low-protein diet the day before the test to achieve an acute tryptophan depletion (ATD) condition.

Results.—Average rates of serotonin synthesis at baseline were approximately 75 and 50 $pmol \cdot g^{-1} \cdot min^{-1}$, respectively, in both men and women. The rate of serotonin synthesis was reduced by ATD by a factor of about 9.5 in the men and about 1.5 in the women. Although men had higher levels of plasma-free tryptophan than women, neither men nor women exhibited significant correlations between plasma-free or total tryptophan levels and rates of serotonin synthesis. Total plasma tryptophan levels were similar in men and women at baseline and after ATD. The effect of ATD on mood ratings was not statistically significant. Only 1 participant, a woman, showed signs of distress by the end of the second scan.

Discussion.—In contrast to the variable serotonin levels measured in different areas of postmortem brains, PET scans in these healthy volunteers showed considerable uniformity in the different areas studied. This finding suggests that the rate of serotonin synthesis depends on factors other than the density of innervation. A marked difference, however, was observed in rates of serotonin synthesis between men and women (average 52% greater in men), and the biochemical effect of ATD was greater in women than in men.

▶ This study clearly establishes that there is an enormously higher rate of serotonin synthesis in men than there is in women. This is in accord with other infrahuman and human data. It is possible that women make up for the lower rate of serotonin synthesis by decreased inactivation or supersensitvie serotonin receptors of various types. Studies involving decreasing serotonin synthesis by tryptophan depletion may be more informative if they focused on women. The method used here will be of great value in further understanding the action of psychotropic drugs on serotonin synthesis in humans.

H. Meltzer, M.D.

5-HT$_{1A}$ Binding Sites in Postmortem Brain Samples From Depressed Suicides and Controls

Lowther S, De Paermentier F, Cheetham SC, et al (St George's Hosp, London; Univ College London)

J Affect Disord 42:199–207, 1997 9–26

Background.—Several lines of evidence indicate a relationship between depressive illness and abnormal serotonergic (5-hydroxytryptamine, or 5-HT) function. There also is documentation of increased serotonergic function during long-term treatment for depression. The effects of 5-HT are mediated through multiple receptors, and 3 classes (5-HT$_1$, 5-HT$_2$, and 5-HT$_3$) are well defined. A post mortem study of depressed suicides examined 5-HT$_{1A}$ binding in the amygdala, hippocampus, and in the frontal and occipital cortex. The 5-HT$_{1A}$ receptor is the best characterized subtype within the 5-HT$_1$ class.

Methods.—A psychiatrist used hospital and coroner's records and interviews with the suicides' medical practitioners to identify those with a diagnosis of endogenous depression or depressive syndrome. Of the eligible suicides, 19 were antidepressant-free and 11 were antidepressant-treated. Controls who had died from causes not involving the central nervous system were individually matched for age and sex to the suicides.

Assays of brain tissue were performed on coded samples blind to subject classification, but arranged so that samples from controls and suicides for each brain area were examined concurrently.

Results.—Tissue storage time did not differ significantly between suicides and matched controls, but time from death to storage of tissue was significantly shorter in antidepressant suicides compared with their controls. The number of 5-HT_{1A} binding sites did not differ significantly overall between suicides and controls after adjustment was made for age, sex, and postmortem delay. This was also true for the 4 regions studied.

Discussion.—Although there is considerable evidence of an association between violent suicide attempts and reduced central 5-HT turnover, violent suicides in this study did not differ from their controls in 5-HT_{1A} receptors. There was a trend toward lower 5-HT_{1A} binding in the hippocampus of nonviolent suicides and toward higher binding in the frontal cortex of antidepressant-treated suicides.

► This study agrees with several others, including one by the author, who failed to find a decrease in the density of 5-HT_{1A} receptors in cortex, hippocampus, and amygdala of patients with major depression or suicide. The several studies that have reported increases used autoradiographic methods. Although more precise in localization, autoradiographic studies are subject to artifactual results caused by methodological complexity. The lack of effect of antidepressant drugs on 5-HT_{1A} receptor density suggests that these agents are not having either a direct or an indirect effect on the 5-HT_{1A} receptor.

H. Meltzer, M.D.

Dopamine-related Genes and Their Relationships to Monoamine Metabolites in CSF

Jönsson E, Sedvall G, Brené S, et al (Karolinska Inst, Stockholm; FORENAP, Rouffach, France; Huddinge Hosp, Sweden; et al)
Biol Psychiatry 40:1032–1043, 1996 9–27

Introduction.—Concentrations of the major monoamine metabolites (MM) in lumbar CSF are widely used as indirect measures of monoamine metabolism and turnover in the brain. Animal studies have shown that a significant portion of CSF homovanillic acid (HVA), 3-methoxy-4-hydroxyphenylglycol (MHPG), and 5-hydroxyindoleacetic acid (5-HIAA) concentrations are determined by genetic mechanisms. A study of healthy volunteers examined genotypes for DNA polymorphisms in the D2 (DRD2), D3 (DRD3), and D4 (DRD4) dopamine receptor and tyrosine hydroxylase (TH) genes and their relationship to CSF MM.

Methods.—A group of 154 healthy controls were screened for potential study participants. Sixty-six agreed to take part in the study, had adequate data available, and had no current or past psychiatric disturbances. All had been controls in previous related investigations and had undergone lumbar puncture (LP) between 1974 and 1982. Their mean age at the time of the present study was 39 years; 37 were men, and 29 were women. Twenty-one had a family history of major mental illness. Samples of CSF MM were obtained by LP for measurements of HVA, MHPG, and 5-HIAA concentrations and genotype analyses. Concentrations of the MM were corrected for back length, a confounding variable.

Results.—No relationships were found between corrected MM levels and age, gender, height, weight, heredity, season of the year, or atmospheric pressure at sampling. A whole series of associations between MM concentrations and monoamine-related genotypes were recorded, primarily between dopamine-related genotypes and levels of HVA and MHPG. Subjects with specific DRD2 and TH allele and genotype configurations significantly differed in their concentrations of HVA and MHPG. The DRD3 homozygotic and heterozygotic genotypes had significantly different levels of CSF 5-HIAA. No relationship was found between DRD4 genotypes and MM concentrations.

Discussion.—Specific DRD2, DRD3, and TH genotypes appear to play a role in the regulation of monoamine turnover in the CNS. Monoamine receptors and synthesizing enzyme genotypes may thus be variance factors influencing MM concentrations in the CSF. Findings support the validity of MM concentrations as biological markers for monoamine transmission in the human brain.

▶ This report intrigued me because it provides, among other things, further evidence for the relationship between the serotonin and dopamine systems. The DRD3 was significantly related to the concentrations of 5-HIAA, the major metabolite of serotonin, in the CSF. The D3 receptor has previously been linked to vulnerability to schizophrenia and tardive dyskinesia. It will be of interest to determine if the DRD3–CSF 5-HIAA relationship also holds for schizophrenia or mood disorders. It remains to be determined which serotonin related genes are important in the determination of CSF 5-HIAA and HVA, the major metabolite of dopamine.

H. Meltzer, M.D.

Diurnal Activity and Pulsatility of the Hypothalamus–Pituitary–Adrenal System in Male Depressed Patients and Healthy Controls

Deuschle M, Scweiger U, Weber B, et al (Clinical Inst, Munich)

J Clin Endocrinol Metab 82:234–238, 1997 9–28

Introduction.—In patients with depression, hypercortisolemia is a frequent endocrine sign. There has also been demonstrated dysregulation of the hypothalamo–pituitary–adrenal stystem. There is still little known about pulsatile secretion of adrenocorticotropic hormone (ACTH) and cortisol or circadian activity in patients with depression. The hypothalamo–pituitary–adrenal system was assessed in medication-free patients and

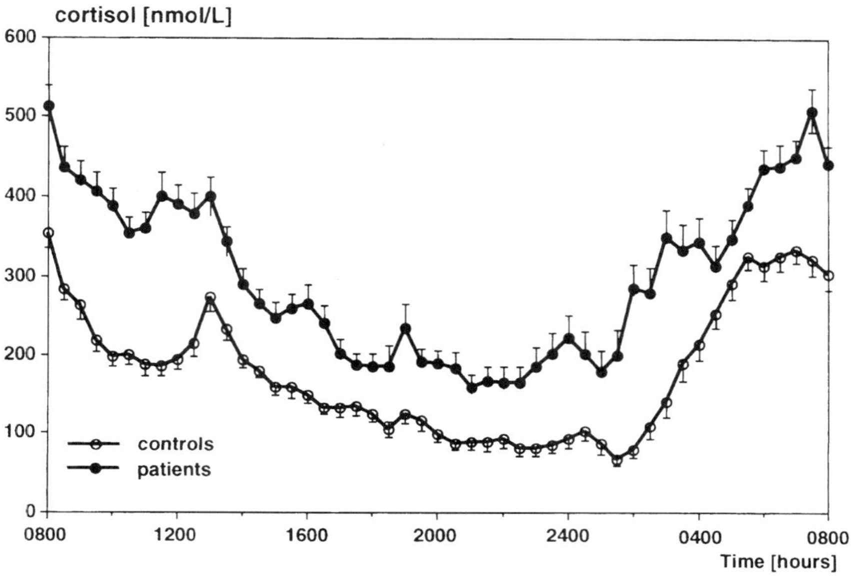

FIGURE 1.—Diurnal profiles of mean plasma cortisol in patients with depression and healthy controls (mean ± standard error of the mean). (Courtesy of Deuschle M, Schweiger U, Weber B, et al: Diurnal activity and pulsatility of the hypothalamus–pituitary–adrenal system in male depressed patients and healthy controls. *J Clin Endocrinol Metab* 81:234–238, 1997. Copyright The Endocrine Society.)

age-matched controls with special regard to pulsatile and circadian features.

Methods.—Fifteen severely depressed men aged 22–72 years, who had a score of 30.4 ± 6.7 on the Hamilton Depression Scale and 22 age-matched male controls were included in the study. Blood sampling was taken every 30 minutes for 24 hours. Circadian rhythm was measured by taking blood samples every 10 minutes from 1800 to 2400 hours.

Results.—In patients with depression, there was a significant increase in 24-hour cortisol (315.9 ± 58.5 vs. 188.2 ± 27.3 nmol/L) (Fig 1) and in mean ACTH (7.82 ± 1.94 vs. 5.79 ± 1.28 pmol/L). In patients with depression the frequency of cortisol (2.6 ± 0.7 pulses per 6 hours) was higher than in controls (1.3 ± 1.0 pulses per 6 hours), and the frequency of ACTH was higher in patients with depression (2.6 ± 1.6 pulses per 6 hours) than in controls (1.6 ± 1.4 pulses per 6 hours). In patients with depression the flattened circadian cortisol variation and the reduced time of quiescence of cortisol secretory activity (140 ± 116 minutes) compared with controls (305 ± 184 minutes) suggest disturbances of circadian functions.

Conclusion.—A greater frequency of episodic hormone release may be behind the increased hypothalamo–pituitary–adrenocortical activity in depression. Altered mineralocorticoid and glucocorticoid receptor capacity and function may partly cause the observed circadian changes. In patients with depression, hypercortisolemia and hypercorticotropinemia may be caused by increased pulsatile hypothalamo–pituitary–adrenal activity at the hypothalamic level, which may reflect an altered feedback at a central site.

► This study provides definitive evidence that the increased activity of the hypothalamo–pituitary–adrenal axis in major depression is caused by increased numbers of pulses of ACTH and cortisol secretion rather than increased amounts of ACTH and cortisol per pulse. The number of pulses in the patients with depression was approximately twice that of the control group. The increase in the number of pulses in patients with depression was particularly evident during the early evening when this system is usually quiescent. The contribution of excessive adrenal corticosteroids to the depressive syndrome is probably substantial and is a current target of antidepressant treatments specifically designed to suppress overactivity of the hypothalamo–pituitary–adrenal axis.

H. Meltzer, M.D.

Pituitary–Adrenal Cortical Axis Measures as Predictors of Sustained Remission in Major Depression

O'Toole SM, Sekula LK, Rubin RT (Hahnemann School of Medicine, Pittsburgh, Pa)

Biol Psychiatry 42:85–89, 1997 9–29

Introduction.—Hyperactivity of the hypothalamic-pituitary-adrenal (HPA) cortical axis is present in up to 50% of patients with major depression and may be predictive of relapse after discontinuation of successful treatment. A study of 35 patients with primary major depression examined the relationship between pretreatment HPA cortical axis measures and relapse.

Methods.—Patients eligible for the study ranged in age from 18 to 64 years and had a score of 17 or greater on the 21-item Hamilton Depression Rating Scale (HDRS). Those who had been treated pharmacologically underwent a 2- to 3-week drug washout period before neuroendocrine testing. Blood samples were analyzed for corticotropin (ACTH) 1-39, immunoreactive ACTH (IR-ACTH), cortisol, and ovine corticotropin-releasing hormone (oCRH). Patients were then treated for depression and underwent repeat neuroendocrine testing after recovery from their depressive episode.

Results.—Twenty-six patients were relapsers, requiring continuing treatment for abatement of symptoms. Eight patients remained in remission after tapering off their medication, and 1 had an apparent spontaneous remission. Relapsers and nonrelapsers did not differ significantly in age, HDRS total score, or number of depressive episodes. Patients who relapsed differed from nonrelapsers in having a longer duration of episode before the initial study and increased baseline ACTH 1-39. Baseline cortisol and cortisol response to ACTH 1-24 was significantly higher in the relapse group. Nine relapsers, but none of the nonrelapsers, were melancholic.

Discussion.—The study hypothesis, that relapsers would have a longer duration of the depressive episode and greater activity of the HPA cortical axis relative to nonrelapsers, was supported in this series of patients with major depression. Increased baseline HPA cortical axis hyperactivity may predict the need for continued medication to sustain remission after successful treatment.

▶ This study suggests that the increased HPA axis activity in major depression may have long-term consequences for the need for maintenance treatment. It is noteworthy that 26 of 35 patients in this study relapsed within 1 month of stopping antidepressant medication. Clinical (e.g. duration of episode before the initial study) and biological predictors of the need for maintenance treatment are of obvious importance. Although it may be impractical to incorporate assessment of HPA axis function into clinical practice, the results reported here suggest that a more severe disturbance in HPA axis function may produce long-term consequences on vulnerability to relapse or that the relative extent of the increase in HPA axis activity may represent a marker for the more recurrent form of major depression. If the former is true, it becomes more important to find ways to decrease HPA axis output in depression as rapidly as possible.

H. Meltzer, M.D.

The Longitudinal Course of Psychopathology in Cushing's Syndrome After Correction of Hypercortisolism

Dorn LD, Burgess ES, Friedman TC, et al (Univ of Pittsburgh, Pa; Natl Inst of Child Health and Human Development, Bethesda, Md; Brown Univ, Providence, RI; et al)

J Clin Endocrinol Metab 82:912–919, 1997 9–30

Introduction.—Depressive symptomatology characterizes Cushing's syndrome, which is diagnosed by low hypothalamic corticotropin-releasing hormone secretion, irritability, hyperphagia, hypersomnia, and increased fatigue. Few studies have examined the psychological profiles of patients with Cushing's syndrome after the correction of hypercortisolism. Patients with Cushing's syndrome were examined after correction of hypercortisolism to determine their longitudinal psychological course for up to a year.

Methods.—At 3 months, 6 months, and 12 months, 33 patients with Cushing's syndrome after correction of hypercortisolism were examined. The patients had their morning cortisol levels and a cortisol response measured in an ACTH stimulation test to determine whether recovery of the hypothalamic-pituitary-adrenal axis was related to psychological recovery. It was also determined whether the psychopathology before or

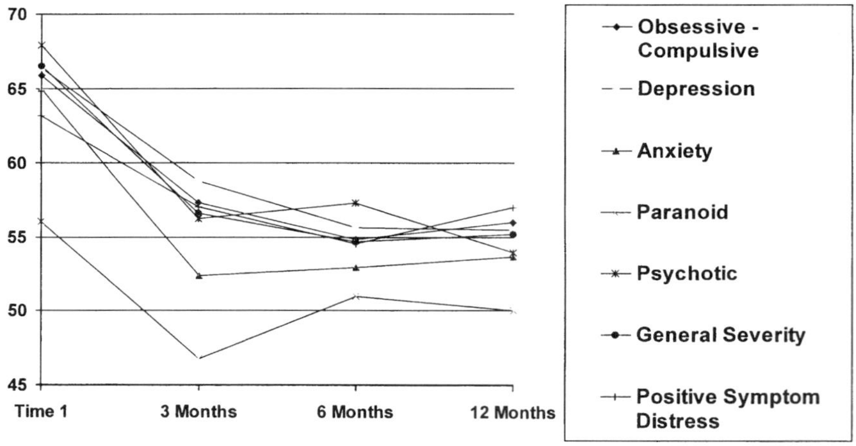

FIGURE 1.—Significant changes in mean T scores of subscales of the Symptom Checklist-90R for patients with Cushing's syndrome during Cushing's syndrome (time 1) and 3, 6, and 12 months post-treatment. (Courtesy of Dorn LD, Burgess ES, Friedman TC, et al: The longitudinal course of psychopathology in Cushing's syndrome after correction of hypercortisolism. *J Clin Endocrinol Metab* 82:912–919, 1997. Copyright The Endocrine Society.)

during Cushing's syndrome was related to the occurrence or intensity of psychopathology after the cure.

Results.—There was significant psychopathology in 66.7% of patients before cure, with the predominant diagnosis of atypical depressive disorder in 51.5% of the patients and a major affective disorder in 12% of the patients. At 3 months after cure, overall psychopathology decreased to 53.6%; at 6 months, it decreased to 36%; and at 12 months, it decreased to 24.1%, as determined by serial morning ACTH stimulation tests (Fig 1). Baseline morning cortisol and psychological recovery had an inverse correlation. After correction of hypercortisolism, atypical depression continued to be the prevailing diagnosis and the frequency of panic and suicidal ideation increased. Glucocorticoid-induced suppression of hypothalamic corticotropin-releasing hormone secretion may be the cause of atypical depression before and after correction of hypercortisolism.

Conclusion.—Atypical symptomatology is associated with Cushing's syndrome, which improves with time after hypercortisolism is corrected. Suicidal ideation and panic attacks occur in a subgroup of patients, and health care providers should be aware of these and other changes in symptomatology.

► This study reminds us that the psychopathology of Cushing's disease, mainly, an atypical depression marked by irritability, hyperphagia, hypersomnia, and increased fatigue, can persist after surgical removal of the pituitary, adrenal, or ectopic source of ACTH, as a result of the replacement therapy with glucocorticoids. The evidence strongly suggests that suppression of the activity of corticotropin-releasing hormone neurons by glucocorticoids before or after surgery may be the cause of the affective syndrome. This raises some interesting questions about the role of these neurons in major depression. The need for close supervision of the mental status even after surgery is made very clear by this important study.

H. Meltzer, M.D.

Hypothalamic–Pituitary–Thyroid-Axis Function in Treatment Resistant Depression

Vandoolaeghe E, Maes M, Vandevyvere J, et al (AZ Stuivenberg, Antwerp, Belgium; Vanderbilt Univ, Nashville, Tenn; Lab of Nuclear Medicine, Antwerp, Belgium; et al)

J Affect Disord 43:143–150, 1997 9–31

Background.—Ultrasensitive radioimmunologic (IRMA) methods of assaying basal thyroid-secreting hormone (TSH) have found serum basal TSH to be significantly lower in patients with major depression during an acute phase of illness than in normal controls or individuals with minor depression. Recent reports also suggest that patients with treatment-resistant depression (TRD) have an increased prevalence of various grades of hypothyroidism. A study of major depressives and normal controls examined whether TRD is accompanied by increased basal TSH levels and decreased thyroxine (T4) levels indicative of hypothyroid disorder.

Methods.—Blood samples were obtained after an overnight fast in the 36 patients and 15 controls. An ultrasensitive IRMA was used to determine basal TSH. At the study institution's laboratory, the euthyroid range for basal TSH–IRMA is 0.10–6.00 μIU/mL. The euthyroid range for T4 values is 5.6 to 11.4 γ%.

Results.—Patient and control groups were similar in age and gender ratio. Of the 36 patients with major depression, 27 had TRD, as defined by a nonresponse to at least 2 trials with antidepressant agents. The length of index episode was significantly greater in patients with TRD, but patients with and without TRD did not differ significantly in duration of illness or number of depressive episodes. Neither basal TSH or T4 levels differed significantly between patients and normal controls or between patients with and without TRD. There was a trend toward lower serum basal T4 concentrations in the TRD group, and 1 of these patients had basal serum TSH levels in the hyperthyroid range. One normal control and 1 patient with TRD had serum TSH values in the subclinical hypothyroid zone, but both had serum T4 values in the euthyroid range.

Discussion.—Ultrasensitive assays failed to detect significant differences in basal TSH or T4 between patients with major depression, with or without TRD, and normal controls. Neither basal TSH or T4 exhibited a relationship with illness severity or duration.

► This article is important because it provides a thorough review of the older literature on thyroid abnormalities in major depression and concludes that new methods of assessment of thyroid function, for example, ultrasensitive TSH radioimmunologic assays, demonstrate lower basal TSH levels in major depression, although most patients are within normal limits. The blunted TSH response to TRH challenge is highly correlated with the lower basal levels, which may be the result of increased T4 levels. In light of this, it is curious that this study of treatment-resistant depression found no difference in serum basal TSH or T4 levels between major depressed subjects and normal controls, or between patients with treatment-resistant depression and nontreatment-resistant depression. There was no relationship between thyroid measures and severity of illness. It may be that thyroid abnormalities are only present during the acute phase of depression. There does not seem to be adequate evidence to support the use of adjunctive thyroid medication to enhance response in treatment-resistant depression.

H. Meltzer, M.D.

Association of Anxiety-related Traits With a Polymorphism in the Serotonin Transporter Gene Regulatory Region

Lesch K-P, Bengel D, Heils A, et al (Univ of Würzburg, Germany; NIH, Bethesda, Md)

Science 274:1527–1532, 1996 9–32

Background.—Serotonin (5-HT) is a neurotransmitter involved in sleep, cognition, and emotional states such as mood and anxiety. The 5-HT effect is modulated by the 5-HT transporter (5-HTT), which is encoded in humans on a single gene on chromosome 17q12. These authors report a polymorphism in an upstream transcriptional control sequence in the 5-HTT gene that was found in both individuals and family members with anxiety-related personality traits.

Methods.—The polymorphism found on the 5-HTT gene was located about 1 kb upstream from the 5-HTT gene transcription initiation site. This 44 base pair mutation resulted in insertions or deletions of repeat elements 6 to 8 (and thus long and short alleles, respectively). Experiments involving transfection of lymphoblast cell lines and ligand binding revealed that the polymorphism had a dominant recessive effect. The associations between this polymorphism and anxiety-related traits were examined in 505 subjects who underwent personality testing. Results of NEO personality inventory indicative of neuroticism were considered to reflect an anxiety-related trait. To confirm these findings, Cattell's 16PF personality inventory and Cloninger's biosocial model were also used.

Findings.—On the NEO test, neuroticism was significantly associated with the 5-HTT gene-linked polymorphic region. Subjects with either 1 or 2 copies of the short allele had higher neuroticism scores than subjects with 2 copies of the long allele. Many submeasures of the neuroticism score were significantly associated with the polymorphism, including anxiety, angry hostility, depression, and impulsiveness. Furthermore, no significant associations were seen between the gene polymorphisms and other aspects measured by the NEO test, such as extraversion, openness, agreeableness, or conscientiousness. These results were corroborated by the other 2 psychometric instruments used. Overall, the 5-HTT polymorphism could account for 3% to 4% of the total variance and 7% to 9% of the genetic variance in anxiety-related personality traits.

Conclusions.—Deletions in this polymorphism reduce the ability of the 5-HTT gene promoter to transcribe 5-HT, thus reducing 5-HT uptake and exacerbating anxiety in some patients. The effects of this gene are only a small part of the complex genetic contribution to anxiety disorders. Nonetheless, identification of this polymorphism may help reveal other genetic events involved in the development of anxiety, and it may eventually help individualize medical therapy for subjects with this polymorphism.

▶ This important study shows a weak but reproducible association between a polymorphism of the 5-HT transporter which is in the upstream regulatory region and the neuroticism trait in 2 large samples of patients. While accounting for less than 10% of total or inherited variation in this trait, it is important to provide additional evidence for the role of serotonin in this trait and to provide an estimate of the contribution of a given gene to such a complex behavioral trait. It will be essential in the future to consider this gene's contribution while others are being evaluated. Ultimately, the interactions between the contributions of different genes will have to be determined.

H. Meltzer, M.D.

Genotype Determining Low Catechol-*O*-Methyltransferase Activity as a Risk Factor for Obsessive-Compulsive Disorder

Karayiorgou M, Altemus M, Galke BL, et al (Rockefeller Univ, New York; Cornell Univ, New York; Lab of Neurogenetics, Natl Inst of Alcohol Abuse and Alcoholism, Rockville, Md; et al)

Proc Natl Acad Sci U S A 94:4572–4575, 1997 9–33

Background.—Dopamine antagonists have been useful in the treatment of a subset of patients with obsessive-compulsive disorder (OCD), indicating that dopaminergic pathways are involved in at least some cases. Catechol-O-methyltransferase (COMT) inactivates dopamine, and its gene maps to chromosome 22q11. Previous studies have shown that deletions in this region result in schizophrenia and OCD. Whether the *comt* gene plays a role in the pathogenesis of OCD was investigated.

Methods.—Blood samples for DNA analysis were drawn from 73 patients with OCD (42 men, 31 women) and 148 subjects without OCD (75 men, 73 women). Because a common polymorphism can decrease COMT enzyme activity by a factor of 3–4, all participants were genotyped to determine any valine (Val)-to-methionine (Met) allele substitutions. Blood samples were genotyped by the use of polymerase chain reaction with amplification.

Findings.—Men with OCD showed a significant correlation between deletions of the *comt* gene and OCD. Male patients with the Met^{158}/Met^{158} genotype had a relative risk for OCD of 5.91 compared to the other genotypes (Val^{158}/Val^{158} and Val^{158}/Met^{158}). Also, more male patients with the Met^{158}/Met^{158} genotype exhibited comorbid tic disorders.

Conclusions.—Men with OCD were significantly more likely to have microdeletions of the *comt* gene, particularly those with the Met^{158}/Met^{158} genotype. Furthermore, previous reports indicate that dopamine antagonists are most effective in patients with OCD who have comorbid tics, and in this study more men with OCD and the Met^{158}/Met^{158} genotype had comorbid tics. These results strengthen the hypothesis that the inactivation of dopamine caused by a microdeletion of *comt* may be active in the pathogenesis of OCD in at least some patients.

▶ This study is a major contribution to our understanding of OCD, although like all genetic studies it needs to be replicated in an independent sample. Nevertheless, it looks promising that a recessive form of the *comt* gene may be a vulnerability factor for OCD, at least in males, leading to decreased inactivation of both norepinephrine and dopamine. Further studies to demonstrate that COMT activity is decreased in OCD would help to confirm this hypothesis. Treatment of OCD with a selective serotonin reuptake inhibitor or a dopamine receptor blocker may serve to decrease the availability of dopamine. If confirmed, this work should be of great value for diagnostic purposes as well as guiding research in pathophysiology and treatment. It might be of interest to try to further disrupt the synthesis of the catecholamines with alpha-methylparatyrosine.

H. Meltzer, M.D.

Tryptophan Depletion in Obsessive-Compulsive Patients

Smeraldi E, Diaferia G, Erzegovesi S, et al (Univ of Milan, Italy)
Biol Psychiatry 40:398–402, 1996 9–34

Background.—Symptoms of obsessive-compulsive disorder (OCD) improve after drug therapy that inhibits serotonin reuptake. It was hypothesized that a reduction in blood levels of serotonin should improve symptoms also. A tryptophan-free mixture of amino acids was used to lower tryptophan and serotonin levels in patients with OCD and changes in clinical symptoms, were examined.

Methods.—Four men and 8 women with OCD who had been drug-free for at least 2 weeks were enrolled in the study. In a double-blind, crossover design, 2 amino acid mixtures (1 with L-tryptophan and 1 without) were administered over 3-day periods. Blood samples were drawn at baseline and at 1, 3, and 6 hours after administration of the mixture. Patients used a 100–point visual analogue scale to describe 11 specific subjective ratings of changes after treatment (including obsession, compulsions, and mood).

Findings.—As expected, the total plasma tryptophan level increased after administration of the amino acid mixture containing tryptophan. Plasma tryptophan levels declined significantly after the administration of the tryptophan-free mixture, and they remained significantly lower over time. However, no significant time × treatment effects were observed based on the patients' visual analogue ratings of any of the 11 measures assessed.

Conclusions.—The depletion of tryptophan did not improve any symptoms of OCD in these 12 patients. This is in contrast to other studies showing a reduction in symptoms after tryptophan reduction in patients with OCD. Although these patients had been drug-free for at least 2 weeks, prolonged use of serotonin reuptake inhibitors may have long-term effects that are not immediately reversed by reducing serotonin levels. Thus, using a longer drug-free period could make a difference in future studies.

► It is disappointing that depletion of tryptophan was without significant effect on OCD symptoms in this group of drug-free patients with OCD. A positive result would have greatly strengthened the argument for the importance of serotonin in the pathophysiology of OCD. These negative data do not rule it out, as discussed by the authors. Further study in patients whose OCD has partially responded to a selective serotonin reuptake inhibitor may be a more informative strategy. It may also be necessary to combine tryptophan depletion with some other pharmacologic intervention, e.g., amphetamine to increase catecholamines, to bring about an exacerbation of the illness.

H. Meltzer, M.D.

Basic Research Related to Biological Psychiatry

Preclinical Characterization of the Potential of the Putative Atypical Antipsychotic MDL 100,907 as a Potent 5-HT$_{2A}$ Antagonist With a Favorable CNS Safety Profile

Kehne JH, Baron BM, Carr AA, et al (Hoechst Marion Roussel Inc, Cincinnati, Ohio; Hoechst Marion Roussel Inc, Strasbourg, France; Univ of Cincinnati, Ohio)

J Pharmacol Exp Ther 277:968–981, 1996 9–35

Introduction.—For schizophrenia, a complex CNS disorder of unknown etiology, much research effort is devoted to developing new pharmacotherapies. Schizophrenia has positive symptoms such as auditory hallucinations, delusions, thought disorders, and it has negative symptoms such as blunted or inappropriate affect and social withdrawal. The goal is to produce a drug that can treat the variety of symptoms. A putative atypical antipsychotic, MDL 100,907, was characterized in vitro as a potent and selective ligand for the serotonin$_{2A}$ (5-HT$_{2A}$) receptor in preclinical studies and was evaluated as a potent (5-HT$_{2A}$) antagonist.

Methods.—MDL 100,907 was compared with benchmark compounds, and it was evaluated for its CNS safety profile and selectivity as a potential antipsychotic agent. Inhibition of a D-amphetamine-stimulated location in mice was used to measure the potential antipsychotic efficacy of MDL 100,907 and was tested against the reference compounds haloperidol, clozapine, risperidone, ritanserin, and amperozide. It was also tested for the side effects of ataxia, general depressant effects, alpha$_1$-adrenergic antagonism, striatal D2 receptor antagonism, and muscle relaxation.

Results.—Low nanomolar or subnanomolar binding in vitro at the 5-HT$_{2A}$ receptor was seen with MDL 100,907 and there was a greater than 100–fold separation for all other receptors measured. As a 5-HT$_{2A}$ antagonist in vitro that reverses 5-HT-stimulated inositol phosphate accumulation in NIH 3T3 cells transfected with the rat 5-HT$_{2A}$ receptor, MDL 100,907 had subnanomolar potency. In mice, in vivo, MDL 100,907 potently inhibited 5-methoxy-N,N-dimethyltryptamine-induced head twitches. In rats, it inhibited 5-hydroxytryptophan-induced head twitches. There was a greater than 500–fold separation between doses that produced 5-HT$_{2A}$ antagonism and doses that produced alpha$_1$-adrenergic or striatal D2 antagonism in in vivo functional tests in mice. MDL 100,907 showed a superior CNS safety index when compared with the reference compounds and in the tests for side effects. The drug may lack extrapyramidal side effect liability as it did not antagonize apomorphine-induced stereotypies in rats. The drug lacked consistent activity in selected rodent models of anticonvulsant, antidepressant, analgesic, or anxiolytic activity and showed selectivity as a potential antipsychotic.

Conclusion.—At the 5-HT$_{2A}$ receptor, MDL 100,907 is a potent and selective ligand. Its activity in preclinical models of antipsychotic potential may be caused by its potent 5-HT$_{2A}$ antagonist activity. The hypothesis that 5-HT$_{2A}$ receptor antagonism is sufficient for antipsychotic activity in humans should be tested with clinical evaluation of MDL 100,907.

▶ It is well known that the new generation of antipsychotic drugs is relatively more potent as serotonin 5-HT2A that as dopamine D2 antagonists, and this may account for their low extrapyramidal side effects. It is not clear what role 5-HT2A antagonism plays in the ability of some of these compounds such as clozamine, olanzapine, risperidone, and quetiapine to control positive or negative symptoms, and to be effective in neuroleptic resistant patients. These and many other important questions will be clarified by MDL 100,907 regarding the role of the 5-HT2A receptor in a variety of behaviors and neuropsychiatric disorders. If it is efficacious on its own in treating schizophrenia, it will be the first drug without any direct-acting dopamine receptor antagonism which is antipsychotic. Amperozide may have been another such compound, but it never had definitive clinical testing.

H. Meltzer, M.D.

Modulation of Learned Helplessness by 5-Hydroxytryptamine$_{2A}$ Receptor Antisense Oligodeoxynucleotides

Paplos DF, Yu Y-M, Rosenbaum E, et al (Albert Einstein College of Medicine, Bronx, NY)

Psychiatry Res 63:197–203, 1996 9–36

Introduction.—Learned helplessness is a behavioral response that is induced by exposure to inescapable shock that is considered to be a reliable animal model for depression. The overall function of serotonin or 5-hydroxytryptamine, 5-HT, is to ward off feelings of depression, helplessness, and fear. Depression may be caused by a reduction in serotonergic activity. A unique antisense oligonucleotide (ASO) was introduced to the 5-HT$_{2A}$ receptor to understand the significance of 5-HT$_{2A}$ receptor-mediated neuronal responses in the pathogenesis of depression and learned helplessness.

Methods.—In all experiments, rats weighting 200–300 g were used. Antisense oligonucleotides were introduced to the 5-HT$_{2A}$ receptor with intracerebroventricular injections in 16 rats. The effect on learned helplessness was determined by an escape–avoidance strategy. These effects were compared with the effects in a control group of 15 rats.

Results.—Eight of 16 rats injected with the 5-HT$_{2A}$ receptor ASO met the criteria for learned helplessness. In the control group 1 of the 15 rats injected with 5-HT$_{2A}$ sense oligonucleotide met the criteria for learned helplessness. Between ASO and control sense oligonucleotides, significant differences were seen in 5-HT$_{2A}$ receptor density in close proximity to the injection site, according to quantitative receptor autoradiography. In the CA_3 hippocampal region, significant decreases in 5-HT$_{2A}$ receptor density caused by oligonucleotide blockade were seen.

Conclusion.—Serotonergic pathways that terminate in this hippocampal subfield may regulate the induction of behavioral depression. Behaviors that are affected by inescapable stress may be regulated by central 5-HT, mediated by the 5-HT$_{2A}$ receptor. Via serotonergic pathways that terminate in the CA_3 region of the hippocampus, the induction of behavioral depression may be specifically regulated.

► Injection of ASOs to knock out the genes that govern the production of specific receptors or other molecules is an elegant means of determining the importance of that protein for a specific process. It differs from knocking the gene out during gestation in that it may be done at any time in the life cycle. The results reported here are consistent with the view that decreasing 5-HT$_{2A}$ receptor activity may promote an animal model of depression called learned helplessness. There is, however, little direct evidence from clinical studies with drugs that block 5-HT$_{2A}$ receptors that they cause or exacerbate depression. On the contrary, drugs such as trazodone, amitriptyline, and clozapine, which are 5-HT$_{2A}$ antagonists, are antidepressants. Because these agents have multiple pharmacologic properties, it may be that their antidepressant effects are based on other actions that overcome the effect of 5-HT_{2A} antagonism. There are new, specific 5-HT_{2A} antagonists e.g., MDL 100,907 in clinical testing that should help clarify the role of this receptor in depression.

H. Meltzer, M.D.

Effect of the *Alpha-2* Adrenoceptor Antagonist Mirtazapine on the 5-Hydroxytryptamine System in the Rat Brain

Haddjeri N, Blier P, de Montigny C (McGill Univ, Montréal)

J Pharmacol Exp Ther 277:861–871, 1996 9–37

Introduction.—A tetracyclic compound with antidepressant activity in humans is mirtazapine, which is an *alpha-2* adrenoceptor antagonist. To characterize the effect of (±)-mirtazapine on presynaptic and postsynaptic *alpha-2* adrenoceptors, in vivo electrophysiologic paradigms were used. Because of its purported selectivity for *alpha-2* adrenergic heteroreceptors, the effects of (–)-mirtazapine were studied.

Methods.—The effects of (±)- and (–)-mirtazapine on the CA_3 dorsal hippocampus pyramidal neurons' responsiveness to microiontophoretic applications of noradrenergic terminals were assessed at the postsynaptic level. The effects of (±)- and (–)-mirtazapine on the endogenous release of 5-HT induced by the electric stimulation of the ascending 5-HT pathway were assessed at the level of the 5-HT terminals, as were their capabilities to antagonize the effects of clonidine on the effectiveness of the stimulation. The effects of (±)- and (–)-mirtazapine on the spontaneous firing activity of dorsal raphe 5-HT and locus ceruleus noradrenergic neurons were investigated.

Results.—By blocking both *alpha-2* adrenergic autoreceptors and heteroreceptors, IV (±)-mirtazapine at 25 μg/kg enhanced the effectiveness of the electric stimulation of the ascending 5-HT pathway. Because of a selective action of (–)-mirtazapine on the *alpha-2* heteroreceptors located on 5-HT terminals, IV (–)-mirtazapine at 10 μg/kg enhanced the effectiveness of these stimulations. The suppressant effect of microiontophoretically applied norepinephrine on the firing activity of CA_3 dorsal hippocampus pyramidal neurons was blocked by IV (±)- and (–)-mirtazapine at 500 μg/kg, indicating their antagonistic effects on postsynaptic *alpha-2* adrenoceptors. In naive rats, the firing activity of the 5-HT neurons was enhanced dose dependently by IV (±)-mirtazapine at 10–250 μg/kg but not in the rats pretreated with 6-hydroxydopamine. The firing activity of locus ceruleus norepinephrine neurons was significantly increased by (±)-mirtazapine. The firing rate of dorsal raphe 5-HT neurons failed to change by administration of IV (–)-mirtazapine at 10–250 μg/kg.

Conclusion.—At postsynaptic *alpha-2* adrenergic receptors, both (±)- and (–)-mirtazapine are antagonists. (±)-mirtazapine is an antagonist of terminal *alpha-2* adrenergic and somatodendritic autoreceptors and heteroreceptors. At *alpha-2* adrenergic heteroreceptors, (–)-mirtazapine is a selective antagonist. Because it is abolished by a 5,7-dihydroxytryptamine pretreatment, the inhibitory effect of (–)-mirtazapine on locus ceruleus noradrenergic neurons appears to be mediated via 5-HT neurons.

► Mirtazapine is the newest antidepressant and the most novel of the agents introduced in the last decade. Its pharmacologic profile includes potent presynaptic *alpha-2* adrenergic antagonist activity and potent 5-HT_{2A} and 5-HT_3 antagonist activity. It does not block serotonin or catecholamine uptake. Because of the central role serotonin plays in depression and in antidepressant drug action, it is important to fully characterize the effect of mirtazapine on the serotonin system. The Montreal group present elegant electrophysiologic evidence that mirtazapine enhances serotonergic neurotransmission by blockade of *alpha-2* adrenoceptors on serotonin terminals. This novel mechanism suggests the possibility that mirtazapine might have synergistic effects with selective serotonin reuptake inhibitors and, thus, be useful in refractory patients and to speed up the response to other antidepressants that enhance serotonergic activity by other mechanisms.

H. Meltzer, M.D.

Cellular Responses to Psychomotor Stimulant and Neuroleptic Drugs Are Abnormal in Mice Lacking the D1 Dopamine Receptor

Moratalla R, Xu M, Tonegawa S, et al (Howard Huges Med Inst, Cambridge, Mass; Univ of Cincinnati, Ohio)

Proc Natl Acad Sci U S A 93:14928–14933, 1996 9–38

Background.—D1 and D2 receptors act both synergistically and independently to exert their effects. A D1-deficient mouse model was used to examine the separate responses of D1 and D2 receptors in a variety of settings.

Methods.—Mutant male mice without D1 receptors were administered cocaine and amphetamine (psychomotor stimulants), hydrobromide (a D1 receptor agonist), haloperidol (a neuroleptic that acts preferentially at D2 receptors), and quinelorane (a D2 receptor agonist). A control group of mice received cocaine or saline. Mice survived 2 hours after drug treatment, after which immunohistochemical analysis was performed to identify rat cFos, rat JunB, and rat dynorphin B_{1-29} peptide. Ligand binding was performed on fresh-frozen sections.

Findings.—D1-deficient mice were practically devoid of dynorphin in the striatum; even large doses of cocaine could not increase their levels of dynorphin. Likewise, large doses of neither amphetamine, cocaine, nor even hydrobromide induced the expression of either cFos or JunB in the striatum of the mutant mice. Mutant mice did not have fewer dopamine transporter-binding sites, which implies that these results are not attributable to fewer dopamine transporters in the striatum. In contrast, haloperidol induced cFos and JunB immunoreactivity in both mutant and control mice. Furthermore, quinelorane blocked expression of cFos and JunB in the striatum in both groups of mice.

Conclusions.—The D1 receptor is needed for the upregulation of dynorphin expression and the induction of cFos and JunB expression in the striatum. The similar effects of haloperidol and quinelorane in both D1-deficient mice and controls indicates that these drugs exert their effects despite the absence of a D1–D2 synergism. Thus, D1 receptors are required in certain situations, but not in others.

► The interaction between various types of dopamine receptors is a murky area that is of great importance for a variety of neuropsychiatric disorders. It has long been known that there are complex and sometimes opposite types of interactions between D1 and D2 receptors for different effects of dopamine. Neuroleptic action predominantly involves D2 receptors, although there is intriguing evidence that cocaine and other psychomotor stimulants may have a predominant action on the D1 receptor. The studies reported here establish that different early intermediate genes are controlled by either D1 or D2 receptors. The mutant mice used in these studies will thus be of great value in determining which effects of drugs such as cocaine, amphetamine, and haloperidol are dependent upon these early intermediate genes, thus moving the locus of inquiry beyond the receptor level.

H. Meltzer, M.D.

Selective Enhancement of Emotional, but Not Motor, Learning in Monoamine Oxidase A–Deficient Mice

Kim JJ, Shih JC, Chen K, et al (Univ of Southern California, Los Angeles; Univ of California, Los Angeles; Centre Natl de la Recherche Scientifique, Orsay, France)

Proc Natl Acad Sci U S A 94:5929–5933, 1997 9–39

Background.—Monoamines such as dopamine, norepinephrine, and epinephrine are involved in emotions and neurologic disorders. Previous reports have indicated that mice deficient in monoamine oxidase A (MAOA) are more aggressive and have higher brain levels of norepinephrine. Whether MAOA-deficient mice also exhibited cognitive defects in learning and memory performance was investigated.

Methods.—Thirteen MAOA-deficient mice underwent fear conditioning (pairing a tone with a footshock), step-down conditioning (administering a footshock when they went from one level of flooring to another), and eyeblink conditioning (pairing a tone with a shock via electrodes implanted in the upper eyelid). After conditioning, mice were killed and the frontal cortex, hippocampus, and cerebellum were dissected and prepared for high-performance liquid chromatographic analysis to determine levels of dopamine, norepinephrine, and serotonin. Maternal nesting, nursing, and pup retrieval behaviors were also examined in first-litter MAOA mice and wild-type mice.

Findings.—The MAOA-deficient mice showed a significantly greater response to fear conditioning (measured by percent who froze in their tracks) compared to wild-type mice. They also were significantly more likely to delay the step-down test (measured by avoidance latencies) than the wild-type mice. However, the groups did not differ in their responses to the eyeblink conditioning, although the mutant mice did require a significantly higher voltage level to elicit a response. Likewise, maternal behaviors did not differ between the groups. The mutant mice had significantly higher levels of norepinephrine and serotonin in the 3 brain regions analyzed.

Conclusions.—The mice deficient for MAOA activity had elevated levels of monoamines and an elevated response to emotional (fear) learning. However, their responses to the eyeblink motor learning task were not changed, nor were their maternal behaviors. These results add further support that elevated catecholamine levels are associated with changes in emotional behavior.

► Decreased MAO was at one time thought to be characteristic of schizophrenia, but subsequent studies have not confirmed this. These MAOA-deficient rats allow a clear determination of what is the role of its substrates, norepinephrine and serotonin, in behavior, at least in the mouse. Previous studies have suggested aggression may be related to deficient MAOA. These studies suggest that enhanced catecholamine function is important for learning during a frightening event. Further pharmacologic studies with selective manipulation of norepinephrine, dopamine, and serotonin should permit increased understanding of the role of each of these monoamines in aggression and fear learning.

H. Meltzer, M.D.

Abnormal Dendritic Spines in Fragile X Knockout Mice: Maturation and Pruning Deficits

Comery TA, Harris JB, Willems PJ, et al (Univ of Illinois, Urbana-Champaign; Univ of Antwerp, Belgium; Erasmus Univ, Rotterdam, The Netherlands)

Proc Natl Acad Sci U S A 94:5401–5404, 1997 9–40

Background.—In humans, the fragile X syndrome is associated with thin, elongated dendritic neuronal spines in the cerebral cortex and with a lack of the fragile X mental retardation protein (FMRP). Now mice have been produced in which the *Fmr1* gene is knocked out, resulting in mice that express no FMRP. Whether the dendritic changes apparent in humans with fragile X syndrome are also found in these knockout mice was investigated.

Methods.—Four mutant mice and 4 wild-type mice underwent Golgi-Cox impregnation of samples from the visual cortex (layer V pyramidal neurons). The spinal lengths of 5 neurons from 5 different tissue sections were examined in each animal, and a mean was calculated. Neuronal spinal density was counted in 25-μm segments from 5 neurons from 5 different tissue sections, and again a mean was calculated.

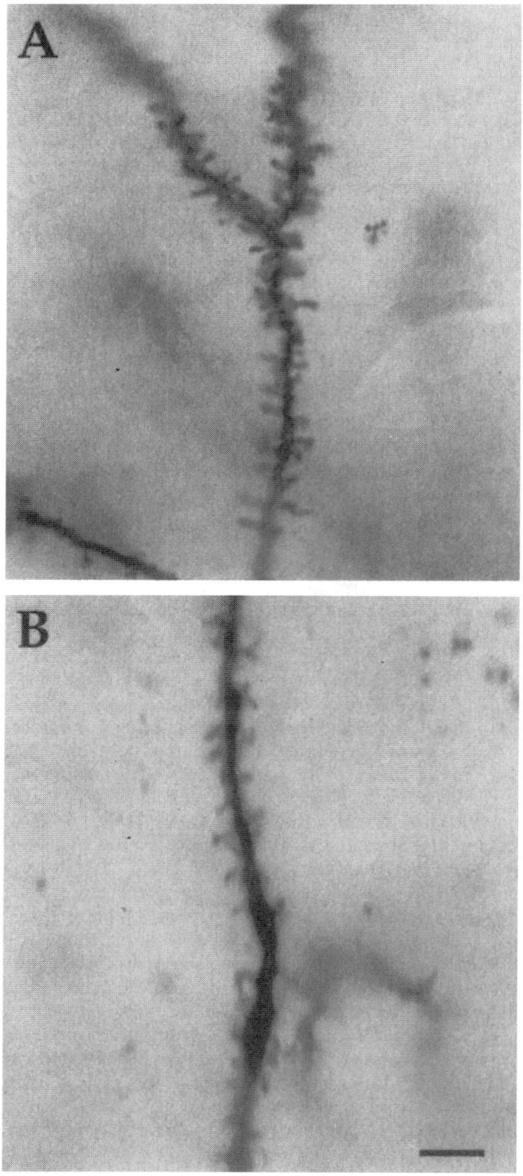

FIGURE 1.—Golgi-Cox impregnated apical dendrites in transgenic and wild-type mice. **A**, Segment of apical dendrite from layer V pyramidal neuron in *Fmr1* knockout mouse demonstrating both the increased incidence of long, thin dendritic spines and the increased spine density. **B**, apical dendrite of layer V pyramidal neuron from wild-type mouse. *Bar* = 10 µm. (Courtesy of Comery TA, Harris JB, Willems PJ, et al: Abnormal dendritic spines in fragile X knockout mice: Maturation and pruning deficits. *Proc Natl Acad Sci U.S.A.* 94:5401–5404, 1997. Copyright 1997 National Academy of Sciences U.S.A.)

Findings.—Compared to those of controls, dendritic spines were significantly longer in the mice lacking the *Fmr1* gene (Fig 1). Spinal density was also greater in the knockout mice compared to the controls.

Conclusions.—The dendritic spine morphologic characteristics in the knockout mice were similar to those seen in early synaptogenesis, and also similar to those seen in humans with fragile X syndrome. These results point to the importance of FMRP in normal adult neuronal morphologic development. The mouse model should be explored as a model for the study of human fragile X syndrome.

▶ This study demonstrates the power of a transgenic animal model of a human disease. The neuropathologic findings of the transgenic mouse that is homozygous for the altered gene which codes for the FMRP closely parallel those found in the human condition. This is a terrific example of what might be possible for other neurodevelopmental disorders. However, for a disorder such as schizophrenia, where multiple genes are involved, the problem will be much more complex. Even the findings reported here may be helpful for schizophrenia insofar as the FMRP may be involved in the process of synaptic stabilization and pruning, processes that may be abnormal in schizophrenia.

H. Meltzer, M.D.

More Hippocampal Neurons in Adult Mice Living in an Enriched Environment

Kempermann G, Kuhn HG, Gage FH (Salk Inst, La Jolla, Calif)

Nature 386:493–495, 1997 9–41

Background.—In mice, environmental enrichment (providing a cage with wheels, tunnels, toys, extra snacks, etc.) can increase hippocampal thickness, dendritic arborization, and the number of glial cells. The effects of environmental enrichment on the number of neurons in the dentate gyrus were examined.

Methods.—Twenty-four female mice 21 days old were maintained under either standard (n = 12) or enriched (n = 12) conditions for 40 days. On days 29–40, all animals received a once-daily injection of bromodeoxyuridine (BrdU), 50 mg/kg, for DNA analysis. On day 41, 5 animals from each group were killed for immunohistochemical analysis. On days 41–45, the remaining animals were tested in a Morris water maze that included a computerized tracking system to measure the swim latency (how long it took to reach the escape platform) and the swim path length. Afterward, they were returned to their environment for an additional 23 days, at which point they were killed and their tissues harvested for analysis. The total number of BrdU-positive cells per granule cell layer was determined by stereology.

Findings.—Enriched mice differed from their control littermates in 4 areas (Fig 2). At 4 weeks after the last BrdU injection, mice living in the

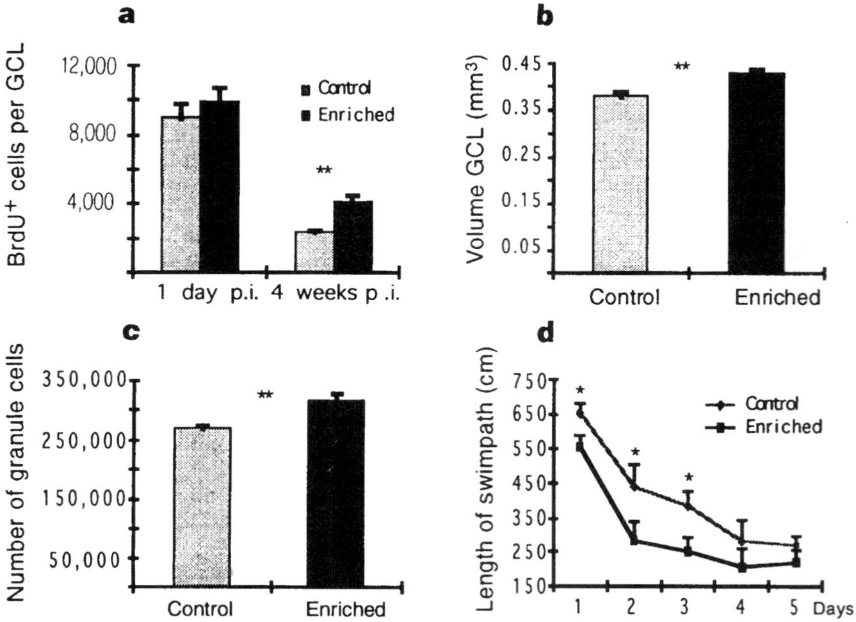

FIGURE 2.—Four parameters in which enriched mice differ from their control littermates. **A**, bromodeoxyuridine number of (BrdU) positive cells per hippocampal granule cell layer (GCL). The density of BrdU-positive cells was determined stereologically (cells per mm^3) and multiplied by the absolute volume of the dentate gyrus. Significance level is $P < 0.005$ (t test). **B**, volume of the dentate gyrus. At 4 weeks after injection (*p.i.*), the volume of the hippocampal dentate gyrus was significantly ($P < 0.005$, t test) increased in the enriched group. **C**, absolute granule cell number in the dentate gyrus. At 4 weeks after injection, enriched mice had significantly more granule cell neurons ($P < 0.01$). The underlying neuronal density was 6.47 ± 0.25 per sample volume in controls and 6.56 ± 0.14 in enriched mice and thus not influenced by environmental enrichment. All data are given as mean ± standard error. No. was 5 per group at 1 day after injection and 7 per group at 4 weeks after injection. **D**, in the spatial learning task (Morris water maze), enriched mice (*lower curve*) have a significantly shorter swim path ($P < 0.05$, t test) on days 1–3 of testing. On day 1 there was no significant difference between the groups in the first 2 trials, indicating equal baselines. The time to reach the platform (latency) paralleled this curve and reached the significance level on day 2. At all time points, no difference in the average swim speed could be found, and on a transfer test without a platform on day 6 no differences between groups were detected (data not shown). (Reprinted with permission from Nature, from Kempermann G, Kuhn HG, Gage FH. More hippocampal neurons in adult mice living in an enriched environment. *Nature* 386:493–495, 1997. Copyright 1997 Macmillan Magazines Limited.)

enriched environment had 57% more labeled cells per gyrus, and the volume of their dentate gyrus was about 15% greater. Neuronal density in the dentate gyrus was also significantly greater in mice from enriched environments (310,000 vs. 270,000 granule cells, or about 15%). Finally, despite similar baselines between the enhanced and standard groups, mice from the enhanced environment performed significantly better on the Morris water maze than their standard-housed littermates.

Conclusions.—Environmental enrichment promoted survival in neuronal precursor cells in the dentate gyrus. This neuronal enhancement occurred in tandem with an improved performance on the Morris water maze. In humans, adult neurogenesis occurs in the subgranular zone of the dentate gyrus, and thus these results may have applicability in adult human neurogenesis. Although a cause-and-effect relationship cannot be confirmed, it is likely that neuronal proliferation indeed contributes to the improved performance brought about by living in an enriched environment.

► This important article provides clear evidence at the cellular level that an enriched environment postnatally has enduring consequences on the number of neurons and hence the structure of the hippocampus, a critical brain area for learning and memory. This is likely to be mediated by the enhanced survival of hippocampal neurons. Further research to determine the effect of timing and type of environmental enrichment should stimulate experiments with primates and guide future observational if not experimental research in man.

H. Meltzer, M.D.

10 Psychopharmacology

Introduction

The field of psychopharmacology is expanding at a rapid rate. There have been important advances in our understanding of anxiety and mood disorders, and issues of compliance and tolerability of treaments. Not so long ago, I thought that long-term treatment was required primarily by individuals with schizophrenia or bioplar disorder. Our increasing awareness of the chronic nature of depression and anxiety disorders has also increased our sensitivity to issues of tolerability and long-term effectiveness. Polypharmacy is no longer a dirty word. We have, at long last, even brought cutting edge psychopharmacology into the area of substance abuse and dependence.

There are several new medications which have recently been introduced, a group of new atypical neuroleptics shows promise as both more effective and less toxic. Several new antidepressants which are safer, more broadly effective and much more tolerable are now part of the armamentarium. These, like the new neuroleptics, offer "better quality of life" benefits—another new area of interest. The newer medications, in other words, may be more "effective" because patients are more willing to take them. New mood-stabilizing uses for older agents are being investigated and appear to have some advantages over the original mood-stabilizing anticonvulsant, carbamazepine, in terms of ease of use. A few anticonvulsants have been or are being studied as treatments for anxiety disorders and non-bipolar depression.

Of course, the flip side of this coin is that there are untoward side effects with these newer agents also, and we are learning more about how to treat or minimize these. The issue of extrapyramidal and sexual side effects of the SSRIs has been recognized as a problem. Drug-drug interactions have been recognized as clinically relevant issues also. The issue of drug discontinuation has appeared in the literature; SSRI withdrawal, and the adverse effects of abrupt discontinuation of lithium vs. tapering are important clinical issues about which we now know more than we did a short time ago.

There are some controversies which will likely never end, such as the long-term use of benzodiazepines, the use of these agents in individuals with a history of alcoholism. The article describing the experience in Chile after benzodiazepines became OTC drugs in an interesting social experiment (contrasting an increasingly restrictive attitude in some areas of the country). Pharmaco-sociology? Pharmaco-economics? I hope there is useful information (or at least some interesting opinions) in this review of topics in psychopharmacology.

R. Bruce Lydiard, M.D., Ph.D.

Mood

Chronological Milestones to Guide Drug Change

Quitkin FM, McGrath PJ, Stewart JW, et al (Columbia Univ, New York)
Arch Gen Psychiatry 53:785–792, 1996 10–1

Introduction.—Thirty percent to 40% of patients do not respond to antidepressant treatment. There is little documentation of when to switch a depressed patient to a new treatment. Some authors maintain that patients who are and are not going to respond can be identified within a short time. This study sought to determine the time when patients not responding to antidepressant treatment are unlikely to benefit and should have their treatment changed.

Methods.—The study used data from 8 antidepressant studies performed at a university-affiliated outpatient clinic over 10 years. Each study included an initial, single-blind placebo run-in period followed by a 6-week double-blind trial. There were 5 drug-placebo comparisons and 3 drug-drug comparisons. Drugs evaluated included monoamine oxidase inhibitors, tricyclic antidepressants, and mianserin. The patients' clinical condition was analyzed by the CGI at the end of the run-in period. The current analysis included 593 patients who did not improve with placebo and proceeded to the double-blind comparison. The course of this 6-week treatment period was analyzed to identify the week at which patients were more likely to respond than patients receiving placebo.

Results.—The percentage of patients who had no improvement in response to treatment by the end of week 3 but were rated as responders by week 6 was 32% in the drug-treated groups and 10% in the placebo-treated groups. Drug and placebo treatment were equally effective in patients who were still unimproved by week 4. Until that point, the prognosis was better with active treatment for drug-treated patients who had not improved significantly but had had minimal improvement at some point.

Conclusions.—Patients who have not had at least minimal improvement in response to 4 weeks of treatment with an adequate dose of antidepressant should have their treatment changed. Such patients account for only about 10% of drug-treated patients in this placebo-controlled analysis. Treatment should also be changed for patients who have previously shown minimal improvement, but not after week 5. In patients with minimal improvement in week 5, treatment should continue for another week.

► Clinicians are frequently faced with the critical decision of when to change medication treatments for patients receiving antidepressants. Most of the time, we "fly by the seat of our pants" and hope that we have made the right decisions to stay the course or to make a switch. This article represents a good attempt to help guide the clinician via a careful analysis of a large research population. Obviously, there are many variables that can affect the decision about switching treatment. It also should be helpful for people who teach psychopharmacology, as well as those who practice it. It is of interest that the type of depression being examined does not significantly alter the authors' suggestions for clinical practice generated in this report. One limitation of this report is that it does not include selective serotonin reuptake inhibitors. The generalizability of findings from an urban research center to the general psychiatric patient population could also be raised as a minor concern. But this also applies to most scientifically solid research. It's likely that patients with clinically significant comorbid anxiety disorders were excluded. Since 40% to 60% of depressed patients have comorbid anxiety, we need to know more about how to optimize treatments.

R.B. Lydiard, M.D., Ph.D.

Serotonin Reuptake Inhibitor Withdrawal

Coupland NJ, Bell CJ, Potokar JP (Univ of Alberta, Canada; Univ of Bristol, England)

J Clin Psychopharmacol 16:356–362, 1996 10–2

Objective.—It is generally recommended that antidepressant treatment with serotonin reuptake inhibitors should continue for months or years. Such long-term treatment may bring out previously unrecognized adverse effects. Symptoms related to the discontinuation of the selective serotonin reuptake inhibitors (SSRIs) have been reported, particularly dizziness and paresthesia but also asthenia, nausea, visual disturbances, and headache. The incidence of withdrawal symptoms and the associated factors were assessed in patients discontinuing treatment with serotonin reuptake inhibitors.

Methods.—The retrospective study included 352 of 380 patients discontinuing treatment with clomipramine or an SSRI—fluoxetine, fluvoxamine, paroxetine, or sertraline. One hundred seventy-one of these patients were monitored closely during the drug discontinuation period. Data collected include effects of restarting medication and whether the patient was considered to have clinical relapse. Cases were identified according to a published definition of withdrawal syndrome, i.e., those with 1 or more new symptoms qualitatively and quantitatively different from their index illness.

Findings.—Many patients experienced adverse effects of drug withdrawal. The most frequent symptoms were dizziness, paresthesia, lethargy, and nausea (Table 2). Some patients with dizziness also had slight eye or head movements associated with jerking or blurred vision. The symptoms started within 5 days of the end of treatment, and sometimes during the dose tapering period. Patients who stopped taking fluvoxamine, paroxe-

TABLE 2.—Frequency (%) of Specific Symptoms During Withdrawal Period

Symptom	Clomipramine (N = 13)	Paroxetine (N = 50)	Fluvoxamine (N = 43)	Sertraline (N = 45)	Fluoxetine (N = 20)
Dizziness	7.7	16.0	9.3	2.2	0.0
Paresthesia	30.8	12.0	2.3	0.0	0.0
Lethargy	7.7	12.0	4.7	0.0	0.0
Nausea	15.4	6.0	7.0	0.0	0.0
Lowered mood	0.0	2.0	7.0	0.0	0.0
Anxiety	0.0	4.0	2.3	0.0	0.0
Vivid dreams	15.4	4.0	7.0	0.0	0.0
Insomnia	15.4	4.0	2.3	0.0	0.0
Headache	0.0	0.0	7.0	0.0	0.0
Irritability	15.4	0.0	4.7	0.0	0.0
Movement-related	0.0	16.0	7.0	0.0	0.0

(Coupland NJ, Bell CJ, Potokar JP: Serotonin reuptake inhibitor withdrawal. *J Clin Psychopharmacol* 16:356–362, 1996.)

tine, or clomipramine were more likely to experience symptoms than those who had taken sertraline or fluoxetine. No patient treated for less than 7 weeks had withdrawal symptoms. The risk of symptoms was not increased by treatment periods of longer than 6 months, however. Most patients did not have relapses.

Conclusions.—Withdrawal symptoms are common after cessation of serotonin reuptake inhibitor treatment. Withdrawal is more likely for patients taking clomipramine or one of the shorter half-life SSRIs. The symptoms occur despite dose tapering and resolve when the medication is restarted; relapses are unusual, however. The occurrence of withdrawal symptoms may be related to serotonin's role in the coordination of sensory, autonomic, and motor activity.

▶ Many of us have read case reports of withdrawal symptoms after discontinuation of an SSRI. Although retrospective, these data suggest that these observations are relatively common across diagnostic groups. They make pharmacokinetic sense also—more adverse events with shorter half-life agents which have no long-acting metabolites—fluvoxamine and sertraline. Clomipramine, both a TCA and SSRI, appears to act more like TCAs. While the discussion of possible mechanisms is interesting, this report underscores the importance of a slow taper of psychotropic medications. This is a nice follow-up of the original observation by Dilsaver[1] who described cholinergic rebound in patients discontinuing tricyclics.

We should all discuss with patients the need for gradual taper of medications. It also suggests that we should be looking for these kinds of symptoms in more severely ill patients (i.e., psychotic patients) being treated with older and newer antipsychotic agents. Since the histories we receive from these patients are often more difficult to interpret, this report provides evidence that we should go on faith that this is probably a common event that may not be as commonly recognized as it should be.

R.B. Lydiard, M.D., Ph.D.

Reference

1. Dilsaver SC, Greden JF: Antidepressant withdrawal syndromes: Evidence for supersensitivity of cholinergic system as an etiologic factor. *J Clin Psychopharmacol* 3:330, 1983.

Decreased Efficacy of Combined Benzodiazepines and Unilateral ECT in Treatment of Depression

Stein JA, Stein G (Mayday Univ, Croydon, England; Farnborough Hosp, Orpington, Kent, England)

Acta Psychiatr Scand 94:101–104, 1996 10–3

Purpose.—Previous studies have suggested that benzodiazepine treatment may reduce the efficacy of unilateral or bilateral electroconvulsive therapy (ECT). Other studies find no such effect. The effects of concomitant benzodiazepine therapy on the efficacy of ECT were assessed.

Methods.—The retrospective study included 124 patients receiving concomitant benzodiazepine and ECT over a 10-year period. Most patients received a 3- to 4-second treatment with an electricity dose of 112 mC to 234 mC. Patients receiving unilateral and bilateral ECT were included. A second shock at a higher level was sometimes administered if the patient did not respond to the first treatment. The efficacy of ECT was assessed from the case notes; the results were compared to those of a matched group of patients who received ECT but not benzodiazepines. DSM-IV criteria were applied where possible.

Findings.—The rate of improvement on ECT was 84% in the patients receiving benzodiazepines and 89% in those not receiving benzodiazepines. However, among patients receiving unilateral ECT, the response was much poorer with benzodiazepines. Hospital stay was longer as well. The response to unilateral ECT was worse with both long- and short-acting benzodiazepines.

Conclusions.—The response to unilateral ECT is not as good in patients taking benzodiazepines. This effect may arise from a benzodiazepine-induced increase in seizure threshold, as well as inadequate energy dosing and insufficient seizure duration. Prospective randomized studies of concomitant benzodiazepine and ECT are needed.

▶ Electroconvulsive therapy in benzodiazepine-treated patients is a common clinical problem. This retrospective report adds support to the clinical impression that benzodiazepines reduce the effectiveness of ECT. One surprising finding was that the benzodiazepine half-life didn't make much difference. While not definitive, it adds significantly to the limited literature regarding this specific problem. One caution is that individuals who are receiving benzodiazepines may be those who are more ill (those who have both anxiety and depression). Comorbidity confers increased resistance to treatment in general. Thus, it's possible that the patients receiving benzodiazepines were instead more treatment-resistant for that reason.

R.B. Lydiard, M.D., Ph.D.

Maintenance Electroconvulsive Therapy and Cognitive Function

Barnes RC, Hussein A, Anderson DN, et al (Whiston Hosp, Prescost, Merseyside; North Mersey Community NHS Trust, Liverpool, England)

Br J Psychiatry 170:285–287, 1997 10–4

Background.—In the past, before the availability of effective drug treatments, electroconvulsive therapy (ECT) was a commonly used form of prophylactic treatment. This raised concerns about its possible adverse effects on cognitive function, although research using standard courses of ECT has shown no such effects. The effects of a protracted course of maintenance ECT on cognitive function in an elderly patient were studied.

Case.—Woman, 74, had a long history of unstable bipolar affective disorder. Numerous approaches to prophylactic drug therapy had failed, and she was placed on twice-weekly ECT maintenance therapy beginning in 1989. All treatments were administered by a standard technique using bifronto-temporal electrode placements. More than 400 treatments were given, most using an Ectron Duopulse constant current device with a visible bilateral motor seizure of 20 to 50 seconds. More recent treatments were performed with a Mecta SR2 ECT device with a mean stimulus dose of 273 mC.

From 1987 to 1996, the patient underwent 5 psychometric assessments, all performed using standard instruments. A clinical psychologist performed all tests, the most recent ones in consultation with a geriatrician. The tests showed no pattern of progressive cognitive deterioration. There were, however, some learning and recall deficits consistent with those observed in the acute period after treatment. Based on the patient's functional status, she appeared to learn and retain important verbal, visual, and visuospatial material, including orientation, people's names, and the days of her treatment. Staff caring for the patient consider her condition improved. The frequency of treatments was successfully reduced to every 2 weeks.

Discussion.—The findings in this case suggest no intellectual impairment associated with a long course of maintenance ECT treatments. There are some cognitive difficulties similar to those associated with acute ECT treatment. It is difficult to generalize these findings because they are drawn from one case and because the patient's premorbid cognitive ability was low.

► The authors present a clinically relevant case report involving a woman treated over several years for recurrent delusional depression. Since this is only a case report, the conclusions cannot be generalized, but the report is still noteworthy. Basically, serial testing of cognitive function in this patient over several years of repeated ECT was not associated with significant cognitive decline. This study sets the stage for further investigations of ECT effects on cognition. Pre-ECT cognitive function testing with repeated assessment of cognitive functioning during the course of ongoing ECT in a larger, representative sample would be informative. One methodologic problem which must be grappled with is the effect of depression on cognitive functioning prior to treatment—how this could be distinguished from ECT-related cognitive disturbance. Obviously, cognitive testing in an individual who is in a normal mood state would be required to discern the effects of subsequent depression on cognitive function, and this is unlikely to occur. Maintenance ECT would be the "next-best" in this regard since posttreatment cognitive function could be followed over time. If ECT truly had an adverse effect, a progressive decline in functioning should be observed.

R.B Lydiard, M.D., Ph.D.

Resistance to Antidepressant Medications and Short-term Clinical Response to ECT

Prudic J, Haskett RF, Mulsant B, et al (New York State Psychiatric Inst, Western Psychiatric Inst, Pittsburgh, Pa; Carrier Found, Belle Mead, NJ)

Am J Psychiatry 153:985–992, 1996 10–5

Objective.—To investigate the clinical response to electroconvulsive therapy (ECT) in patients who are resistant to antidepressant medication and in patients who have not failed prior medication trials.

Background.—Electroconvulsive therapy was used to treat major depression well before antidepressant medications were introduced, and early studies reported a response rate of 80% to 90%. Currently, a lack of response to pharmacological treatment is the most common indication for ECT. It is important to know if resistance to antidepressant medication will affect a patient's response to ECT. Uncontrolled studies have reported that resistance to antidepressant medication is not predictive of outcome of ECT, but these studies did not compare patients resistant to medication and patients who had not failed adequate medication trials.

Methods.—There were 100 patients with primary, unipolar, nonpsychotic major depression who were treated with ECT at 3 sites. The patients scored at least 20 on the Hamilton Depression Rating Scale. Medication resistance was evaluated with the Antidepressant Treatment History Form. Patients were assessed immediately after and 1 week after ECT.

Results.—Analysis showed that 91.4% of patients with inadequate pharmacotherapy before ECT had a response immediately after cessation of ECT, whereas 63.1% of patients who were resistant to medication had a response immediately after cessation of ECT. This was observed at all 3 sites. Patients who were medication-resistant scored higher on the Hamilton Depression Rating Scale immediately after ECT. Immediately after cessation of ECT, scores on the Hamilton Depression Rating Scale decreased less than 40% in 10 patients who were medication-resistant. From baseline to immediately after cessation of ECT, there was a significant, inverse relation between scores from the most potent medication trial and the percentage change in scores on the Hamilton Depression Rating Scale.

Discussion.—The predictive value for outcome of ECT of various antidepressant medications may vary. A lower response rate to ECT was predicted by resistance to heterocyclic or bupropion medications. Resistance to an adequate SSRI or monoamine oxidase inhibitor trial had no predictive value. Medication resistance was most common for SSRIs. Heterocyclic antidepressants, SSRIs, and monoamine oxidase inhibitors are all effective for major depression, but may act through different mechanisms. These findings show that the mechanisms of action of heterocyclic antidepressants and ECT may be more similar than the mechanisms of action of SSRIs or monoamine oxidase inhibitors and ECT. SSRIs are being used more frequently for major depression, and it is important to distinguish between SSRI-resistance and resistance to other classes of antidepressants.

► The decision to move to ECT after a failure in antidepressant medication treatment has always been complicated. Given the relative lack of information regarding the use of ECT, this sophisticated clinical study is welcomed. The bad news is that medication-resistant depression is relatively more resistant to ECT. It also suggests caution in conveying too much optimism regarding the likelihood of response to ECT, especially for patients who have been resistant to adequate pharmacological trials of heterocyclic agents. Surprisingly, this finding wasn't found in individuals receiving monoamine oxidase inhibitors (MAOIs) or SSRIs. We still lack information on the outcome of depressed individuals who failed to respond to an SSRI, then fail a heterocyclic, and then an MAOI, which is the usual clinical path toward ECT. Only a small percentage (10%) had failed an MAOI in this study, defined as equivalent to ≥60 mg phenelzine for at least four weeks. However, selegiline and moclobemide may not be "equivalent" at any dose. This means also that *less* than 10% had failed an MAOI such as phenelzine or tranylcypromine. I am surprised that 90% of these treatment-resistant patients had not received an MAOI. This study represents one of the best objective assessments of outcome after ECT in patients who had been treated with antidepressants. Another important area in which scientifically based clinical information appears to be lacking is which agents are best to use in maintaining those individuals who have been fortunate enough to gain a therapeutic response from ECT. The current clinical wisdom is that some individuals who did not respond prior to ECT could then be successfully *maintained* on an agent that would not have provided antidepressant efficacy before. Although the report leaves the reader hungry for more information on the longer-term picture, this is a clinically noteworthy step forward in our knowledge about the ultimate short-term outcome of individuals who are medication resistant and then receive a course of ECT.

R.B. Lydiard, M.D., Ph.D.

Fluoxetine Versus Phenelzine in Atypical Depression

Pande AC, Birkett M, Fechner-Bates S, et al (Univ of Michigan, Ann Arbor; Lilly Research Centre, Surrey, England)

Biol Psychiatry 40:1017–1020, 1996 10–6

Background.—Although monoamine oxidase inhibitors (MAOIs) are effective antidepressants, certain medications and foods must be restricted to prevent hypertensive crises, which limit MAOI use. Fluoxetine, an effective and well-tolerated antidepressant with serotonergically mediated effects on mood and appetite, may be an alternative for atypical depression. Previous research has shown that the presence of atypcal features in a depressive illness predicts a better response to fluoxetine. The efficacy and safety of fluoxetine and phenelzine in patients with atypical depression were compared.

Methods and Findings.—Forty-two patients were enrolled in the randomized, double-blind trial. All met the criteria for major depressive disorder (MDD), dysthymic disorder, or depressive disorder not otherwise specified (NOS) in the DSM-III-R; all met the Columbia criteria for atypical depression; and all scored 10 or more on the 17-item Hamilton Depression Rating Scale (HDRS). After a single-blind placebo lead-in, patients were given fluoxetine 20–60 mg/day or phenelzine 45–90 mg/day for 6 weeks. Thirty-eight patients completed the 6-week study. Response rates between treatment groups did not differ. Phenelzine produced more frequent adverse effects than fluoxetine, with a few exceptions (such as tremor) (Table 3).

Conclusions.—In this group of patients with atypical depression as defined by the Columbia criteria, fluoxetine and phenelzine both effectively reduced depressive symptoms. Response and remission rates did not

TABLE 3.—Response and Remission Rates

	Fluoxetine (*N* = 20) [*n*(%)]	Phenelzine (*N* = 20) [*n*(%)]
Response (HDRS-17)	17 (80)	17 (85)
Response (CGI-1)	17 (85)	17 (85)
Remission	16 (80)	14 (70)

(Reprinted by permission of Elsevier Science Inc. from Pande AC, Birkett M, Fechner-Bates S, et al: Fluoxetine versus phenelzine in atypical depression. *Biol Psychiatry* 40:1017–1020, copyright 1996 by the Society of Biological Psychiatry.)

differ between groups. The frequency of adverse effect was greater with phenelzine, but both treatments were fairly well accepted.

► The clinical lore is that the selective serotonin reuptake inhibitors (SSRIs) will eventually replace the MAOIs. If it were shown that these newer agents were as effective as the MAOIs in certain patient subgroups, including those with atypical depression as defined by the Columbia group, the favorable side effects and safety profile would make the SSRIs the treatment of choice. Additionally, the nagging restrictions associated with the low tyramine diet as well as the intermediate and long side effects associated with MAOIs treatment can occasionally tilt the risk/benefit scale. The study lacks a placebo, but there was a robust and similar clinical response in atypical depressions receiving fluoxetine or phenelzine. In this study, only dizziness and asthenia, somnolence, and arthralgia were significantly more frequent with phenelzine than fluoxetine. However, had this study been carried out to present a more "real life" (i.e., long-term treatment) situation, weight gain, sexual dysfunction, and other side effects would have likely appeared in the phenelzine group at a greater frequency than in the fluoxetine-treated group. While this study has methodologic limitations, it does provide some evidence that the SSRIs may provide a safer alternative—for at least some patients—to MAOIs. Long-term data on patients receiving an SSRI vs. phenelzine for atypical depression could inform the clinician more completely about the optimal treatment options recommended, at least as the first line. This study represents a good start.

R.B. Lydiard, M.D., Ph.D.

A Comparison of Fluvoxamine and Fluoxetine in the Treatment of Major Depression

Rapaport M, Coccaro E, Sheline Y, et al (Univ of California, San Diego; Med College of Pennsylvania, Philadelphia; Washington Univ, St Louis; et al)

J Clin Psychopharmacol 16:373–378, 1996 10–7

Background.—Selective serotonin reuptake inhibitors (SSRIs) are generally as effective as tricyclic antidepressants (TCAs) but have a better safety profile, perhaps especially in medically unstable or elderly patients with depression. Whether the incidence and severity of adverse events differ with the different SSRIs has not been established. The efficacy and tolerability of fluvoxamine and fluoxetine were compared.

Methods.—By random assignment, 51 patients received fluvoxamine and 49 received fluoxetine, for 7 weeks. Eighty-four percent of each group completed treatment.

Findings.—Both treatment groups had a 60% improvement in Hamilton Rating Scale for Depression scores after the trial. The 2 groups did not differ significantly on any efficacy parameter. Only 2 patients in each group quit the study because of adverse effects. The side-effect profiles associated with the 2 treatments did not differ. Less nausea occurred with fluvoxamine than with fluoxetine.

Conclusions.—Fluvoxamine and fluoxetine were equally effective in decreasing depressive symptoms in these patients. The side-effect profiles of the 2 drugs differed slightly.

► Rapaport and colleagues at 5 other sites conducted a head-to-head comparison of fluvoxamine and flouxetine in depressed outpatients over a 7-week period. Studies of this nature are useful for clinicians in helping to sharpen the potential differences in clinical side effects profiles between the SSRIs. In this 7-week study, demographically similar groups received either fluvoxamine (averaging 100 mg by the end of the study) or fluoxetine (averaging about 35 mg at study end). One puzzling aspect was that the fluvoxamine was administered as a daily evening dose and fluoxetine was administered in the morning, while the double-blind was maintained by the placebos. The most striking finding was that the drugs were not particularly different in terms of effectiveness or in side effects profiles. This was not explained by the admixture of comorbid diagnoses in the groups (which was surprisingly small in both groups) or in gender distribution. Interestingly, the incidence of insomnia between the 2 groups was not different despite the differences in dosing strategies. The incidence of agitation was not different between the groups (although a slightly, but not significantly higher percentage of fluoxetine recipients experienced it). Akathisia was not observed as a significant problem in either group. While short-term studies such as the one reported by Rapaport and colleagues are important in helping clinicians choose agents for acute treatment, long-term comparative studies are going to be necessary to really discriminate between the agents meaningfully. For example, what is the incidence of sexual side effects over the longer term? Weight gain/weight loss?

R.B. Lydiard, M.D., Ph.D.

Lack of Advantage for Imipramine Combined With Lithium Versus Imipramine Alone in the Treatment of Major Depression: A Double-blind Controlled Study

Shahal B, Piel E, Mecz L, et al (Technion Israel Inst of Technology, Haifa)
Biol Psychiatry 40:1181–1183, 1996 10–8

Background.—Lithium's role in the treatment of major depression (MD) responsive to antidepressants has not been clearly defined. A previous report has suggested that lithium combined with nortryptiline results in a more rapid effect than that of nortryptiline alone. The possible advantages of initiating treatment with a combination of lithium and a tricyclic antidepressant (TCA) in patients with nonresistant MD compared with TCA alone were explored.

Methods.—Twenty-two consecutive inpatients with MD were included in the study. By random assignment, 12 received imipramine plus lithium and 10 received imipramine plus placebo. The initial imipramine dose of 50 mg/day was gradually increased to 150 mg/day in the first week, maintained between 150 and 175 mg/day. Lithium was begun at 300 mg and gradually increased based on plasma levels, with the goal of maintaining 0.7–0.9 mEq/L throughout the study. Levels of imipramine and its metabolites were not measured in serum.

Findings.—Eleven patients in the imipramine plus lithium group and 9 in the imipramine plus placebo group completed 5 weeks of therapy. The daily dose of imipramine was 168 and 167 mg in the 2 groups, respectively, at the end of the study. Weakness was more common in the patients receiving imipramine and lithium.

Conclusions.—Adding lithium to imipramine yielded no therapeutic benefits in the rapidity of the antidepressant effect onset or in treatment outcomes. Lithium augmentation during an active depressive episode should probably be reserved for patients with resistant depression.

▶ Shahal and coworkers address the clinical question of whether adding lithium to imipramine in the treatment of major depression would provide a significant advantage in terms of more rapid onset of antidepressant effect. Based on some open label studies, there was a suggestion that accelerated treatment response may be possible by initially using a combination of lithium and a tricyclic. The study was small (22 patients, 19 with prior depression, none resistant). Over the course of 5 weeks, Hamilton ratings dropped from the mid-20s to approximately 6 in each of the groups; the imipramine dose was approximately 170 mg per day in each treatment group but no levels were drawn. The authors did follow lithium levels and maintained in the range of 0.7–0.9 mEq/1 throughout the study. The bad news is we can't really tell if this was a negative study; the authors estimate that over 5,000 subjects would have been required to detect (if actually present) an early difference. There was no information on depressive subtype and there was no placebo treatment group. However, the study is clinically relevant in that it does not suggest any large effect for coadministration of lithium with a tricyclic. In today's world, a similar comparison in conjunction with a serotonin selective uptake inhibitor would be of interest.

R.B. Lydiard, M.D., Ph.D.

Nefazodone and Akathisia

Eberstein S, Adler LA, Angrist B (New York Univ.)
Biol Psychiatry 40:798–799, 1996 10–9

Background.—Previous reports have described akathisia in association with serotonin-specific reuptake inhibitors (SSRIs), including fluoxetine, sertraline, and paroxetine. A case of akathisia after nefazodone treatment was reported.

Case Report.—Man, 64, was admitted for the treatment of major depression characterized by somatic preoccupation. A previous episode had been successfully treated with bupropion and low-dose mesoridazine 1 year earlier. The patient refused mesoridazine treatment and so was treated with venlafaxine, up to 300 mg/day, and then bupropion, 200 mg/day. The patient eventually refused both of these agents, complaining of light-headedness and weakness. Treatment with nefazodone, 200 mg/day, was started. After 4 days, the patient complained of restlessness and difficulty remaining still when seated or lying down. When standing, he rocked from foot to foot. Akathisia was diagnosed and improved somewhat with propranolol, up to 80 mg/day, and clonazepam, 1 mg/day. Two days later, the nefazodone dose was increased to 300 mg/day, causing no discomfort to the patient. After 4 weeks of inpatient treatment, the patient was discharged with nefazodone, propranolol, and clonazepam.

Discussion.—The development of akathisia after nefazodone treatment could lead to dose limitation or noncompliance if not promptly recognized and treated. Physicians should be aware of the possibility of akathisia in patients receiving SSRIs. The drugs for treating akathisia have little potential for harm in patients without contraindications, so treatment should be started if akathisia is suspected.

► This case report reminds us that the new serotonin-selective agents, including nefazodone, can cause side effects which we do not expect. Nefazodone–which has enjoyed a reputation as an agent that causes very little agitation—is capable of producing what appears to be akathisia. This is probably a relatively rare adverse effect of nefazodone, as it has postsynaptic serotonin receptor–blocking activity. The case described appears to be akathisia, and the akathisia-like symptoms responded to treatments which we would expect to be helpful.

Another relevant issue this report brings to mind is that clinical trials often exclude patients with more than 1 disorder. We may expect side effects in our patients to be the same as those reported, but the neurobiology of a patient with 2 or more disorders may be different from that of "pure culture" patients. It is not surprising that the complicated patients we see may have different side effects than we anticipated. Nefazodone *is* different from the SSRIs in many ways. This report underscores the need for clinicians to have a heightened awareness of unexpected side effects when prescribing newer agents.

R.B. Lydiard, M.D., Ph.D.

Combining Serotonin Reuptake Inhibitors and Bupropion in Partial Responders to Antidepressant Monotherapy

Bodkin JA, Lasser RA, Wines JD Jr, et al (Harvard Med School, Boston; Massachusetts Gen Hosp, Belmont, Mass)

J Clin Psychiatry 58:137–145, 1997 10–10

Objective.—A significant number of patients with affective disorders fail to achieve full remission of symptoms or improvement in all symptoms in controlled trials. Possibly these patients may benefit from combinations of antidepressants. Records of 27 patients treated with combinations of serotonin reuptake inhibitors (SRIs) and bupropion were reviewed. Five cases were discussed.

Methods.—Between February 1991 and April 1996, 27 incompletely recovered patients (16 women) aged 20–83 years, were treated with a combination of an SRI and bupropion for an average of 11 months. Mood, energy level, anxiety or panic, obsessive-compulsive symptoms, sleep disturbance, motivation, cognitive function, and sexual dysfunction were analyzed clinically. Responders and nonresponders to combination therapy were compared.

Results.—Patients received diagnoses of unipolar major depression (n = 9), dysthymic disorder (n = 6), bipolar disorder type II (n = 5) or type I (n = 3), attention deficit-hyperactivity disorder (n = 3), and generalized anxiety disorder with obsessive-compulsive disorder (n = 1). Twenty patients had at least 1 additional comorbid psychiatric disorder. Nineteen (70.4%) patients were considered responders to a mean daily dose of 243 mg of bupropion and a mean daily fluoxetine-equivalent dose of 31 mg. At least 10% of patients had adverse events including sexual dysfunction (40.7%), insomnia (22.2%), reduced energy level (14.8%), and tremor (11.1%). Adverse events were similar to those encountered with monotherapy. Treatment of 4 patients was discontinued because of adverse events.

Conclusion.—Combinations of SRIs and bupropion can be beneficial in incompletely recovered patients with affective disorders. Drug selection and dosing must be done carefully and closely monitored.

► This interesting clinical report from Bodkin and colleagues suggests a novel use for combination antidepressant treatment—SSRIs with bupropion. One might speculate that adding a selective serotonin agent to a dopamine uptake inhibitor may add up to a monoamine oxidase inhibitor profile. The monoamine oxidase inhibitors have broad effects on neurotransmitter metabolism, including dopamine. Combining the serotonin uptake properties of fluoxetine and the dopamine uptake inhibitor properties of bupropion appears to benefit many patients. Also, the price is right in terms of adverse effects (although there were some). It appears that the days of monotherapy may be over, and clinical wisdom is gradually beginning to appreciate the need for a broader spectrum of effects in mood disorders, at least in part because of the heterogeneity of the illness itself. We now are beginning to appreciate comorbidity as well. Clinical reports like this one are a welcomed addition to the knowledge base relating to treating patients who suffer from chronic recurrent mood disturbances. Hopefully, a controlled trial will confirm this clinical report.

R. Bruce Lydiard, M.D., Ph.D.

A Placebo-controlled, Randomized Clinical Trial Comparing Sertraline and Imipramine for the Treatment of Dysthymia

Thase ME, Fava M, Halbreich U, et al (Univ of Pittsburgh, Pa; Massachusetts Gen Hosp, Boston; State Univ of New York, Buffalo; et al)

Arch Gen Psychiatry 53:777–784, 1996 10–11

Purpose.—Dysthymia is a common and chronic mood disorder that carries substantial social dysfunction, disability, and comorbidity. Despite these considerations, dysthymia has generally been underrecognized and undertreated. Several studies have shown the effectiveness of drug therapy for dysthymic patients, but these trials have been limited by a variety of factors. A randomized, controlled, multicenter trial evaluated the safety and efficacy of sertraline hydrochloride and imipramine hydrochloride for patients with dysthymia.

Methods.—The study included 416 outpatients who met *Diagnostic and Statistical Manual of Mental Disorders*, ed III, revised, criteria for early-onset, primary dysthymia. There were 271 women and 145 men, (age range, 25 to 65 years). All were free of concurrent major depression. The patients were randomized into 3 treatment groups: sertraline, up to a maximum dose of 200 mg/day; imipramine, up to a maximum dose of 300 mg/day; or placebo. The results were evaluated using the Hamilton Rating Scale for Depression, (HAM-D), the Montgomery-Asberg Depression Rating Scale, the Hopkins Symptom Checklist, and the self-rated version of the Inventory of Depressive Symptoms. A positive response was defined as a Clinical Global Impressions improvement score of 1 or 2, corresponding to very much or much improved.

Results.—Three hundred ten patients completed the study; the completion rate was 84% with sertraline, 67% with imipramine, and 76% with placebo. Adverse events were significantly more likely to cause discontinuation of imipramine treatment. Both sertraline and imipramine significantly reduced scores on all efficacy measures used. On the HAM-D, the mean reduction from baseline score was 5.6 points with sertraline, 5.9 points with imipramine, and 3.9 points with placebo. Clinical response rates were 59% with sertraline, 64% with imipramine, and 44% with placebo. At the time of the initial response, the modal dose was 50 mg for sertraline and 100 mg for imipramine; the median doses were 50 and 150 mg, respectively.

Conclusions.—In patients with early-onset primary dysthymia, sertraline and imipramine both offer significant symptomatic relief, compared with placebo. Sertraline causes fewer adverse effects, which is an important consideration given the chronicity of dysthymia. Evidence from previous studies suggests that patients with dysthymia will maintain their response to drug treatment over the long term.

► Dysthymia is a common disorder which only recently has been appreciated as being an important cause of functional disability. The Rand Medical Outcome Study provided some of the first evidence of the significant disability associated even with only a few depressive symptoms. Not too many years ago, dysthymia was seen as a "personality disorder." This placebo-controlled study demonstrates nicely that dysthymia is a treatable disorder. The study was scientifically sound and sufficiently powered to find a difference between active sertraline and placebo. Once again, the issue of poor compliance with tricyclics is revealed in this study. The study suggests that—like patients with major depression—patients with more chronic, low-grade mood disturbance are unwilling to suffer through the considerable side effects associated with these older agents.

R.B. Lydiard, M.D., Ph.D.

Maintenance Treatment of Major Depression: A Review of the Literature

Blacker D (Massachusetts Gen Hosp, Boston)

Harvard Rev Psychiatry 4:1–9, 1996 10–12

Background.—Beliefs regarding the proper treatment for major depressive disorder are diverse. This article reviews the current literature on the long-term treatment of depression to determine which drugs work best for which patients.

Methods.—A database search from 1971 through 1991 identified articles that discussed depression, antidepressant drugs, lithium, or electroconvulsive therapy. Another database and psychiatric journals search from 1991 to 1994 uncovered articles on depression prevention and control. The term *major depressive disorder* refers to a depressed or irritable mood with typical neurovegetative changes, regardless of a specific diagnosis. Three phases of illness are used: the goal of the acute phase is to achieve remission of the current episode; that of the continuation phase is to prevent relapse of the current episode; and that of the maintenance phase is to avoid future episodes.

Findings.—One British study reported the need for 4–6 months of continuous drug treatment after acute symptoms resolved; most relapses occurred within the first 3 months. Recurrence rates after 2 years were 48% for amitriptyline and 43% for lithium. A U.S. study also confirmed this need for continuation treatment, reporting that most relapses occur within the first 4 months. Recurrence rates after 2 years were 73% for lithium and 56% for imipramine. In another U.S. study, maintenance treatment with lithium had a 57% recurrence rate, imipramine had a 44% recurrence rate, but their combination had only a 34% recurrence rate.

This study indicated that the severity of the depression affected outcome, and that imipramine was superior to lithium in patients with severe disease. Finally, a fourth study (from the United States) used imipramine or interpersonal psychotherapy over 3 years. Combined treatment with imipramine and interpersonal psychotherapy had marginally the best results, then imipramine alone, then psychotherapy alone. Furthermore, these authors reported a significantly longer delay before recurrence with the use of full-dose (135 weeks) rather than half-dose (75 weeks) imipramine.

Conclusions.—Any patient with recurrent major depression should receive maintenance drug therapy. Patients most likely to benefit are those with severe episodes, severe disruption of social and work life, and an inability to recognize the early signs of their illness. Amitriptyline and imipramine have proven efficacy, whereas lithium should probably be reserved for patients who cannot tolerate antidepressants. The optimal length of maintenance therapy seems to be between 2 and 2.5 cycle lengths (measured from the start of one episode to the start of the next one). Psychotherapy by itself is not indicated, but its combination with drug therapy should provide benefit.

► Blacker's thoughtful and comprehensive review of the literature on maintenance treatment for bipolar disorder is clearly a noteworthy gathering of the current clinical wisdom, which appears to be surprisingly limited. For example, we know practically nothing about long-term treatment with the SSRIs beyond the few studies that have appeared in the literature. She argues convincingly that the available database suggests that there should be a lower threshold for initiating longer-term treatment of mood disorders, especially since we have agents with acceptable side effect profiles and low toxicity. Clearly, more work is needed in this area. One last note—it is informative that the number of patients left in the large maintenance study conducted by Kupfer et al.[1] was only 20 patients after 3 years. Half of these were randomly assigned to receive imipramine, the half of the group received placebo. Thus, although we do know that "the dose that gets you well keeps you well," it appears that the price patients have to pay for taking long-term tricyclics may ultimately prove to be too high for them. Despite their history of recurrent depression, patients are unwilling to continue taking necessary and effective treatment. Similar studies with the SSRIs and other newer compounds are urgently needed.

R.B. Lydiard, M.D., Ph.D.

Reference

1. Kupfer DJ, Frank E, Perel JM, et al: Five-year outcome for maintenance therapies in recurrent depressions. *Arch Gen Psychiatry* 49:769–773, 1992.

Antidepressant Treatment During Breast-Feeding

Wisner KL, Perel JM, Findling RL (Case Western Reserve Univ, Cleveland, Ohio; Western Psychiatric Inst, Pittsburgh, Pa)

Am J Psychiatry 153:1132–1137, 1996 10–13

Objective.—To review the literature for studies on the use of antidepressant medication during breast-feeding.

Background.—The number of new psychiatric episodes in women during the 3 months after childbirth has increased dramatically. At least 80% of these episodes are affective episodes, and the most common diagnosis is depression. The rate of minor or major depression in this population is between 10% and 15%. Treatment of depression with medication creates a dilemma for women who are breast-feeding, with some being reluctant to wean their infants. There is no critical review of the literature on the use of antidepressant medication in women who are breast-feeding. Complete information is critical to physicians and women if they are to make informed risk-benefit decisions.

Methods.—A search was made of MEDLINE for articles with individual names of all antidepressant drugs used during breast-feeding from 1966 to 1995. Only articles that stated infant serum levels were included.

Results.—Information on 29 mothers who were breast-feeding and being treated with tricyclic antidepressants was available. With the exception of doxepin, tricyclic parent drugs were not detected at levels as low as 1 ng/mL to 10 ng/mL in infant serum. There were no reports of adverse effects. In one study, doxepin was detected at 3 ng/mL. There was no evidence of accumulation of tricyclics in infant serum, and infants older than 10 weeks appear to have a low risk of adverse effects from tricyclics. There was only one instance of an adverse effect from a tricyclic in which the mother was taking doxepin, and respiratory depression in association with high concentrations of the metabolite *N*-desmethyldoxepin occurred in the nursing infant. In another study, a mother was taking twice the dose of doxepin as in the first study, but the infant had no adverse effects. There were reports of colic and high infant serum levels during treatment with fluoxetine, which now carries labeling that recommends it not be used in women who breast-feed.

Discussion.—After the physician presents the risks and benefits of drug treatment for depression, the mother must ultimately make the treatment decision. The physician should never suggest that there are no risks associated with antidepressants. It is impossible to generalize the findings from a few studies to all infants. The metabolic processing of these drugs is bound to vary from infant to infant, and it is theoretically possible for any infant to react to even minute amounts of a drug. The following should be documented in the medical record: all discussions with the mother or parents and pediatrician regarding drug and alternative treatment, the mother's competence to consent to treatment, indications for treatment, and improvement in the target symptoms or a lack of response. The authors favor the use of these drugs to treat depression in women who are breast-feeding: amitriptyline, nortriptyline, desipramine, clomipramine, dothiepin, and sertraline. The mother and infant should be carefully monitored while the mother is being treated. Although unlikely, it is possible that long-term very low doses of antidepressant medication could affect the behavioral function of the infant.

► It is surprising that so little is known about the effects of antidepressant treatment on infants of mothers who received antidepressant therapy. This report synthesizes the available literature gathered from case reports over the years. It is amazing that the very population at greatest risk for depression (women of child-bearing potential) has received so little attention about this common dilemma to date. The lack of information probably feeds the anxiety of both mothers and doctors who are faced with the emergence of postpartum depression or depression that develops during the course of pregnancy. While we will all continue to wring our hands until more definitive studies appear, this report nicely walks the reader through the decision-making process and provides some reassurance (as welll as published informations) to make the case for treatment. The appropriate caveats are included in the report, and the important clinical decision-making process is advised thoughtfully. The good news is that there is relatively little information to suggest that it is dangerous to treat symptomatic mothers and the authors point out the danger of not treating depressed mothers. It may well provide reassurance to hesitant new mothers who are depressed and already have inappropriate guilt. The report also addresses the effects of maternal depression on infant development as another factor in the equation for planning treatment. The article will be useful when consulting primary care physicians who face the same dilemma.

R.B. Lydiard, M.D., Ph.D.

Treatment of Bipolar Depression With Carbamazepine: Results of an Open Study

Dilsaver SC, Swann SC, Chen Y-W, et al (Univ of Health, Houston)

Biol Psychiatry 40:935–937, 1996 10–14

Background.—Antidepressants may adversely effect patients with bipolar disorder (BPD), inducing rapid cycling or mixed states. New strategies for treating BPD are needed. The efficacy of carbamazepine in 1 patient series was investigated.

Methods.—Thirty-six men and women, aged 19–50 years, were included in the open study. All were inpatients at a psychiatric center and had been depressed for at least 2 weeks. Carbamazepine was given for up to 21 days. Initial dose was 400 mg, given orally. Between treatment days 4 and 10, serum levels were obtained. If the serum level was less than 10 μg/ML and side effects were not limiting, the dose was increased in 200 mg increments to a maximum of 1,000 mg daily. No adjustments were made after day 10. Oral or IM lorazepam, 1–2 mg, was given every hour or more for anxiety.

Findings.—Sixty-three percent of patients with BPD entered remission. Remission occurred after 7 days of treatment in 4 patients, after 14 days in 9, and after 21 days in 4. Seventy-two percent of patients with psychotic features entered remission, as did 55.6% without. The mean HDRS scores of remitting patients declined by 88.7%. Of 9 patients with depressive mania (6 women and 3 men), 22.2% entered remission after 14 days of treatment. Remission was less likely to occur in patients with depressive mania than in those with BPD.

Conclusions.—In this study, patients with BPD had a 79% median reduction in HDRS scores with carbamazepine treatment, compared with 43% in patients with depressive mania. Though carbamazepine appears to be ineffective for depressive mania, an exacting definition of remission was used in the current study. Although the drug was unrelated to remission among the patients with depressive mania, it was associated with a decrease in symptom severity.

► Studies assessing the antidepressant effects of carbamazepine (CBZ) in unipolar depression have not been encouraging. This open study suggests that CBZ may be useful in treatment of depression associated with bipolar disorder (BPAD). Dilsaver and colleagues treated 36 patients with BPAD—either depressed or with depressive mania (both mania and depression simultaneously). Plasma levels were monitored to ensure both compliance and adequacy of treatment (levels greater 10 µg/mL for most patients). Approximately two thirds of patients with bipolar depression had psychotic symptoms. Seventy-two percent of these responded to treatment and approximately 63% of the total sample experienced remission. An additional group of 9 individuals (3 men and 6 women) with concurrent depression and mania were treated in a similar fashion. Two thirds of these patients also had psychotic features but only 2 of the 9 patients achieved remission. These data suggest that CBZ may be a useful treatment for bipolar depression but probably not mixed mania (concurrent mania and depression). It also underscores the relative paucity of data available for clinicians to treat patients with BPAD, depressed subtype. Of particular interest, the proportion of psychosis was approximately the same in both these samples, but the response rate in those with the mixed syndrome was much less. Of course, I should note that this was an open-label study, and remission and response rate were not well defined. The study was otherwise described well and utilized a standard depression rating scale. The study suggests that it would be useful to conduct prospective studies during standard treatments for bipolar depression.

R.B. Lydiard, M.D., Ph.D.

How Safe Are Serotonin Reuptake Inhibitors for Depression in Patients With Coronary Heart Disease?

Sheline YI, Freedland KE, Carney RM (Washington Univ, St Louis)

Am J Med 102:54–59, 1997 10–15

Purpose.—Patients with coronary heart disease (CHD) are at risk of depression, which carries significant risk of additional cardiac morbidity and mortality. However, for unclear reasons, patients with CHD are rarely treated for depression. Although the cardiac effects of the tricyclic antidepressants are well documented, little is known about the potential cardiac effects of the selective serotonin reuptake inhibitors (SSRIs). Available data on the cardiac effects of the SSRIs are reviewed, including recommendations for their use in patients with coronary heart disease.

Findings.—All articles on the cardiac effects of SSRIs from 1986 to 1996 were analyzed. Case reports have suggested some cardiac effects of SSRIs in patients without known cardiac disease. These include arrhythmias—such as atrial fibrillation and flutter, bradycardia, and supraventricular tachycardia—and heart block. However, the rate of arrhythmias and other cardiovascular effects of SSRIs seems to be very low—less than 5,000 reported out of an estimated 15 million treatment cases. In overdose, these drugs have a remarkable safety record. Through their effects on metabolism, however, they have the potential to affect plasma levels of other drugs. Interactions with tricyclic antidepressants and type IC antiarrhythmic agents are possible.

In SSRIs administered to CHD patients with depression, the risks associated with drug interactions must be assessed against the benefits of treating depression. However, there are few data on the effectiveness of SSRIs in elderly patients or in patients with cardiac disease. The lack of data would suggest the need for caution in using SSRIs for cardiac patients, especially elderly patients receiving certain types of antiarrhythmic drugs. On the other hand, as long as due consideration is given, the risks of not treating depression in patients with CHD probably exceed the risks of SSRI treatment. More study is needed to compare the antidepressant effects of tricyclic antidepressants and SSRIs in patients with cardiovascular disease.

Summary.—Depression is a common and serious problem in patients with CHD. The SSRIs appear to have very few adverse cardiovascular effects, although they do have the potential for interaction with other drugs, including certain antiarrhythmic drugs. There are insufficient data on the effects of SSRIs in elderly patients and in patients with CHD.

▶ The authors examined the MEDLINE database for a 10-year period (1986–1996) to assess the frequency of cardiac effects of SSRIs. Based on the recent awareness that depression can complicate the recovery from acute cardiac events such as myocardial infarction, examination of the incidence of cardiac effects of these presumably safe agents was conducted. Because patients with no cardiac pathology who have overdosed on these agents experience arrhythmias including atrial fibrillation and flutter, bradycardia, and superventricular tachycardia, as well as an association with heart block, the question was raised as to whether they may be less safe than presumed in individuals with preexisting cardiac disease. The main findings of the study were that the SSRIs appear to be quite safe. The incidence of *any* cardiac event was extremely low (0.003%). This included even relatively benign events such as change in EKG and even some incidents which may have little or nothing to do with the treatment itself. Thus, it appears that the SSRIs are a safe treatment alternative for individuals with cardiac disease. Unfortunately, the authors did not include a comparison of a similarly large group of individuals treated with tricyclics, which would have been nice. The authors do caution of the potential of SSRIs to interfere with the metabolism of important agents such as antiarrhythmic agents of the IC class and others. Thus, the clinical risks of drug interaction should be included in the clinical decision picture. However, given the clear cardiovascular effects of the tricyclics on cardiac conduction and blood pressure, the SSRIs clearly have a place near the front of the line as therapeutic agents used to treat depression in people with cardiovascular disease. As always, clinicians must remain informed about potential drug interactions with other special situations in which traditional agents still may be preferable.

R.B. Lydiard, M.D., Ph.D.

Low Use of Neuroleptic Drugs in the Treatment of Psychotic Major Depression

Mulsant BH, Haskett RF, Prudic J, et al (Univ of Pittsburgh, Pa; Columbia Univ, New York; Carrier Found, Belle Mead, NJ)

Am J Psychiatry 154:559–561, 1997 10–16

Introduction.—Based on the available research, an antidepressant/neuroleptic combination is recommended for the treatment of patients with major depression and psychotic features. The frequency and adequacy of antidepressant/neuroleptic treatment for patients with psychotic major depression was evaluated.

Methods.—The prospective, multicenter study included 187 patients referred for electroconvulsive therapy (ECT). The patients' mean age was 62 years, and the median duration of the depressive episode before ECT was 25 weeks. The patients had received a median of 4 medication trials. Episodes with psychotic features occurring at any time were classified as psychotic. Fifty-three patients had psychotic depression while 134 had nonpsychotic depression.

Drug therapy given before ECT was assessed and classified for adequacy. For example, a treatment trial with an antidepressant alone for psychotic depression was classified as clearly or probably inadequate. A combination of 4 weeks of antidepressant therapy plus at least 3 weeks of neuroleptic treatment with a daily dose of 400 mg of chlorpromazine equivalents was regarded as adequate. Drug trials for patients with psychotic and nonpsychotic depression were compared for adequacy.

Findings.—The patients with psychotic depression were significantly less likely to have received at least 1 adequate trial of drug therapy than those with nonpsychotic depression. Forty-seven percent of the patients with psychotic depression received either no neuroleptic treatment or less than 3 weeks of neuroleptic treatment. When at least 3 weeks of neuroleptic treatment was given, the dose was usually too low. Just 4% of patients with psychotic depression received an adequate trial of antidepressant/neuroleptic therapy before referral for ECT.

Conclusions.—Patients with psychotic depression may be especially likely to receive inadequate drug therapy. Perhaps because their psychotic features go unrecognized, many patients do not receive neuroleptic therapy, or receive less than the minimum effective dose. The results suggest the need for additional education in the recognition and treatment of psychotic depression.

▶ The authors systematically studied the medication treatments of 125 patients who subsequently received ECT over a 4-year period. Patients were involved in a multicenter study examining whether medication treatment resistance has a prognostic relationship on post-ECT course of illness. The finding that nearly half of the patients with psychotic depression received no neuroleptics prior to ECT raises concerns about current standards of treatment of psychotic depression. These patients were all being seen by clinicians in sophisticated university-based treatment centers. One might surmise that individuals in the general community may receive even less adequate pharmacotherapy for delusional depression. Given the considerable expense and time required for administering ECT, it should not be undertaken before optimal pharmacotherapy has failed. The authors considered the appropriate factors which may have potentially biased these results. For example, the patients already being considered for ECT may have received less aggressive pharmacotherapy as a result. This study suggests that efforts to educate mental health providers about the need for adequate levels of pharmacotherapy, including both neuroleptics and antidepressants in individuals with psychotic depression, are needed.

R.B. Lydiard, M.D., Ph.D.

Dosing Strategies and Time Course of Response to Antimanic Drugs

Bowden CL (Univ of Texas, San Antonio)

J Clin Psychiatry 57:4S-9S, 1996 10–17

Background.—Early response is important in the treatment of mania. Manics can be dangerous to themselves and others and require costly care. Dosing strategies and the rapidity of response to lithium, valproate, and carbamazepine were reviewed.

Discussion.—Only recently have the diagnoses of hypomania, mixed mania, and rapid cycling become possible. Many forms of mania respond poorly to lithium (Tables 1 and 2). Lithium treatment for patients with

TABLE 1.—Improvement in Manic Syndrome at Day 5 in Randomized, Double-blind Comparison of Lithium, Divalproex, and Placebo

Treatment	N	% Improvement	Effect Size
Divalproex	67	26	0.86
Lithium	35	19	0.49

(Courtesy of Bowden CL: Dosing strategies and time course of response to antimanic drugs. *J Clin Psychiatry* 57:4S–9S, 1996. Copyright 1996, Physicians Postgraduate Press. Reprinted by permission.)

uncomplicated mania may be initiated at 15 mg/kg of body weight, with dose increases every 3–4 days until a response, complicating adverse effects, or a 1.2–1.4 mEq/L serum level is noted. Divalproex may be more effective in mixed mania, rapid cycling, secondary mania, and mania with comorbid substance abuse. Divalproex may be about equally effective in pure, mixed, secondary, rapid cycling, and psychotic forms of acute mania. The initial dosage of divalproex is 20 mg/kg of body weight. Though predictors of response to carbamazepine have not been well studied, results with this agent may be more positive in lithium-refractory patients. A slow dosage escalation is needed for carbamazepine, beginning with 200 mg once or twice daily. Combining drugs may be more effective than monotherapy. Also, some patients with mixed mania may improve faster with the concurrent administration of an antidepressant.

Conclusions.—Aggressive treatment is indicated for manic patients. The 3 antimanic agents differ in rapidity of onset and adverse effects. The most favorable appears to be divalproex. Adjunctive agents may help facilitate an early response. However, finding the best regimen will require substantial, relatively early modification to minimize the risks of adverse effects, increase functional status, and reduce eventual poor compliance.

► Dr. Bowden, one of the nation's experts in the treatment of bipolar disorder presents a brief review of the 3 currently available antimanic agents: lithium, valproate, and carbamazepine (CBZ). Carbamazepine, which has not been approved as an antimanic agent appears to be a useful mood

TABLE 2.—Comparative Adverse Effects of Divalproex and Lithum in Acute Mania Which Were at Least Twice as Frequent as for Placebo

Adverse Event	Divalproex N = 69 (%)	Lithium N = 36 (%)
Asthenia	13	19
Constipation	10	17
Dizziness	16	8
Fever	1	14
Nausea	23	31
Twitching	3	8
Vomiting	14	25

(Courtesy of Bowden CL: Dosing strategies and time course of response to antimanic drugs. *J Clin Psychiatry* 57:4S–9S, 1996. Copyright 1996, Physicians Postgraduate Press. Reprinted by permission.)

stabilizer which has been used widely for the treatment of bipolar disorder and was the first anticonvulsant to be used in this fashion. The main focus of this paper was to suggest that there may be more rapid onset of action with divalproex sodium when a loading dose of 20 mg/kg is utilized and a plasma level of ≥50 μg/mL is generated. Citing limited evidence which suggests that levels over this may be associated with a positive early response (if one were to occur), Dr. Bowden suggests that patients who have not responded completely to doses which yield a level of approximately 50 μg/mL should have their dose increased so that approximately twice this plasma level is achieved (100–125 μg/mL). In general, plasma levels of anticonvulsants for use in psychiatry have not typically been helpful. This article suggests that it may be useful to determine divalproex sodium (if assays are readily available) during acute treatment of mania to hasten acute response and earlier discharge from inpatient treatment. Further, it provides the hypothesis which can be tested prospectively. If it were shown there was a differential onset of action among the 3 standard antimanic treatments currently used, it would represent a significant advance in the acute stabilization of this difficult patient population.

R.B. Lydiard, M.D., Ph.D.

Reduced Morbidity After Gradual Discontinuation of Lithium Treatment for Bipolar I and II Disorders: A Replication Study

Baldessarini RJ, Tondo L, Floris G, et al (Internatl Consortium for Bipolar Research)

Am J Psychiatry 154:551–553, 1997 10–18

Introduction.—An earlier report demonstrated that the median time to recurrence of affective symptoms after lithium discontinuation in 64 patients with bipolar I and II disorders was 4.7 times as great for gradual discontinuation over 2–4 weeks, compared to rapid discontinuation over less than 2 weeks. This trial is repeated in a different group of 78 patients with bipolar I and II disorders in well-matched discontinuation groups.

Methods.—All patients had been receiving effective lithium maintenance treatment for more than 1 year with at least a 75% decrease in the time they were ill. Lithium treatment was discontinued with or without medical advise either rapidly (1–14 days) or gradually (15–30 days). Survival analysis of time to first recurrence was compared for the 2 discontinuation schedules.

Results.—Lithium treatment was discontinued rapidly in 35 patients and gradually in 29 patients. Sixty patients (76.9%) discontinued lithium because of prolonged well-being. Eighteen patients (23.1%) discontinued therapy because of side effects or pregnancy. The median time to recurrence was 14 months and 2.5 months for patients who underwent gradual and rapid discontinuation, respectively. Between-group median survival times were similar for I and II subtypes and for depression and mania. The polarity of the first recurrence after lithium was discontinued was 83.6% concordant.

Conclusion.—The median time to recurrence was 5.6 times longer for patients with gradual discontinuation of lithium, compared to patients with rapid discontinuation. Patients should be advised not to discontinue lithium treatment without psychiatric supervision. Elective discontinuation should be performed gradually and under close clinical observation.

▶ As a follow-up to a retrospective chart review of abrupt vs. gradual discontinuation of lithium in bipolar disorder patients, Baldessarini and colleagues prospectively studied this phenomenon in 78 patients with bipolar disorder who were receiving lithium. Contrary to the current clinical wisdom that lithium is one of the few agents that can be discontinued abruptly, the retrospective report suggested that lithium, like other psychotropic agents, should be withdrawn gradually. This prospective follow-up study, which was carefully done, supports this finding. Perhaps most surprising was that a period of only a few weeks (less than 2 weeks vs. 2–4 weeks for discontinuation) made a difference in the risk of relapse in both bipolar I and bipolar II patients. Thus, clinicians overseeing the treatment of individuals with bipolar disorder may want to alter their patterns of medication treatment and warn patients of the risks of abrupt discontinuation as well. It would be most interesting to see if even more gradual discontinuation of lithium (months rather than weeks) would reduce the risk of early relapse even further.

R.B. Lydiard, M.D., Ph.D.

Lithium Versus Carbamazepine in the Maintenance Treatment of Bipolar Disorders: A Randomised Study

Greil W, Ludwig-Mayerhofer W, Erazo N, et al (Univ of Munich, Germany; Psychiatric Hosp of the RWTH Aachen, Germany; Univ of Tübingen, Germany; et al)

J Affect Disord 43:151–161, 1997 10–19

Introduction.—Lithium is the current drug of choice for maintenance therapy in patients with bipolar affective disorder. However, lithium may be unsatisfactory in up to 40% of patients. Carbamazepine has become a viable alternative for long-term therapy of bipolar disorders and other affective disorders. A randomized comparison of lithium and carbamazepine for maintenance therapy of bipolar disorders was reported.

Methods.—The study included 144 patients with bipolar disorder at 9 centers. They were randomized to receive either lithium or carbamazepine maintenance therapy. The average lithium dose was 27 mmol/day (serum level, 0.63 mmol/L); the average carbamazepine dose was 621 mg/day (serum level, 6.4 µg/mL). The patients were followed for 2.5 years. Study definitions of treatment failure were hospitalizations, recurrences, need for concomitant psychotropic medication, and adverse effects prompting drug discontinuation.

Results.—Assessed in terms of hospitalizations and recurrences, there were no significant differences between drugs. However, for the combined outcomes of recurrence and/or co-medication and/or severe side effects, the results were superior with lithium. Nine patients taking carbamazepine had adverse effects requiring drug discontinuation, compared with just 4 taking lithium. However, 61% of lithium-treated patients had slight-to-moderate side effects, compared with 21% of carbamazepine-treated patients. Among patients who completed the study, the recurrence rate was 28% with lithium vs. 47% with carbamazepine.

Conclusion.—For patients with bipolar disorders requiring maintenance therapy, lithium appears to be superior to carbamazepine. The advantages of lithium are particularly apparent when the outcomes assessment includes the need for concomitant psychotropic medication and severe side effects. Carbamazepine offers fewer slight-to-moderate side effects over the long term and, thus, could be considered an alternative to lithium for preventive treatment of bipolar disorder.

► This large cohort of patients with bipolar disorder was observed for 2½ years. Despite the relatively low (0.63 mmol/L) lithium serum levels, the results favored lithium over carbamazepine. This study differed from many others in that several different outcome measures were included, all of which are relevant to clinical practice. Thus, reporting simple recurrence of a mood disturbance in the absence of assigning some clinical relevance can sometimes be misleading. This study—which included outcomes of hospitalization, recurrence, use of concomitant medications, or some combination of these—was an interesting study design variation which merits some attention.

As might be expected, there were more side effects with lithium treatment than with carbamazepine treatment, which parallels current clinical wisdom. The field has now moved beyond single mood-stabilizer treatment for many patients, and a useful extension of a study like this would be to compare monotherapies with various combination therapies, including valproate and, hopefully, some of the newer anticonvulsant agents.

R.B. Lydiard, M.D., Ph.D.

The Anticonvulsant Lamotrigine in Treatment-resistant Manic-Depressive Illness

Sporn J, Sachs G (Massachusetts Gen Hosp, Boston)

J Clin Psychopharmacol 17:185–189, 1997 10–20

Purpose.—Patients with bipolar disorder commonly receive anticonvulsant drugs. The standard mood stabilizers have limited antidepressant effects, whereas the antidepressants tend to induce mania or decrease cycle length. These considerations can complicate the treatment of depression in bipolar disorder. The new anticonvulsant drug lamotrigine (LTG) has few side effects. It may offer both mood-stabilizing and antidepressant properties. The results of LTG treatment for patients with resistant bipolar disorder were reported.

Patients.—Sixteen treatment-resistant patients (13 with bipolar disorder I and 3 with bipolar disorder II) were treated. Many patients had had previous psychotic symptoms, substance abuse, and/or hospitalization. All had had a less-than-satisfactory response to standard mood stabilizers. They were treated with an LTG dose of 50–250 mg/day. The results were assessed an average of 5 weeks after the start of LTG therapy, including a symptom rating and Clinical Global Impressions (CGI) and Global Assessment of Functioning (GAF) scores.

Outcomes.—Eight patients were considered responders, with a GCI score of 2 or less. This group had a mean 16-point increase in their GAF scores. The mean LTG dose was 141 mg/day in responders vs. 103 mg/day in nonresponders. The responders reported a sense of well-being, intellectual sharpness, and improved energy. Marked anxiety symptoms persisted in 2 of the responders.

Discussion.—Lamotrigine has mood-stabilizing, antimanic, and antidepressant effects in patients with treatment-resistant bipolar disorder. The agent could become a useful treatment for patients with bipolar disorder with residual depressive symptoms or those in whom there are concerns regarding the use of standard antidepressants. There is some concern that the drug could precipitate a switch to mania. The results must be confirmed in randomized, controlled trials.

► Attaining adequate mood stabilization via pharmacotherapy for bipolar disorder remains a significant clinical problem. Many patients are lithium-resistant, and the high comorbidity of substance abuse within this patient group is an additional headache for the treating physician. Sporn and Sachs report beneficial effects of LTG in patients with bipolar depression, mixed mania, and (in one patient) mania. Considering the cost to the individual and to society of uncontrolled bipolar disorder, every new step toward optimal treatment is welcome.

Lamotrigine is one of the newer anticonvulsants that has been used for some time in treatment-resistant seizure disorder. It also appears—like carbamazepine, valproate, and, possibly, gabapentin—to have a place in the treatment of these poorly responsive patients with bipolar disorder who have multiple psychiatric disorders and an unstable course of illness. As the authors point out, more investigation of long-term treatment and combination treatment with anticonvulsants plus lithium for bipolar patients will provide valuable information for the clinician on the front line. One last thought is that the unique ability of some of these anticonvulsants to inhibit kindling suggests that the course of bipolar illness may be improved by early intervention with multiple mood stabilizers in a substantial number of patients with bipolar illness.

R.B. Lydiard, M.D., Ph.D.

Anxiety

Efficacy of Buspirone in Generalized Anxiety Disorder With Coexisting Mild Depressive Symptoms

Sramek JJ, Tansman M, Suri A, et al (California Clinical Trials, Beverly Hills, Calif; Univ of Pennsylvania, Philadelphia; Univ of California, San Diego; et al)

J Clin Psychiatry 57:287–291, 1996 10–21

Background.—Anxiety and depression frequently occur together; most patients with generalized anxiety disorder (GAD) also have depressive symptoms. There are conflicting data about the anxiolytic efficacy of buspirone in patients with GAD and coexisting depressive symptoms. This issue was assessed in a randomized, placebo-controlled trial.

Methods.—The multicenter study included 222 adult patients with GAD and mild depressive symptoms. All scored at least 18 on the Hamilton Rating Scale for Anxiety (HAM-A) and a score of 12 to 17 on the Hamilton Rating Scale for Depression (HAM-D). After a placebo lead-in phase, 162 patients were randomized to receive 6 weeks of treatment with buspirone or placebo. The dose of buspirone was titrated from 15 to 45 mg/day. The anxiolytic effects of treatment were determined by weekly measurement of the HAM-A.

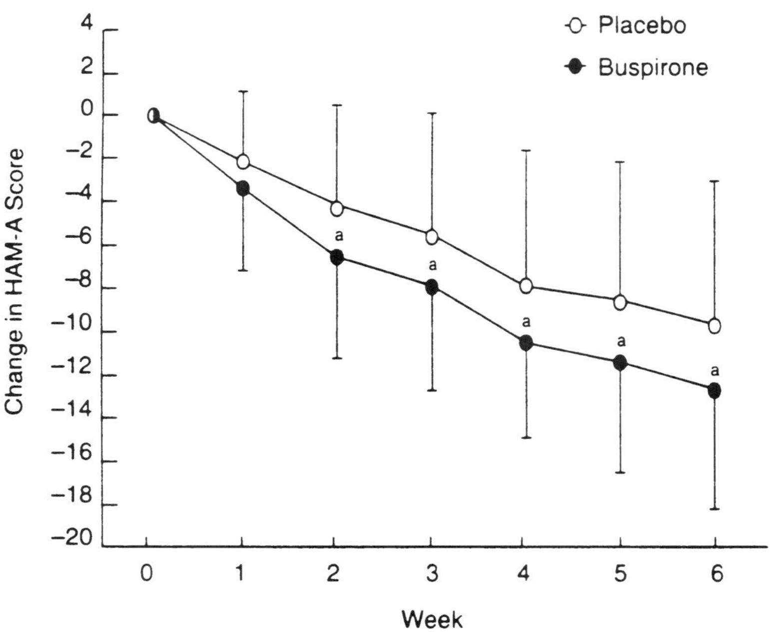

FIGURE 1.—Mean ± SD change in HAM-A total score during treatment for all patients who completed the study at four sites.* *Buspirone, N = 52; placebo, N = 61; statistical significance from ANOVA. [a]$p < .05$. (Courtesy of Sramek JJ, Tansman M, Suri A, et al: Efficacy of buspirone in generalized anxiety disorder with coexisting mild depressive symptoms. *J Clin Psychiatry* 57:287–291, 1996. Copyright 1996, Physicians Postgraduate Press. Reprinted by permission.)

Results.—One hundred twenty-one patients completed the study. Compliance rates were similar in the 2 groups, the average number of tablets taken per day was about 6 in both groups. The HAM-A score decreased by 12.4 points in the buspirone group vs. 9.5 points in the placebo group, a significant difference (Fig 1). There was also a significantly greater reduction in the HAM-D score with buspirone, average 5.7 vs. 3.5 points. Physician and patient ratings both suggested patients receiving buspirone were more likely to have a clinically significant improvement, by about 55% to 35%.

Conclusions.—In patients with GAD and coexisting mild depression, buspirone is superior to placebo in improving both types of symptoms. The depressive symptoms show rapid and sustained improvement with buspirone treatment. Buspirone is well tolerated, though it may cause nausea, dizziness, somnolence, and sweating.

► This article makes an attempt to assess the antidepressant effectiveness in patients with generalized anxiety disorder (GAD), with moderate levels of anxiety, some depressive symptoms, but not major depression. Because GAD is commonly associated with depressive symptoms or major depression, the issue of whether to prescribe an azapirone, a benzodiazepine, or an antidepressant for patients with GAD is still a murky one. While the usual multicenter variability was evident in this large trial, it appears that GAD patients with some depression are likely to experience a benefit from buspirone. What we still *don't* have is a head-to-head comparison of buspirone, benzodiazepines, and an antidepressant in this same patient group. Unlike many of the earlier studies examining buspirone, this one achieved an average dose of nearly 30 mg per day, which we now know is a more appropriate level of treatment for patients with GAD. It adds an incremental piece of information on treatment for those clinicians who see anxious patients with depressive symptoms.

R.B. Lydiard, M.D., Ph.D.

The Effect of Citalopram in Panic Disorder

Wade AG, Lepola U, Koponen HJ, et al (Clydebank Health Centre, Dunbartonshire, Scotland; Kupio, Finland; Moisio Hosp, Mikkeli, Finland; et al)
Br J Psychiatry 170:549–553, 1997 10–22

Background.—Panic disorder is a chronic and often disabling illness. Benzodiazepines, tricyclic antidepressants, and, more recently, serotonin reuptake inhibitors have been used to treat the disease. This study compares the efficacy of the serotonin reuptake inhibitor citalopram with that of clomipramine and placebo in treating panic disorder.

Methods.—Patients with panic disorder who met DSM-III-R criteria and who had experienced a panic episode during the trial's 1-week screening period were enrolled in this 8-week trial. Most (70%) were women and all were white patients, with a mean age of 38 years. Panic disorder occurred in conjunction with agoraphobia in 355 patients (75%). All patients had been free of psychotropic drugs (except benzodiazepines), monoamine oxidase inhibitors, and fluoxetine for ≥1, ≥2, or ≥5 weeks, respectively. Those taking oxazepam were weaned from the drug by week 5 of the study. Drug doses used were placebo (n = 96), 10–15 mg of clomipramine (n = 98), and citalopram at 3 doses, with higher doses titrated over 3 weeks: 10–15 mg (n = 97), 20–30 mg (n = 95), and 40–60 mg (n = 89). Physical examinations, blood chemistry tests, and adverse effect assessments were performed regularly.

Findings.—The efficacy of placebo, citalopram, and clomipramine was still increasing by the last week of the study. Compared with placebo, citalopram at all 3 doses was significantly better in controlling panic attacks by 4 weeks. In particular, the 20–30 mg dose of citalopram was the most effective. Clomipramine was also significantly better than placebo, but the citalopram dose of 20 to 30 mg was always more effective than clomipramine. Side effects occurred in all groups, with nausea, sweating, dizziness, and anorgasmia occurring with equal frequency in the 2 drug groups; dry mouth, insomnia, tremor, and constipation slightly less frequent in the citalopram group; and headache and abdominal pain slightly less frequent in the clomipramine group. Anorgasmia in the citalopram group was dose related and more frequent at higher doses. One patient committed suicide during the run-in placebo period, and 2 others attempted suicide (both fully recovered). One patient died of coronary atheroma, 1 had a diagnosis of schizophrenia, and depression developed in 1 patient after 46 days of placebo.

Conclusions.—Citalopram at a dose of 20–30 mg was the most effective treatment for panic attacks and was slightly more efficacious than 10–15 mg clomipramine. Side effects were tolerable, and side effects with citalopram did not differ significantly from those with clomipramine. Further improvement could have been seen had the trial extended beyond 8 weeks.

► Citalopram is an agent that has been marketed in Europe as an antidepressant for some time. Interest in this compound have reemerged as a treatment for panic disorder. This report found that citalopram is efficacious in the treatment of panic disorder. Moreover, it appears to be as effective as clomipramine, but with fewer side effects. The study design was somewhat unusual, as was the unfortunate suicide by 1 patient with new-onset schizophrenia. This suggests that not all the patients may have been evaluated as carefully as would have been desirable. An interesting finding in this study was that the lower dose of citalopram (20–30 mg) was better than higher doses. The most frequent adverse effect, headache, was somewhat lower in the clomipramine group (probably because it protected against headache). Overall, the side effect profile of citalopram was favorable and the response rate robust. The reader should also be reminded that this was a short-term study and panic is a long-term disorder. Thus, yet another agent, citalopram, appears to be an alternative for treating patients with panic disorder. Not surprisingly, clomipramine exhibited the usual array of adverse effects, and clomipramine recipients were more likely to withdraw from the treatment study because of adverse events. Further comparative studies such as this one will be welcomed, and comparison of citalopram with other selective serotonin reuptake inhibitors will also provide a useful clinical appraisal of their comparative pharmacologic spectra of efficacy and tolerability.

R.B. Lydiard, M.D., Ph.D.

Developments in the Drug Treatment of Panic Disorder: What Is the Place of the Selective Serotonin Reuptake Inhibitors?

Westenberg HGM (Univ Hosp, Utrecht, The Netherlands)

J Affect Disord 40:85–93, 1996 10–23

Introduction.—The reported incidence of panic disorder has increased as awareness of its clinical manifestations has grown. Recent studies have reported a lifetime prevalence of 3.8% to 4.2% for panic disorder and 5.6% to 15.0% for panic attacks. The consensus panel of the United States National Institutes of Health and the National Institutes of Mental Health issued a statement in 1991 that panic disorder is a distinct condition that can be treated by pharmacological and cognitive-behavioral methods. There is evidence that dysregulation of noradrenaline and serotonin systems are involved in the production of anxiety, and that antidepressant medication that affects these systems is effective in treating panic disorder. Selective serotonin reuptake inhibitors (SSRIs) may have an important role in panic disorder.

Comorbidity.—Comorbidity strongly affects the choice of drug treatment. The most common comorbid condition in patients with panic disorder is depression. Panic disorder and unipolar depression seem to coexist more often than chance would predict. There is an association between panic disorder and major depression, seasonal depression, and bipolar disorders. Agoraphobia, other anxiety disorders, and drug and alcohol abuse may also exist.

Selective Serotonin Reuptake Inhibitors.—There is evidence that serotonergic pathways have a role in the pathogenesis of anxiety disorders. The main pharmacological difference between the effective tricyclic antidepressants and the ineffective tetracyclic maprotiline is that tricyclics have serotonin uptake blocking properties. The first drug with serotonin reuptake inhibitory properties that was approved for use in Europe was clomipramine. Because it is a tricyclic, it has the same disadvantages of other tricyclics. Studies have shown that zimeldine, fluoxetine, and fluvoxamine are very effective in patients with panic disorder and panic disorder with agoraphobia. Side effects include a transient initial increase in anxiety or general increase in agitation with fluvoxamine or fluoxetine. A meta-analysis comparing SSRIs and imipramine and alprazolam showed that they were all more effective than placebo, and that the SSRIs were more effective than imipramine and alprazolam. Paroxetine is a more selective serotonin reuptake inhibitor and may cause fewer side effects than tricyclics. It has been used to treat depression and has been approved to treat panic disorder. There has been no evidence of initial increased anxiety.

Discussion.—Currently, there is much epidemiological and pharmacological interest in panic disorder. There is a great need for safe and effective treatments. The evidence to date suggests that SSRIs may be effective in treating panic disorder. They are faster-acting and better-tolerated than tricyclics and are not associated with dependence and the discontinuation syndromes of benzodiazepines.

► Panic disorder is now recognized as being as disabling as major depression. Like depression, panic often has a chronic course and requires long-term maintenance treatment. We also know that panic disorder frequently coexists with depression and other anxiety disorders, and that comorbidity confers significantly more morbidity and mortality for affected individuals. This report reviews the traditional medication treatments for which efficacy in panic has been shown, as well as some that have provided less benefit. Because of the chronic nature of the disorder, the need for treatments which are tolerable and effective longer term is discussed. Interestingly, a group of experts convened a few years ago at the NIMH International Psychopharmacology Algorithm Project to discuss treatment algorithms for various disorders, including panic disorder. At that time, there were few data on the efficacy of the SSRIs. Surprisingly, the majority of the experts indicated that the SSRIs were the first-line treatment for panic disorder in the majority of their patients. Subsequently, the scientific literature has supported the usefulness of the SSRIs in the treatment of panic disorder. Some clinicians are still unaware of the efficacy of the SSRIs in treating panic, and this report reviews the advantages and disadvantages of the various agents available, including the newer SSRIs. We now know that the newer agents paroxetine, fluvoxamine, sertraline, (and probably fluoxetine) are all effective treatments as a first line. Given the likelihood of the emergence of depression in patients at some point, the use of antidepressants in this group of patients is preferable, whether used alone or in combination with an anxiolytic. Information regarding the usefulness of combining a benzodiazepine and an antidepressant from the outset is needed. Anecdotally, most clinicians appear to use the combination more often than monotherapy with either a benzodiazepine or an antidepressant. Controlled studies should provide us with useful information in (hopefully) the near future.

R.B. Lydiard, M.D., Ph.D.

Anxiogenic Effects of Pentagastrin in Patients With Social Phobia and Healthy Controls

van Vliet IM, Westenberg HGM, Slaap BR, et al (Univ Hosp Utrecht, The Netherlands)

Biol Psychiatry 42:76–78, 1997 10–24

Background.—Social phobia is defined by DSM-IV as marked and persistent fear in social situations in which embarrassment may occur. It has recently been determined that administration of fragments of the neuropeptide cholecystokinin (CCK) or its synthetic analog pentagastrin, elicits panic in patients with panic disorder. To investigate the specificity of the pentagastrin test as a model of panic attacks, social phobics and healthy controls were exposed to this agent intravenously and their responses monitored.

Study Design.—Four women and 3 men, with an average age of 32 years, who met the DSM-IV criteria for social phobia and 5 women and 2 men, with an average age of 26 years who served as healthy controls, comprised the study group. There was no significant difference in age, sex, height, or weight distribution between these 2 groups. In this double-blind, placebo-controlled study, all subjects received pentagastrin and saline on 2 separate occasions 1 week apart in a random sequence. Vital signs were automatically recorded at baseline, just prior to and at 5, 20, 30, and 60 minutes after injection. The response to challenge was assessed by the Panic Symptom Scale (PSS) and the Profile Mood Scale (POMS).

Findings.—Five of the 7 social phobics and 2 of the 7 healthy volunteers had an increase in DSM-IV panic attack symptoms, which peaked within 5 minutes of injection of pentagastrin. No panic attack symptoms were observed after injection of placebo in either group. This difference between patients and controls did not reach statistical significance.

Conclusions.—Pentagastrin injection produced panicogenic properties in both social phobic patients and healthy controls. Although social phobics appeared to be more responsive to this challenge, the difference did not reach statistical significance, and requires larger studies for confirmation. These results demonstrate that the pentagastrin challenge panic model is not specific for the induction of panic attacks in patients with panic disorder.

▶ It appears that social phobia is an extremely common disorder, affecting as many as 13% or more of the general population over the lifespan. Little is known about the neurobiology of this disorder, especially compared with other disorders such as panic disorder or obsessive-compulsive disorder. The hypothesis that cholecystokinin may play a role in the neurobiology of anxiety disorders has focused primarily on panic disorder. This report is an extension of those findings which have suggested, among other things, that panic disorder patients are particularly sensitive to the administration of CCK-4. Due to the small number of patients, there were no statistically significant differences in anxiety generated by the challenge, but this was probably a power issue. Unfortunately, the authors did not include information as to whether the patients had generalized or nongeneralized social phobia. However, the finding that the infusion caused anxiety similar to that which was felt under nonexperimental conditions is of some interest. Further exploration of these types is useful, since there have been some agents which block cholecystokinin receptors, but which unfortunately have not made it to the marketplace. Hopefully, there are some in the pipeline which can allow the hypothesis that blocking cholecystokinin receptors will be an effective therapeutic approach toward treating pathological anxiety.

R.B. Lydiard, M.D., Ph.D.

Obsessive-Compulsive and Spectrum Disorders: Overview and Quality of Life Issues

Hollander E, Kwon JH, Stein DJ, et al (Mount Sinai School of Medicine, New York)

J Clin Psychiatry 57 (suppl 8):3–6, 1996 10–25

Purpose.—Obsessive-compulsive disorder (OCD) is the most common psychiatric disorder, affecting 2% to 3% of the United States population. However, unless specifically looked for, the diagnosis may be missed. In recent years, obsessive-compulsive spectrum disorders (disorders that include the obsessive thinking and compulsive behaviors associated with OCD) have been identified as well. A review of OCD and obsessive-compulsive spectrum disorders, including quality-of-life issues, was reported.

The Obsessive-Compulsive Spectrum.—Psychiatric disorders that share features with OCD include the somatoform disorders, dissociative disorders, eating disorders, impulse control disorders, and certain neurologic disorders such as Tourrette's syndrome and Sydenham's chorea. These can be clustered into groups in terms of a focus on bodily appearance and sensations, neurologic disorders, and impulse disorders. Estimation of risk may provide a useful dimension for classifying these disorders; there may be a risk-aversive or "compulsive" end point that overestimates the probability of future harm, as well as a risk-seeking or "impulsive" end point in which actions are taken without consideration of the negative consequences. Features in common between OCD and obsessive-compulsive spectrum disorders include clinical symptoms, associated features, etiology, and response to treatment, including serotonin reuptake inhibitors. Although relationships between the 2 are not uniform, the presumed relationship will be of interest to primary care practitioners, who often have the first chance to recognize obsessive-compulsive spectrum disorders.

Quality of Life.—Obsessive-compulsive disorder is a chronic and often disabling condition. A recent survey suggests that obsessions and compulsions cause the patient considerable distress, including negative effects on relationships and career. Patients may become socially isolated because of their time-consuming rituals and peculiar behavior. Obsessional thoughts may make it difficult to concentrate. Some patients may attempt suicide.

Treatment.—Patients with OCD often take great pains to hide their affliction. They may not know that treatment is available for their symptoms. As a result, treatment-seeking is often delayed—by an average of 10 years in one study. Further delays in treatment are possible if the condition is misdiagnosed as anxiety and/or depression. Recently, effective treatments for OCD have been recognized, including serotonergic medications, reading about OCD, and behavioral therapy. Other medications, psychoanalysis, and hypnosis appear to be of little benefit.

Costs.—Obsessive-compulsive disorder is a very expensive problem. One estimate of total yearly costs was $8 billion in 1990, including $6 billion in indirect costs. Lifetime indirect costs arising from lost wages may total $40 billion.

Discussion.—The OCD spectrum concept may prove helpful in identifying and treating a broad range of disorders. Primary care practitioners should be aware that patients will not readily discuss their symptoms unless specifically asked. Prompt, appropriate treatment can bring significant improvements in quality of life, relationships, and work or school performance.

► Hollander and colleagues review the concept of obsessive-compulsive spectrum disorders. Obsessive-compulsive disorder was the anxiety disorder of the 1980s; obsessive-compulsive "spectrum" disorders—all of which had been described in 1 form or another over the years—have been revisited in this unique review. Hollander and colleagues have contributed a great deal to our ability to treat many of these disorders. The literature regarding the OCD spectrum suggests that this theoretical framework may be clinically useful. Compulsive disorders (paraphilias, compulsive gambling, compulsive shopping, and distorted body image [body dysmorphic disorder]) have all been shown to be responsive to the antiobsessional agents (serotonin-specific reuptake inhibitors). Not too many years ago, these disorders, as well as OCD, were treated primarily by psychotherapy or incarceration. Fortunately, this new perspective has allowed us to consider new treatments—antiobsessional agents—for some of these disorders.

R.B. Lydiard, M.D., Ph.D.

Compulsive Buying: A Review

Black DW (Univ of Iowa, Iowa City)

J Clin Psychiatry 57:50–55, 1996 10–26

Objective.—Compulsive buying has long been recognized as a problem; it was described a century ago by Kraepelin. Recent reports have suggested that compulsive buying is a very common problem with characteristics of a psychiatric disorder. It appears to be a chronic disorder affecting mainly young to middle-aged women, usually with considerable psychiatric comorbidity. Responses to antidepressant medication have been reported. Current knowledge of compulsive buying is reviewed, including preliminary results of fluvoxamine treatment.

Compulsive Buying.—Compulsive buying has been defined as a maladaptive preoccupation with shopping, with potentially harmful thoughts and behaviors. Impairment can occur in the form of personal distress, marital or job problems, or financial or legal troubles. Consumer behavior research suggests a 2% to 8% prevalence of compulsive buying. The causes is unknown; psychoanalytic and sociocultural explanations have been proffered, whereas biologically oriented researchers have focused on its similarity to obsessive-compulsive disorder. Many affected patients meet the criteria for other axis I disorders, such as mood, anxiety, and eating disorders and substance abuse.

Complusive buying is usually chronic, sometimes episodic. The patients have irresistible urges to buy things and have tried—but failed—to control their impulses. Shopping may make them feel happy or powerful; this is usually followed by a letdown. Most, but not all, patients prefer to shop alone. Remorse may cause patients to return or hide their purchases. The most commonly purchased items are clothes, shoes, jewelry, and makeup; it is not the cost of the individual items but the quantity purchased that causes problems. Compulsive buyers rely heavily on credit cards.

Treatment.—There have been no controlled trials of treatment for compulsive buyers. Support groups such as Debtor's Anonymous have been formed and may be helpful. Prompted by recent reports of successful antidepressant treatment, the authors considered trying antiobsessional medication. Ten patients with moderate-to-severe compulsive buying were treated with the serotonin reuptake inhibitor fluvoxamine. Treatment continued for 9 weeks on a flexible dose schedule. Nine of the 10 patients had at least a 50% improvement on the Yale-Brown Obsessive Compulsive Scale—Shopping Version. They reported fewer thoughts and preoccupations regarding shopping and went shopping less. Spending decreased and the ability to resist the urge to shop increased. The improvement was comparable to that seen in obsessive-compulsive patients but occurred earlier and at a lower dosage (mean, 205 mg/day).

Discussion.—The available information suggests that compulsive buying is a common and definable clinical syndrome. Affected patients are significantly distressed and have considerable psychiatric comorbidity. The authors are conducting a double-blind, placebo-controlled study of fluvoxamine for the treatment of compulsive disorders. Other possibly useful treatments include cognitive-behavioral psychotherapy and group therapy.

► Hollander et al.[1] paid attention to symptom patterns rather than DSM diagnostic groups of symptoms. This has clearly been a valuable new perspective. Ritualistic or compulsive behaviors and intrusive thoughts or desires are symptoms that are not exclusive to obsessive-compulsive disorders (OCD). This novel approach to paraphilias, autism, nail-biting, and other habits has opened up a series of disorders now called "OCD-spectrum" disorders. Yet another OCD spectrum disorder has been identified. Although not a new disorder by any means, viewing it from a new perspective—an OCD "spectrum" disorder—has led to some advances in our ability to treat it.

Like other OCD spectrum disorders, compulsive buying may not be necessarily associated with "ego-dystonic" symptoms. The patient may seek treatment because of spousal complaints or other adverse effects of the compulsive shopping. Fortunately, antiobsessional agents such as fluvoxamine and other selective serotonin reuptake inhibitors appear to have significant potential therapeutic effects. Thus, another potentially serious behavioral disturbance, which only a few years ago would have been treated with intensive psychotherapy may be amenable to biological treatments initially developed for obsessive-compulsive disorder.

R.B. Lydiard, M.D., Ph.D.

Reference

1. Hollander E, Kwon JH, Stein D, et al: Obsessive-compulsive and spectrum disorders: Overview and quality of life issues. *J Clin Psychiatry* 57:3–6, 1996.

Body Dysmorphic Disorder: Diagnosis and Treatment of Imagined Ugliness

Phillips KA (Brown Univ, Providence, RI)

J Clin Psychiatry 57 (Suppl 8):61–65, 1996 10–27

Background.—Patients with body dysmorphic disorder (BDD) believe they have a defective appearance— such as an overlarge nose, thinning hair, scarred skin. Although BDD is a common obsessive-compulsive disorder, it often goes unrecognized. This article examines the symptoms, diagnosis, and treatment of BDD.

Symptoms of BDD.—Typically, most patients believe that more than 1 aspect of their appearance is defective. Preoccupations with these perceived defects are very hard to resist, and many patients become obsessive about them. Some patients realize that they are being obsessive, whereas others are delusional and are convinced that the defect is real. Most patients with BDD repetitively check their perceived defects by looking in mirrors, continuous grooming, questioning others about their appearance, and picking at the skin. Functionality may or may not be affected (it typically is), and many patients with BDD also experience depression, social phobia, and substance abuse disorders.

Diagnosis of BDD.—Physicians should be alert to the symptoms described above, particularly mirror checking, obsessive grooming, and paranoia that other people think patients are unattractive. Requests for cosmetic or dermatologic surgery are a particular clue to the illness. Directly asking a patient how he or she feels about his or her appearance is often the only way to recognize BDD.

Treatment of BDD.—Patients with BDD rarely seek psychiatric treatment, opting instead for cosmetic or dermatologic surgery. However, surgical treatment does not improve their self-image, and in fact surgery may make them more unhappy with their appearance—even to the point of getting angry with the surgeon. Serotonin reuptake inhibitors have been successful in treating patients with BDD, with a reduction in distress and preoccupation and an improvement in functionality. Some patients treated with these drugs even report that the perceived defect has disappeared. Serotonin should be used in high doses for at least 3 months before deciding whether it is helpful. For patients who do not respond, the addition of buspirone (a partial serotonin agonist), clomipramine, or an antipsychotic may be successful. If these drug combinations do not work, then a monoamine oxidase inhibitor should be considered. Finally, psychotherapy may be useful as an adjunctive treatment.

► This article reviews an obsessive-compulsive spectrum disorder, BDD, which has features of obsessive-compulsive symptoms (obsessional concern with a perceived defect, repetitive checking in reflective services) with some aspects of social anxiety (fearing or believing that others will see them as deformed or ugly, much like patients with social phobia believe that they lack social skills, intelligence, and so on). In fact, patients with obsessive-compulsive disorder or social phobia are more likely to have body dysmorphic disorder than patients with other anxiety disorders. There is an important message here for psychiatrists—BDD dysmorphic disorder is clinically relevant and is often detected only by inquiring about the specific problem. It appears to be relatively responsive to antiobsessional agents such as fluvoxamine (even in some patients with delusional BDD). Finally, in our role as consultants to our primary care and surgical colleagues, the possibility of BDD existing in patients who request unnecessary cosmetic surgery or other questionable treatments should clearly be considered.

R.B. Lydiard, M.D., Ph.D.

Are Fluoxetine Plasma Levels Related to Outcome in Obsessive-Compulsive Disorder?

Koran LM, Cain JW, Dominguez RA, et al (Stanford Univ, Calif; Univ of Texas, Dallas; Univ of Miami, Fla)

Am J Psychiatry 153:1450–1454, 1996 10–28

Background.—The relationship between blood levels of serotonin reuptake inhibitors and clinical outcome is unclear in obsessive-compulsive disorder (OCD). The association between steady-state plasma levels of fluoxetine and norfluoxetine with clinical outcomes was studied.

Methods.—Two hundred adult outpatients with moderately severe OCD were included. Sixty-eight were treated with 20 mg/day of fluoxetine; 64 received 40 mg/day; and 68, 60 mg/day. Symptom severity ratings were obtained at baseline and after 13 weeks.

Findings.—Mean plasma levels of fluoxetine and norfluoxetine were significantly higher with greater doses. Plasma levels did not significantly predict end point percent change in OCD scores. Plasma levels of responders were comparable to those of nonresponders. There was no evidence of a therapeutic window or a relationship limited to 1 gender or within the lowest dose group. However, the absence of chiral assays in this study limits the findings.

Conclusions.—Steady state plasma concentrations of fluoxetine and norfluoxetine are unassociated with clinical outcome in patients with OCD. The optimum fluoxetine dose for an individual is the dose that produces the greatest therapeutic effect with the smallest side effect burden.

► This study examines whether there is a relationship between steady state plasma levels of fluoxetine and norfluoxetine. After at least 6 weeks of treatment, plasma samples were obtained at 8 sites participating in a multicenter study of the efficacy of fluoxetine in OCD. As has been the observation in depression, there was no relationship between clinical response, as evidenced by change in YBOCS ratings and plasma levels of the parent drugs, its metabolite, or the combination. Nearly 200 patients participated in this study and one would assume that if there were a strong relationship, it would have been observed. One interesting observation was that 6 patients who had been assigned to active drug treatment exhibited plasma levels of 0, reminding us that the ultimate pharmacokinetic variable may be compliance. Of note, the authors mention in the discussion that magnetic resonance spectroscopy studies have indicated that levels of fluoxetine and metabolite in the brain correlate only modestly with plasma levels. The bottom line, however, is that plasma levels are of little or no use in determining the adequacy of treatment of patients with OCD. However, since 6 patients who were supposedly taking active drugs had no evident plasma levels, it may be that fluoxetine levels in this patient population may provide a useful index of compliance.

R.B. Lydiard, M.D., Ph.D.

Schizophrenia

Medical Complications of New Antipsychotic Drugs

Umbricht D, Kane JM (Hillside Hosp, Glen Oaks, NY)

Schizophr Bull 22:475–483, 1996 10–29

Introduction.—Although they are effective, antipsychotic drugs cause some adverse effects in most patients. The most difficult-to-manage side effects have been neurologic in nature, such as tardive dyskinesia (TD) and neuroleptic malignant syndrome (NMS). The "new generation" of antipsychotic drugs, clozapine and risperidone, are less likely to produce adverse neurologic effects. The clinically significant medical complications of these drugs are reviewed.

Neurologic Side Effects.—The available data suggest a linear relationship between the dose of risperidone and the likelihood of extrapyramidal side effects (EPS). Given a similar dose, risperidone is probably less likely to cause EPS than haloperidol. Few cases of clozapine-related TD have been reported; clozapine may even be an effective treatment for patients with severe TD or tardive dystonia. Further study is needed to be sure that the improvement in movement disorders after clozapine treatment represents true improvement or a "masking" effect. Clozapine can cause NMS, the possibility of which must be considered whenever the patient is seen with fever. However, clozapine is probably less likely to cause NMS than conventional antipsychotics. Two cases of NMS associated with risperidone have been reported.

Other Side Effects.—Hypotension occurs at the start of risperidone treatment in about one third of patients. This complication may be prevented by starting with a low dose and titrating upward. As with conventional antipsychotics, clozapine may cause weight gain. In one study, more than half of patients on long-term clozapine treatment became at least 20% overweight. There are few data on the prevention and treatment of this side effect. Risperidone has also been associated with weight gain, although the problem is not as severe or as frequent. The drug dose appears to be related to weight gain for risperidone, but not for clozapine. Clozapine is associated with a high incidence of agranulocytosis. Seventy-nine deaths related to this complication have been reported, although there have been fewer such deaths in recent years. Risperidone does not appear to cause agranulocytosis or other blood dyscrasias. Clozapine increases seizure risk, especially at higher doses; risperidone does not appear to affect seizure risk.

Withdrawal Effects.—Gradual cessation of antipsychotic treatment is always preferred to abrupt stoppage, but withdrawal may be a particular problem with clozapine. Several reports have described the return of psychotic symptoms after abrupt discontinuation of clozapine, although the extent of this risk is unclear. Risperidone poses no special withdrawal problems, although it too should be stopped gradually if possible.

Discussion.—Clozapine and risperidone are valuable antipsychotic drugs. Their medical side effects are usually manageable and rarely life-threatening, the exception being clozapine-induced agranulocytosis. It is hoped that the newer antipsychotic drugs becoming available will improve the benefit-to-risk ratio even further.

► Clinical wisdom comes slowly with each new agent released. Clozapine represented a major step forward in our ability to treat the sickest of the sick, but it came with more potential for serious adverse events. The same doubts about risperidone as an improvement over the other high-potency agents remain, but it is clear from this report that the accumulated literature suggests the relative safety and benign side effects profile of risperidone. Clozapine causes less acute EPS and a much lower risk of TD, but it increases risk for seizures, weight gain, and hematologic effects. A reduction in clozapine-related deaths undoubtedly has resulted from increased monitoring of hematological side effects. This thoughtful review suggests the need for head-to-head comparisons of clozapine with the newer agents. If they were safer and equally effective as clozapine, it would change practice patterns. Given the devastation of chronic psychosis, even relatively significant risks associated with agents such as clozapine still appear to be worth taking. It will be interesting to see how olanzapine and the other newer agents stack up as long-term information accrues.

R.B. Lydiard, M.D., Ph.D.

Negative Symptoms: A Path Analytic Approach to a Double-blind, Placebo- and Haloperidol-controlled Clinical Trial With Olanzapine

Tollefson GD, Sanger TM (Lilly Research Lab, Indianapolis, Ind)
Am J Psychiatry 154:466–474, 1997 10–30

Introduction.—It has been suggested that the negative symptoms of schizophrenia have an independent pattern of evolution that should be evaluated during clinical treatment trials. Three-hundred thirty-five patients who met the DSM-III-R criteria for schizophrenia were evaluated to determine whether primary negative symptoms of schizophrenia are enduring or treatment-responsive.

Methods.—All patients were experiencing an acute exacerbation of schizophrenia. They were randomized in double-blind fashion to receive either: olanzapine (5, 10, or 15 mg/day), placebo, or haloperidol (10–20 mg/day) for up to 52 weeks. Patients were evaluated at baseline and end point using summary scores of the Scale for the Assessment of Negative Symptoms (SANS) and other secondary measures.

Results.—High-dose olanzapine provided significantly greater improvement, compared to haloperidol and placebo. With the exception of anhedonia-asociality, olanzapine had a significantly greater direct effect than placebo on SANS dimensions. Olanzapine had a significantly greater direct effect than haloperidol on negative symptoms, particularly on the dimensions of affective flattening and avolition-apathy. The superior effects of olanzapine were duplicated in a subgroup of 116 patients with SANS-defined prominent symptoms and a subgroup of 117 patients with a Brief Psychiatric Rating Scale-defined cross sectional proxy for the deficit state.

Conclusion.—Findings suggest that negative symptoms in patients with schizophrenia can become directly responsive to treatment. The dopaminergic, serotonergic, muscarinic, and adrenergic activities of olanzapine may explain the significantly greater direct and indirect effects on the negative symptoms of schizophrenia. It may be that negative symptoms are under the influence of several neurotransmitters within one or more neuroanatomic circuits.

▶ The quest for superior treatments for schizophrenia continues, and the new generation of "atypical" antipsychotics has provided encouraging results in the search for agents which are more tolerable, as well as more effective. This path analysis report attempts to focus specifically on negative symptoms of schizophrenia (affective flattening, alogia, anhedonia/asociality, etc.). The analysis indicated that "high-dose" olanzapine (averaging 16.3 mg per day) vs. an equivalent dosage of haloperidol (16.4 mg average) was superior in reducing negative symptoms in chronic schizophrenia. The appropriate discussion and cautions were provided by the authors, as was a call for additional studies to more specifically focus on this important issue. The reason the newer agents are more effective than the older agents, such as haloperidol, raise at least two possibilities. First, the agent may be superior to the older agents because of its broader spectrum of events on the core symptoms of schizophrenia. Another possibility is that this additional pharmacological activity may be effective in treating accompanying psychopathology, which is commonly minimized in schizophrenia research (anxiety, depression, and others). Although the authors include this idea to some extent in their discussion, the concept of comorbidity of psychiatric disorders in individuals with schizophrenia has received too little attention. The take-home message, however, is that the newer agents may be more effective against negative symptoms than the traditional agents. Whether this improves the course over the longer term, specifically with respect to psychosocial functioning, is an area of much-needed investigation. Hopefully, this study will encourage further evaluation of the effectiveness of the new generation of antipsychotic medications including assessment of comorbid psychiatric illnesses.

R.B. Lydiard, M.D., Ph.D.

Cholinergic Rebound and Rapid Onset Psychosis Following Abrupt Clozapine Withdrawal

Shiovitz TM, Welke TL, Tigel PD, et al (California Clinical Trials, Beverly Hills; Sandoz Pharmaceuticals, East Hannover, NJ; Worldwide Clinical Trials, Beverly Hills, Calif)

Schizophr Bull 22:591–595, 1996 10–31

Introduction.—Sudden cessation of clozapine treatment can lead to nausea and vomiting, diarrhea, headache, restlessness, and other symptoms attributed to cholinergic rebound. There have been some reports of clozapine withdrawal psychosis or early relapse. Abrupt clozapine withdrawal is sometimes necessary because of white blood cell count abnormalities; it is, therefore, important to understand possible withdrawal effects. The effects of sudden withdrawal of clozapine in schizophrenic inpatients were reported, including 1 case of rapid-onset psychosis.

Methods.—The study included 30 patients with a *Diagnostic and Statistical Manual of Mental Disorders*, ed III, revised diagnosis of schizophrenia, residual type, or schizophrenia in remission. All had participated in a 28-day inpatient bioequivalent study of clozapine. At the end of that study, the patients were abruptly removed from their regimen of clozapine,

200 mg/day. For the next 7 days, they with monitored for symptoms of clozapine withdrawal. Twenty-eight patients completed the study.

Results.—Eleven of the 28 patients had no symptoms of clozapine withdrawal, and 12 had only mild adverse effects such as agitation, headache, or nausea. Four patients had moderate withdrawal effects, including nausea, vomiting, and diarrhea. One of these patients was successfully treated with trihexyphenidyl. One patient had a rapid-onset episode of psychosis requiring prolonged hospitalization. In that case, clozapine withdrawal was thought to have unmasked an underlying affective component of illness.

Conclusion.—Patients in whom low-dose clozapine treatment is abruptly withdrawn can experience mild, moderate, and even severe withdrawal effects. The mild-to-moderate symptoms probably result from cholinergic rebound and can be treated with an anticholinergic agent. The episode of rapid-onset psychosis observed in this study may have involved mesolimbic supersensitivity, as well as specific properties of clozapine. This and previous reports underscore the need for close follow-up of patients who have abruptly stopped taking clozapine.

► This study was intended to investigate the effects of withdrawal of low-dose clozapine and represents a methodical assessment of this phenomenon. Just under one half of patients experienced mild withdrawal symptoms; 5 the initial 28 patients experienced severe cholinergic rebound, and psychosis developed in 1. The findings, which were observed in patients who received a relatively low dose of clozapine for a relatively short time, indicate that gradual withdrawal of clozapine (as is the case with most psychotropic drugs that have been used chronically) makes good clinical sense. For patients who have received clozapine, a gradual taper may be even more important than is the case with other psychotropic drugs. A small but predictable number of patients will have blood dyscrasias, which require abrupt discontinuation of clozapine.

It might be wise to consider adding an agent with anticholinergic properties (diphenhydramine [Benadryl] and others) if the patient is switched from clozapine to a less anticholinergic agent. Incorrect attribution of new symptoms to a change in the course of the disorder may also be avoided if the clinician is aware of the possible effects of clozapine discontinuation.

R.B. Lydiard, M.D., Ph.D.

Large Variations of Plasma Levels During Maintenance Treatment With Depot Neuroleptics

Tunninger E, Levander S (Malmö Lund Univ, Sweden)

Br J Psychiatry 169:618–621, 1996 10–32

Objective.—Plasma drug monitoring in patients taking neuroleptics can be used to confirm drug compliance or to assess drug metabolism. Neuroleptic medication has better clinical effectiveness and fewer side effects when plasma levels are stable, and depot neuroleptic administration is thought to improve stability. Variations in plasma neuroleptic drug levels were assessed in patients receiving maintenance therapy.

Methods.—The study included 30 patients with schizophrenia receiving depot neuroleptic treatment at a Swedish psychiatric outpatient clinic. The patients were 16 men and 14 women; perphenazine was the most commonly used drug, followed by fluphenthixol and haloperidol. Over 3 years of follow-up, the patients were assessed by repeated measurements of plasma drug level. The samples were taken on the same day as scheduled administration of the depot drug. At the same times, ratings of clinical symptoms and side effects were assessed. A total of 120 blood samples were analyzed.

Results.—For all 3 drugs, plasma levels were highly unstable over time. In 29% of samples, the plasma neuroleptic levels measured deviated from expected values by more than 2 SD in either direction. Only 36% of samples were within 1 SD. The percentage of deviant blood samples was 46% with perphenazine vs. 25% with haloperidol and 12.5% with flupenthixol. Significant intra-individual variation was evident as well, even under seemingly stable long-term conditions. Medication side effects were apparently unrelated to fluctuations in plasma levels.

Conclusion.—Plasma neuroleptic medication levels vary considerably, even with depot drug administration. The findings suggest that at least 3 samples obtained at separate injection intervals are needed to make a valid assessment of plasma level during depot neuroleptic maintenance therapy. Clinical effects and side effects do not vary with plasma neuroleptic levels, so these clinical findings cannot be used to adjust the maintenance dose.

► The concept of depot neuroleptics was specifically intended to assure consistent plasma levels and compliance with neuroleptic treatment regimens for patients who need these treatments. Large variations in plasma levels were a surprise to the authors and a surprise to me. That there were no differences among different depot neuroleptic preparations indicates that this is not a drug-specific phenomenon, but rather a clinical phenomenon which likely occurs in our patients as well.

Even more surprising is the finding that patients who smoke had less variability in their drug levels over time. This raises the interesting possibility that smokers may have consistent (and perhaps maximal) enzyme induction which allows for constant metabolic activity. Those who do not smoke may have more fluctuations because of intervening variables that could alter metabolism briefly but significantly. Speculation aside, this is a "heads up" for treating psychiatrists who must consider pharmacokinetic variability as at least 1 cause for instability in patients receiving these depot neuroleptics.

R.B. Lydiard, M.D., Ph.D.

Tardive Dyskinesia as a Result of Long-term Prochlorperazine Use

Alberts VA, Catalano G, Poole MA (Naval Med Ctr, San Diego, Calif; Univ of South Florida, Tampa)

South Med J 89:989–991, 1996 10–33

Background.—The centrally acting dopamine receptor antagonist prochlorperazine is commonly used to treat nausea and vomiting. This drug, like other dopamine antagonists, can cause extrapyramidal reactions in susceptible patients. There have been few reported cases of tardive dyskinesia caused by long-term prochlorperazine use. The case of such a patient was reported.

> *Case.*—Woman, 48, was evaluated for long-standing gastrointestinal complaints with intermittent nausea, vomiting, and abdominal pain. Despite several evaluations, no cause of this complaint had been found. The patient had an alcohol dependence problem for which she refused treatment. She had been using prochlorperazine almost daily for 6 to 7 years. Two days after admission, a new movement disorder developed, including frequent blinking, writhing, and choreiform movements of the neck. The patient had had no previous movement disorder and had never received a psychiatric diagnosis or treatment. She was not given prochlorperazine in the hospital; promethazine for nausea control was started instead. A neurologic consultation resulted in a diagnosis of tardive dyskinesia, probably related to long-term antiemetic use. The patient did not improve with diphenhydramine treatment. Ondansetron was substituted for promethazine.
>
> Beginning on the eighth hospital day, the patient's condition deteriorated rapidly, including respiratory, hepatic, and renal failure. Sepsis was presumptively diagnosed; autoimmune phenomena were considered as well. The patient died in the ICU at 31 days; the movement disorder never resolved.

Discussion.—It is important to remember that tardive dyskinesia is a potentially irreversible side effect of antipsychotic medications used as antiemetics. The authors recommend the newer effective antiemetics—such as ondansetron and granisetron—which lack the serious side effects of the phenothiazines.

► Prochlorperazine is a phenothiazine which is used to treat nausea. This case report emphasizes that patients without psychotic illnesses who receive chronic phenothiazine antiemetic medications are at risk for the dreaded irreversible neurologic side effect of tardive dyskinesia. This case is reminiscent of a case I saw while I was in training. A successful businessman who had intractable nausea (probably anxiety related) had disabling tardive dyskinesia as a result of long-term prochlorperazine use. This report underscores the need for vigilance and sensitivity to the observation that patients without psychotic illnesses are also vulnerable to tardive dyskinesia. With the advent of the newer agents such as ondansetron and those that have followed it, we may be able to avoid this tragic side effect in the future. However, the pressure of cost control in managed care organizations and formulary committees is likely to require that we continue to make the case for using the best and safest available agents.

R.B. Lydiard, M.D., Ph.D.

Benzodiazepines in Schizophrenia
Stimmel GL (Univ of Southern California, Los Angeles)
Pharmacotherapy 16:148S-151S, 1996 10–34

Background.—There is a long history of debate over the use of benzodiazepines in the treatment of psychiatric disorders. They were widely used for nonspecific indications during the 1970s, but concerns about dependence and withdrawal led to severe cutbacks in their use during the 1980s. With recent advances in the diagnosis of anxiety disorders, benzodiazepines have come to be viewed as a specific treatment option for specific indications. The current use of benzodiazepines for schizophrenia was reviewed.

Benzodiazepines for Schizophrenia.—There are many problems with the conventional antipsychotic drugs for schizophrenia, including permanent disabling symptoms, poor response, and intolerance. As a result, many different agents are used as adjunctive therapy, including the benzodiazepines. Benzodiazepines are commonly used to reduce agitation and behavioral symptoms. They may be effective in lessening relapse in the early phase or in minimizing stress-induced psychotic exacerbations. Research suggests that these drugs may have a direct antipsychotic effect through inhibiting dopamine neurotransmission via γ-aminobutyric acid–enhancing activity.

Several studies have examined the use of benzodiazepines as sole agents or as adjuncts to antipsychotic drugs. These studies have generally shown excellent responses in a few patients, with little or no response in the majority. In about half of controlled trials reported, benzodiazepines had antipsychotic effects. When positive responses occur, there is improvement in the core psychotic symptoms, including anxiety, agitation, and positive and negative symptoms of schizophrenia. Almost all benzodiazepines have shown antipsychotic efficacy. No particular agent is best, although low-potency benzodiazepines with long elimination half-lives are recommended. No dose-response pattern has been established, yet higher doses appear to yield a more favorable response. Adverse effects are possible, including sedation and cognitive impairment; behavioral disinhibition; exacerbation of psychotic symptoms; and potential for problems of dependence, withdrawal, and abuse. Because they are not as effective as antipsychotic drugs, benzodiazepines should be used only as adjunctive therapy. There is no way to predict which patients will respond. The patients must be monitored closely during the first 2 weeks of treatment; tolerance may develop within 4 weeks. With the availability of newer, atypical antipsychotic drugs, there is less need to consider using benzodiazepines beyond the initial treatment of agitation in psychotic episodes.

Summary.—Extensive studies suggest that benzodiazepines are unpredictably effective for schizophrenia. There is continuing concern regarding their adverse effects and addictive potential. Beyond initial use in psychotic episodes, the sedation and cognitive impairment caused by benzodiazepine treatment would offset any long-term benefits.

▶ This review is interesting in light of the availability of several new treatments for chronic psychotic illnesses. Whereas Dr. Stimmel recommends that benzodiazepines may be "dinosaurs" with respect to their usefulness as an adjunctive treatment for schizophrenia, he also provides a thoughtful review of the available evidence suggesting that some patients do benefit from concomitant use of benzodiazepines. It is helpful to remind ourselves that our schizophrenic patients are not immune to the array of other disorders that affect the general population, such as the highly prevalent anxiety disorders. Because social phobia or panic disorder, for example, may be quite frightening and limiting for schizophrenic patients (even, at times, compromising their ability to participate effectively in treatment), one should not throw these babies out with the bathwater. Dr. Stimmel also points out that the treatment of some side effects of antipsychotics, such as akathisia, may be responsive to the benzodiazepines.

Thus, although his advice to the clinician appears to discourage the use of benzodiazepines, it is reasonable to periodically reevaluate the need for any adjunctive treatments, including benzodiazepines. There will be at least a minority of schizophrenic patients who may benefit from benzodiazepines over the longer term because of a comorbid anxiety disorder or treatment-related adverse effects which could significantly interfere with ongoing pharmacologic and psychosocial treatments which are now available.

R.B. Lydiard, M.D., Ph.D.

Other

Tyramine Content of Previously Restricted Foods in Monoamine Oxidase Inhibitor Diets

Walker SE, Shulman KI, Tailor SAN, et al (Univ of Toronto)
J Clin Psychopharmacol 16:383–388, 1996 10–35

Objectives.—To determine the tyramine content of various foods and beverages that have been restricted from the diets of individuals taking monamine oxidase inhibitors (MAOIs), but whose tyramine content is unclear or unknown, and to evaluate the effect of freshness on the tyramine content of some foods.

Background.—Monoamine oxidase inhibitors are important in the treatment of refractory depressive illnesses, anxiety, and eating disorders. They have been associated with hypertensive crisis resulting from an

TABLE 1.—Tyramine Content of Foods Per Serving Based on the Stated, Assumed Serving Size*

	Serving Size (g)	Tyramine Content Per Serving (mg)
Air-dried meats		
Mini pepperoni (Piller Sausages)	30	0.11
Pepperettes (Springer)	30	0.19
Pepperoni (Mastro)	30	0.78
Pepperoni (Fortinos) skin	30	1.88
Pepperoni (Fortinos) inside	30	0.41
Cacciatore sausage mild (Siena)	30	4.50
Cacciatore (Venetian)	30	7.57
Salami cacciatore (Mastro) skin	30	5.40
Salami cacciatore (Mastro) inside	30	4.58
Salami genoa (Mastro) skin	30	2.20
Salami genoa (Mastro) inside	30	1.16
Salami calabrese (Mastro)	30	1.58
Nostrano chub (Venetian) skin	30	0.99
Nostrano chub (Venetian) inside	30	7.16
Beverages		
Chianti Ruffino (Italy)	120 mL	0
Beck's 330-mL bottle (Germany)	500 mL	0.50
Soy milk	250 mL	0.50
Soy sauce (Kimlan)	15 mL	**14.12**
Pickled herring juice	30 mL	0.24
Cranberry juice	250 mL	
Miscellaneous		
Tofu	100	0.80
Sauerkraut	250	7.75
Chocolate (Toblerone)	35	0
Aspartame (0.45 g/packet)	0.45	0
Monosodium glutamine	?	0
Sliced meats and meat products		
Pastrami (Shopsy's)	30	0.30
Pastrami (Ziggy's)	30	2.08
Cooked sliced ham	30	0.13
Waxed bologna (Maple Leaf)	30	0.11
Wieners (Maple Leaf)	45	0.36
Bacon (Maple Leaff)	30	0.75
Sliced chicken	30	0.25
Chicken liver, fresh	200	1.27
Chicken liver, aged 9 days	30	**63.84**
Pickled herring (Feature)	30	2.45
Lasagna (Chef Boyardee)	212	0
Ravioli (Chef Boyardee)	212	0.21
Spaghetti and meatballs (Chef Boyardee)	212	0.54
Fruits		
Raspberries, fresh (Fruticola, Chile)	100	0
Raspberries, 4 days in refrigerator, no mold	100	1.00
Raspberries, 4 days in refrigerator, mold	100	0.90
Raspberries, 4 days, room temperature	100	0.20
Raspberries, frozen	100	2.10
Raspberries, jam	30	0.12
Banana (black), pulp	100	1.30
Banana (black with mold), pulp	100	0.40
Banana (black with mold), skin	30	2.58
Cheese-related products		
Mozzarella, processed, part skim	30	0.30
Mozzarella, 5 days, room temperature	30	0.30
Kraft dinner		0

*Manufacturer given in parentheses.

(Courtesy of Walker SE, Shulman KI, Tailor SAN, et al: Tyramine content of previously restricted foods in monoamine oxidase inhibitor diets. *J Clin Psychopharmacol* 16:383–388, 1996.)

interaction with foods containing tyramine. The list of restricted foods linked to hypertensive crisis has grown to more than 70 items. The danger of over-inclusive diets is that if a patient ingests a prohibited food and has no negative reaction, he or she may become careless and indulge in other restricted foods that may be more dangerous. The restricted foods and beverages have now been classified as containing high or low amounts of tyramine. The authors have received requests for information on specific foods for which there is little or no reliable information.

Methods.—The tyramine content of various foods and beverages was tested by liquid chromatography; 51 samples were tested, including samples of the inside and skin or peel of sausages and bananas.

Results.—Foods with dangerously high levels of tyramine include chicken liver aged 9 days, air-dried sausage, soy sauce, and sauerkraut (Table 1). No tyramine was found in Italian Chianti wine. Part-skim mozzarella cheese had extremely low amounts of tyramine. Although only one beer was analyzed and found to have small amounts of tyramine, alarmingly high amounts of tyramine were found in 4 tap beers in a previous report. This indicates that storage and hose contamination may encourage the production of tyramine. The pulp of bananas, even overripe bananas, had acceptable levels of tyramine. Raspberries contained low concentrations of tyramine.

Discussion.—The hypertensive response is variable and depends on many factors. Therefore, patients may be able to ingest 6 mg or more of tyramine and not have a response, but the danger of an increase in blood pressure is always present and may occur the next time a restricted food or beverage is ingested. The amount of ingested tyramine should remain below 6 mg. Most of the reported fatal and nonfatal hypertensive reactions associated with MAOIs have involved the ingestion of cheese. Although all aged cheese has traditionally been restricted, not all cheeses need be prohibited. Tap beer should be avoided. Foods that have been improperly stored or are spoiled may contain higher amounts of tyramine. Only foods with dangerously high levels of tyramine should continue to be restricted. All other foods are safe or safe in moderation. Patients should be given a diet that clearly identifies these two groups of foods. These findings should be combined with findings from similar studies to develop accurate and comprehensive lists of foods that must be absolutely restricted for these individuals.

► Psychiatric practitioners who use monoamine oxidase inhibitors are all familiar with the "white-knuckle" approach to treating those patients. Since the selective MAO-A inhibitors failed to make it to the marketplace, we still have to rely on these old agents at least occasionally. This article nicely revisits the issue of tyramine content as a risk factor in the MAOI diet restriction. Psychopharmacologists almost uniformly attest to the effectiveness of these agents for patients who have failed standard treatments. This article gives objective information about the danger of many foods that we have advised patients to avoid. (I have never had any patients, by the way, who ate banana peels.) This article should allow many of us to modify our food restriction lists and the advice we give to patients. It is also probably worth noting that the explosion of "microbreweries" creating new beers every week will continue to make our lives interesting. Caution is probably indicated until we have information about these newer brews (which we are not likely to get any time soon). This report is a useful clinical article for practitioners and patients who already have enough problems on their plate (pun intended).

R.B. Lydiard, M.D., Ph.D.

Effects of Tryptophan Depletion in Drug-free Adults With Autistic Disorder

McDougle CJ, Naylor ST, Cohen DJ, et al (Yale Univ, New Haven, Conn)
Arch Gen Psychiatry 53:993–1000, 1996 10–36

Background.—Evidence suggests that dietary depletion of the essential amino acid tryptophan (TRYP), the precursor of 5-HT, may specifically decrease brain 5-HT function. In animal experiments, increases and decreases in dietary TRYP intake have resulted in corresponding changes in brain TRYP and 5-HT levels. Dietary TRYP depletion also changes behavioral indexes of 5-HT function. The behavioral and biochemical responses to acute TRYP depletion in drug-free adults with autistic disorder were investigated in a double-blind, placebo-controlled, randomized crossover study.

Methods.—Sixteen men and 4 women, all drug free, underwent short-term TRYP depletion. A 24-hour, low-TRYP diet was followed by an amino acid drink the next morning. Periodic behavioral ratings were obtained. Active and sham testing were performed 7 days apart.

Findings.—Sixty-five percent of the 17 patients completing both test days had a significant global worsening of behavioral symptoms with short-term TRYP depletion. None showed any significant change in clinical status from baseline after sham depletion. Depletion of TRYP resulted in significant increases in behaviors such as whirling, flapping, pacing, banging and hitting self, rocking, and toe walking. Plasma total TRYP levels were reduced by 86% and free TRYP levels by 69% 5 hours after the TRYP-deficient amino acid drink.

Conclusions.—Consistent with previous findings, these data implicate a dysregulation in serotonin function in some autistic patients. Continued study of the role of 5-HT in the pathogenesis and treatment of autistic disorder may be beneficial.

▶ McDougle and colleagues utilized a biologic probe to explore the potential role of serotonin function is autistic disorder. This carefully controlled and conducted study adds to the literature suggesting there is serotonin dysfunction in individuals with autistic disorder. The lack of any effect of the sham depletion contrasts sharply with a 65% rate of worsening in patients with short-term tryptophan depletion. The authors did not observe any change in social relatedness, repetitive thoughts, or stereotypic behavior, but this short-term procedure may not have been sufficient to acutely observe these findings. This study and others like it set the stage for additional clinical studies, one of which is also reviewed below (Abstract 10–37). Given the serious nature of autistic disorder, neurobiological studies like this one are important in focusing on the biological aspects of this autism. These studies move away from older theories which implicated, at least to some extent, early developmental experiences as contributing to the etiology of this disorder.

R.B. Lydiard, M.D., Ph.D.

A Double-blind, Placebo-controlled Study of Fluvoxamine in Adults With Autistic Disorder

McDougle CJ, Naylor ST, Cohen DJ, et al (Yale Univ, New Haven, Conn)
Arch Gen Psychiatry 53:1001–1008, 1996 10–37

Background.—Patients with autistic disorder are impaired in social functioning and communication and have a markedly restricted repertoire of activities and interests. Some patients have abnormalities in their serotonin neurotransmitter system. Currently there are no consistently effective, safe drugs for treating the symptoms of autism. Fluvoxamine was tested in a double-blind, placebo-controlled trial.

Methods.—Thirty adults with autistic disorder completed the 12-week trial. Behavioral ratings were obtained before treatment and after 4, 8, and 12 weeks of therapy.

Findings.—Fifty-three percent of the 15 patients receiving fluvoxamine responded, compared with none receiving placebo. Fluvoxamine was better than placebo in decreasing repetitive thoughts and behavior, maladaptive behavior, and aggression. Active treatment was also superior in improving some aspects of social relatedness, especially language usage. Treatment response was unassociated with age, level of autistic behavior, or full-scale IQ. Fluvoxamine was well tolerated; a few patients experienced mild sedation and nausea.

Conclusions.—In adults with autistic disorder, fluvoxamine is more effective than placebo in the short-term treatment of symptoms. Further studies of this agent and other potent selective serotonin uptake inhibitors appear to be warranted in autistic children and adolescents.

► Building on the literature suggesting that serotonergic abnormalities in autistic disorder and few case reports suggesting positive response of autistic patients to serotonin uptake inhibitors, McDougle et al. conducted a controlled study of fluvoxamine in patients with autistic disorder. One of the most remarkable aspects of this study was there was a 0% response to placebo, while over half the patients receiving fluvoxamine were considered globally improved by stringent a priori criteria. While many studies have shown statistical differences and experimental designs, the clinical significance of these findings is sometimes less than dramatic. In this study, however, 2 of the 15 patients were able to move from group settings to individual living arrangements, and another was able to obtain and keep a full-time job without supervision. Given the tremendous limitations experienced by individuals with autism, this study shows that theoretical findings such as abnormal serotonin function can generate testable hypotheses and ultimately suggest very clinically useful treatments for individuals with severe, unremitting mental illnesses. This controlled study, which clearly demonstrates for the first time that selective serotonin uptake inhibitors may have a therapeutic role in individuals suffering from autism, is an important milestone in research relating to this disorder. It should encourage additional exploration of the role of neurobiological abnormalities in autistic disorder.

R.B. Lydiard, M.D., Ph.D.

Blunted Serotonin Response to Fenfluramine Challenge in Premenstrual Dysphoric Disorder

FitzGerald M, Malone KM, Li S, et al (Columbia Univ, New York; New York State Psychiatric Inst)

Am J Psychiatry 154:556–558, 1997 10–38

Objective.—Previous reports have linked premenstrual dysphoric disorder (PDD) to abnormal serotonergic function. However, all the evidence to this point is indirect. The role of serotonergic deficiency in premenstrual dysphoric disorder was studied by measuring the prolactin response to the serotonin-releasing agent fenfluramine.

Methods.—The study included 9 drug-free women with PDD and 11 healthy controls. The diagnosis of PDD was based on DSM-IV criteria and was established using the Premenstrual Assessment Form and a daily rating form for 2 cycles. All subjects underwent a fenfluramine challenge test, which measured the serum prolactin response to a 60 mg oral dose of fenfluramine. The tests were performed during the luteal phase of the menstrual cycle.

Results.—The prolactin response to fenfluramine was significantly blunted in the women with premenstrual dysphoric disorder.

Conclusions.—The findings support the hypothesis that serotonergic deficiency may play a role in the pathogenesis of PDD. The results are limited by the history of depression in the patients with PDD, although none had a major depressive disorder at the time of the study. The effects of drug therapy for depression on the prolactin response to serotonergic challenge are unknown. The findings are consistent with reports of successful tryptophan, fenfluramine, and selective serotonin reuptake inhibitor treatment for PDD.

► The authors showed that females with PDD, compared with 11 healthy women (all of whom were in the same menstrual phase) showed an abnormally blunted response to oral fenfluramine challenge. Added to the pre-existing evidence regarding serotonin dysfunction in women with PDD, this in vivo challenge goes one step further by using a pharmacologic challenge strategy to study CNS serotonin function. Recent information suggests the usefulness of serotonin reuptake inhibitor agents in the treatment of PDD. This study adds to the literature by demonstrating serotonergic abnormalities in women with PDD. The authors cautioned that all of the women with PDD had a prior history of major depression, and noted that their findings may be related to the mood disorder history. However, the study was conducted in nondepressed PDD patients. Additional carefully designed biological studies in this important area are warranted.

R.B. Lydiard, M.D., Ph.D.

Development and Evaluation of a Clinical Psychopharmacology Educational Curriculum

Naranjo CA, Shulman RW, Özdemir V (Univ of Toronto)

J Clin Pharmacol 37:474–479, 1997 10–39

Background.—Researchers have shown that clinical psychopharmacology training is inadequate in United States and Canadian psychiatric residency programs. The current authors developed and evaluated a Clinical Psychopharmacology Educational Curriculum at the University of Toronto to complement the education provided to trainees and staff.

Clinical Psychopharmacology Educational Curriculum.—The 2-year program, consisting of journal clubs, case rounds, and didactic research tutorials and lectures, was attended by staff, fellows, psychiatry residents, graduate pharmacology students, medical students, and pharmacists. Program participation offered no course or continuing medical educational credits. Anonymous evaluation forms, collected after each session, asked for participants' assessment of content, presentation style, and educational value on a scale from 1 (unsatisfactory) to 5 (excellent). Ratings were close to excellent for each curriculum component. Presentation style and educational value were rated slightly higher for the case rounds.

Conclusions.—This experience suggests that similar programs, especially using case-based methods, should be implemented in other teaching hospitals. Qualified faculty and funding are needed for such an effort.

Ejaculation-retarding Properties of Paroxetine in Patients With Primary Premature Ejaculation: A Double-blind, Randomized, Dose-response Study

Waldinger MD, Hengeveld MW, Zwinderman AH (Leyenburg Hosp, The Hague, The Netherlands; Leiden Univ, The Netherlands)

Br J Urol 79:592–595, 1997 10–40

Background.—A previous placebo-controlled study reported that the selective serotonergic antidepressant paroxetine, 40 mg/day, significantly delayed intravaginal ejaculation in men with premature ejaculation. However, there were problems with fatigue and, in three patients, bursts of frequent, severe yawning. This randomized trial compared the effects of a 20 and 40 mg/day dose of paroxetine on ejaculatory latency.

Methods.—The study included 34 men with primary premature ejaculation. For 1 week, all patients received a 20 mg/day dose of paroxetine. They were then randomized to 7 weeks of treatment with 20 or 40 mg/day. Outcomes were assessed in double-blind fashion in separate interviews with the men and their female partners.

Results.—Twenty-seven patients completed the study; the results were unchanged on intent-to-treat analysis. Both dose groups had a statistically significant and clinically meaningful increase in ejaculation latency. Median time to ejaculation improved from 10 seconds from intromission to 4 to 5 minutes from intromission within 3 weeks, with no significant difference between groups. The improvement could not be explained by decreased anxiety. Side effects occurred in both groups but became less intense during the trial.

Conclusion.—Paroxetine, 20 mg/day, is a clinically effective treatment for men with primary premature ejaculation. If the patient desires a further delay in ejaculation, it may be helpful to increase the dose to 40 mg/day. At either dose, failure of ejaculation is rare.

▶ This study points out the wisdom of turning adversity into opportunity. Delayed ejaculation or orgasm are common side effects of the selected serotonin reuptake inhibitors (SSRIs). Here we see the use of a potential side effect as a *treatment* for men with ejaculatory latency—a non-psychiatric use for a psychotropic medication. As we get more clinical experience with the SSRIs, more non-psychiatric uses will undoubtedly emerge as psychopharmacology and neuropharmacology overlap.

Other novel uses for SSRIs include weight control, treatment of premenstrual disorders, alcohol consumption, attention deficit disorder, agitation, and anger. Of course, we ought to see convincing placebo-controlled studies before we accept enthusiastic endorsements. As my previous teacher, Jerrold Rosenbaum, M.D., told me: "Sometimes you have to be blind to see accurately."

R.B. Lydiard, M.D., Ph.D.

Benzodiazepine Use in Chile: Impact of Availability on Use, Abuse, and Dependence

Busto UE, Ruiz I, Busto M, et al (Addiction Research Found, Toronto; Universidad de Chile, Santiago; Corporación de Salud y Políticas Sociales, Santiago, Chile)

J Clin Psychopharmacol 16:363–372, 1996 10–41

Introduction.—There are questions regarding the health and social consequences of benzodiazepine misuse and dependence, leading to uncertainty regarding how these drugs should be used and their potential for abuse and dependence. In most developed countries, benzodiazepines can be sold by prescription only. In Latin America and many Asian countries, they are available over the counter (OTC). This study sought to determine whether the ability to obtain benzodiazepines OTC is a major risk factor for benzodiazepine substance use disorders, abuse, and dependence.

Methods.—The study was conducted in Chile, where about half of all benzodiazepines sold are purchased OTC. A stratified population sample of 1,500 households was surveyed by trained interviewers. The interviews included data on demographic factors, drug use, psychoactive substance use disorders, and other psychosocial factors. The study hypothesis was that OTC benzodiazepine users would have higher rates of benzodiazepine abuse and dependence than prescription users.

Results.—Thirty-one percent of respondents had used benzodiazepines in the past year, and 6% had used them on a daily basis for 1 year or longer. About 3% of the sample met the *Diagnostic and Statistical Manual of Mental Disorders*, ed III, revised criteria for benzodiazepine dependence. The most commonly used benzodiazepine was diazepam; the main indications were anxiety and insomnia. Of benzodiazepine users, 74% obtained the drugs on an OTC basis at least some of the time. None of the respondents reported using benzodiazepines recreationally or met the criteria for benzodiazepine abuse. Prescription and OTC benzodiazepine users were similar in their use and long-term use of benzodiazepines and in benzodiazepine dependence.

Conclusion.—Being able to obtain benzodiazepines on an OTC basis appears to increase their use and daily, long-term use. However, OTC availability of the drugs is not a major risk factor for benzodiazepine abuse or dependence. Even when benzodiazepines are widely available, abuse and dependence appear to be rare. Continuing education appears to be a better alternative than strict regulatory limitations on these drugs.

► This report sheds an interesting light on a common clinical dilemma for treating clinicians. One of the biggest problems in treating anxious patients is convincing them to take enough medication. We also have another factor to deal with: public opinion and the questionable clinical wisdom that long-term use of benzodiazepines is inappropriate. The American Psychiatric Association Task Force on Benzodiazepines report states that long-term benzodiazepine treatment *is* appropriate for patients who have severe anxiety disorders. In the interesting situation reported here, benzodiazepines are freely available. It does not appear that this easy access contributed significantly to increased use or abuse as prescription-based use and OTC use were not different. Given the difficulty caused by restriction of benzodiazepine prescription by practicing clinicians and the inconvenience for patients, we might want to rethink the questionable triplicate prescription policy in New York State and pay more attention to empirical data such as these. A last point: the data suggested that the prevalence of usage was high in Chile. The subgroup who used benzodiazepines chronically, however, was small. This "social experiment" will provide information on the true abuse potential of the benzodiazepines. In my opinion, there has been a lot of heat and very little light generated during the ongoing controversy regarding abuse of this clinically useful class of anxiolytics.

R.B. Lydiard, M.D., Ph.D.

Dose-Related Efficacy of Levomethadyl Acetate for Treatment of Opioid Dependence: A Randomized Clinical Trial

Eissenberg T, Bigelow GE, Strain EC, et al (Johns Hopkins Univ, Baltimore, Md)

JAMA 277:1945–1951, 1997 10–42

Purpose.—Levomethadyl acetate hydrochloride (LAAM) is a long-acting μ-opioid agonist approved for use for the treatment of opioid dependence. It can be given 3 times per week, avoiding the need for daily clinic visits or take-home medications. There have been no systematic studies of the relationship between the dosage and clinical efficacy of LAAM. A randomized, dose-response study of LAAM for the treatment of opioid dependence was reported.

Methods.—The randomized, double-blind trial included 180 opioid-dependent patients attending a treatment-research clinic. Patients were assigned to low-, medium-, and high-dose groups. In all 3 groups, treatment consisted of a dose induction phase from weeks 1 to 4, a maintenance phase from weeks 5 to 17, and a dose reduction phase from weeks 18 to 29. Oral LAAM was given on Monday, Wednesday, and Friday in doses of 25/25/35 mg, 50/50/70 mg, or 100/100/140 mg. Patients were offered counseling as well. The outcome measures were treatment retention rate, patient-reported heroin use, and testing of urine specimens for opioids.

Results.—The treatment retention rate was unaffected by patient sex or LAAM dose. The greater the dosage, the greater the reduction in self-reported heroin use. At last follow-up, the reported number of days of heroin use was 2.5/30 days in the high-dose group, compared with 4.1/30 days in the medium-dose group and 6.3/30 days in the low-dose group. The dose-response relationship was also apparent in the urinalysis results. The rate of opioid abstinence for 4 consecutive weeks was 34% in the high-dose group, compared with 14% in the medium-dose group and 11% in the low-dose group. The outcomes data suggested that patients in the high-dose group achieved more than a 90% reduction in illicit opioid use.

Conclusion.—For patients with opioid dependence, the clinical efficacy of LAAM treatment is dose related and not sex specific. This agent can be used for opioid substitution therapy to reduce illicit opioid use. Basing LAAM dosages on clinical data may help to maximize its therapeutic efficacy in opioid-dependent patients.

► Psychiatry has largely ignored substance abuse until the relatively recent past. It is clear that there is a substantial overlap between psychiatric disorders and alcohol and substance abuse and dependence. Given this overlap, it is important that investigations which take into account psychiatric status be conducted in substance-abusing populations. This study represents an important step in that direction.

The research comes from a group that has had considerable experience with substance abuse in human subjects. This new agent appeared to reduce opiod use in a dose-dependent fashion. As the authors point out, the study is the first double-blind clinical trial of LAAM to include women. It also excluded certain psychiatric subgroups such as schizophrenics and patients with bipolar disorder, patients who ought to be studied in separate cohorts. One of the more intriguing findings was that there was a non–dose dependent reduction in cocaine use across 3 different dosage groups; this should yield additional hypotheses, which could then be tested.

One critical comment is that the psychiatric statuses of these subjects, beyond the exclusion criteria, were not mentioned; it would be interesting to know whether the presence of a coexisting psychiatric illness had any effect on treatment outcome. The stratification design included antisocial personality but essentially ignored other psychiatric conditions. However, this is a relatively small weakness, at worst, for this extremely well-conducted and well-designed scientific trial.

Hopefully, further controlled studies such as this will include stratification techniques and large numbers of individuals with coexisting psychiatric and opioid/polysubstance abuse. Given the tremendous cost to the individual and to society at large, we cannot afford to ignore either substance abuse or the overlap between substance and psychiatric disorders.

R.B. Lydiard, M.D., Ph.D.

Subject Index

A

B

C

D

E

I

M

N

O

P

Q

R

S

T

U

V

Author Index

A

B

C

Q

R

S